GHK COPPER
for Skin and Hair Beauty

RESETTING YOUR GENES TO YOUTH TODAY

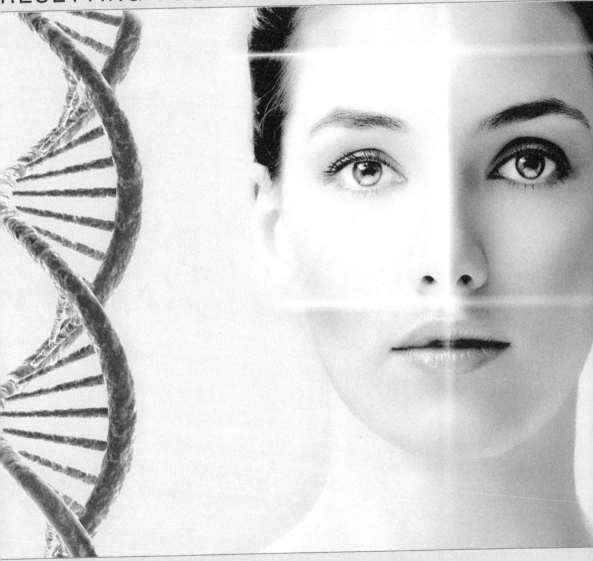

- Tighten loose skin & Thicken older skin
- Repair protective skin barrier proteins
- Reduce fine lines and depth of wrinkles
- Improve hair growth and thickness
- Improve overall appearance
- Act as anti-inflammatories
- Inhibit numerous cancer metastasis genes

- Repair damaged DNA at cellular level
- Reduce spots, photodamage and hyperpigmentation
- Help adult stem cells produce new skin cells
- Control or affect over 6,000 human genes
- Reset cells from COPD patients to repair
- Strongly suppress NFKB - primary cause of aging

First Edition – July 2005
Second Edition – December 2011
Third Edition – March 2015
Fourth Edition – July 2017

Published by
Cape San Juan Press
Summit Associates International
4122 Factoria Boulevard – Suite #200
Bellevue, WA 98006
425-644-0160
www.ReverseAgingwithGHK.com
ghkcopperpeptides@gmail.com

ISBN 978-0-9771853-0-6 (HB)
ISBN 978-0-9771853-1-3 (PB 2nd Edition)
ISBN 978-0-9771853-2-0 (epub 2nd Edition)
ISBN 978-0-9771853-3-7 (PB 3rd Edition)
ISBN 978-0-9771853-4-4 (epub 3rd Edition)
ISBN 978-0-9771853-5-1 (PB 4th Edition)
ISBN 978-0-9771853-6-8 (epub 4th Edition)

Cartoon Scientist graphic used with the permission of Brad Fitzpatrick Illustration.

These products are trademarks of the following companies: Neova, Tricomin, Graftcyte (Procyte Corporation); Active Copper, Visibly Firm, Retin-A, Renova (Johnson & Johnson); Propecia (Merck Corporation); Rogaine (Pharmacia & Upjohn Consumer Healthcare).

In memory of my mother,
Grace Pickart,
who started all of this long ago
by taking me to see dinosaurs at museums.

— Loren Pickart

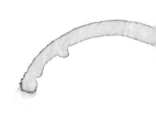

CONTENTS:

This book began over 55 years ago with my rather naive idea of finding a way to reverse human aging. Over the years, this quest led me to laboratories in Minneapolis, Santa Barbara, San Francisco, Seattle, and finally to my home on San Juan Island where I am writing today. During the course of this journey, I was more successful than I had ever imagined in discovering a human molecule that helps to turn back the clock on many types of aging.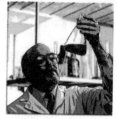

Today this molecular gem, derived from copper peptides, can be found in many cosmetic and dermatological products. Copper truly rejuvenates damaged skin. But it took me until now to truly understand how the body's aging reversal system works. This book details my findings.

The topics explored on the following pages arose from the thousands of questions I have received through the years. Most of these individuals who contacted me focused on their quest for healthier, more beautiful skin and hair.

However, people have also asked me about a variety of topics such as pheromones, diets, supplements, suntanning, and the actual published science behind Skin Remodeling Copper Peptides (SRCPs), the skin's natural renewal signals. If you would like to quickly learn the best ways to benefit from SRCPs, read Chapters 3-11 that were written as "how-to" chapters.

I would like to thank Anna Margolina PhD, Idelle Musiek MFA, and Germaine Pugh BA who helped bridge the gap between pedantic science and emotions (such as the thoughts that arise while sitting at a vanity table applying lip plumper).

And a special thanks to Cassia McClain, who expertly formatted the manuscript and illustrated most of the graphics within the book.

I also would like to thank all of the scientists, clinicians, and veterinarians around the world whose work finally enabled a biochemical understanding of the mode of action of remodeling copper peptides.

I also appreciate the many clients who have been enthusiastically sharing their experiences with GHK and copper peptides over the years (often with detailed diaries and "before and after" photographs) to help me better understand what is possible to achieve.

Finally, a big thanks to my beautiful, gracious, and talented wife Charlene for all her help and support.

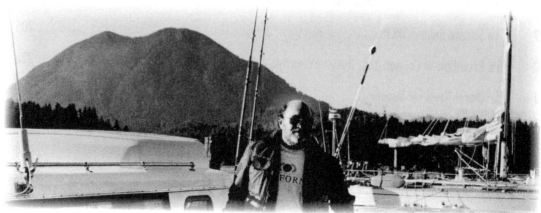

1

WHAT GHK COPPER PEPTIDES CAN DO FOR YOU
AND WHO AM I?

The most important question for any serious and honest scientist is: "What is true?" I've been asking this question all my life. I was fortunate to discover a molecule, the human copper peptide GHK, which has a profound effect on skin and many other organs and tissue.

I have spent decades researching it, not satisfied with knowing only a part of the truth. In today's cosmetic industry, the pursuit of truth is not always a priority. And even for scientists, it is sometimes too easy to start riding a wave of hype and fairy tales.

We are witnessing many cosmetic ingredients rising to the peak of fame only to be thrown off their pedestal a few years later. GHK, a molecule you will learn about from this book, is very different.

Today, after decades of intensive research, I am convinced that this simple molecule can fulfill one of the most desirable dream of humanity—reversing skin aging and preserving youth and beauty.

Interestingly, it all started with a prayer.

The Story of My Science Life
and a Prayer for a Molecule

When I was young, there were 21 Protestant ministers in the family, mostly in the Evangelical United Brethren Church (EUB), and all residing within small Minnesotan farm towns. The most distinguished, in a worldly sense, was Reuben Mueller, who moved the EUB into the Methodist Church to form the United Methodist Church. Reuben was also the President of the National Council of Churches from 1963-1966, during the days of the Vietnam War, and gave many talks on ending the war. Two Pickart men, of a total of 400 in the USA, died fighting in Vietnam. My uncle also talked and wrote about improving race relations in the USA (needed: a nice home, a good neighborhood, a good job). The overall message from the family was that each person should have a mission in life.

My maternal grandmother died in great pain and misery of aggressive metastatic colon cancer in 1940. My mother often talked about her mother and lived in fear of such a death. So, at age five, I told my mother, "Don't worry, Mom, I will become a scientist and cure cancer". Later in life, I found that electronics in the US Army and physics at the University of Minnesota were very easy for me; one learns a little and can guess the rest. But I stuck to my promise and obtained degrees in Chemistry and Biochemistry, both of which are not especially logical, and spent my life working on human aging and its diseases. Yet, my mother suffered and died in the same pain and misery of aggressive metastatic colon cancer in 1997. In 2012, researchers at the Singapore General Hospital, using patient gene data and Broad Institute data, found that the Broad computers recommended GHK, out of 1,309 molecules, as the best potential treatment for aggressive metastatic colon cancer. What are the statistics on this happening? Grandmother, mother, and finding GHK: together?

Penicillin and insulin were two molecules that fascinated me. For two weeks, when I was 10 years old, I was bedridden with a serious and painful streptococcus throat infection. A physician drove out to our farm and gave me a shot of penicillin; in two hours, all the pain vanished. Similarly, older adults talked of the slow and painful deaths of young people with juvenile diabetes before insulin was used. But after four months spent working at a research laboratory, I realized how difficult it would be to discover a new molecule that would help in the treatment of difficult human diseases. So I did what our family's ministers always recommended and prayed to God to lead me to a a new miraculous health molecule. This was GHK, which I isolated in 1973, but whose importance only began to be understood after 2010.

However, I did not start my research on cancer. In 1960, I talked with health research scientists at the University of Minnesota Medical Center. They all told me that cancer and heart disease would be cured in 10 years, and they doubted that their health science graduates would be able to even obtain employment. But I reasoned that people would still age, and this would generate new diseases. So, I found a laboratory in Minneapolis that worked on heart disease and aging. It was a rather dysfunctional laboratory, but this very fault gave me a lot of freedom to do strange experiments.

All in all, over the past 55 years, my work has gone better than I expected. And the use of GHK for cosmetic skin care has become established. But things have been difficult because of all the attacks on me and my work by many one-dimensional academics and the US Government, which has had the effect of slowing and even stopping my research projects for human healing. Now, at age 78, my goal is to inform the world of GHK's possible uses to improve human health and reduce human diseases before the Forces of Evil can bury the GHK work.

"I am who I am." -Exodus 3:14

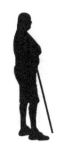 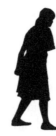 

FIGHT AGING AND STAY YOUNG Those of us over 35 are all too aware that time takes a cruel toll on our skin. As we age, our skin becomes thinner and accumulates imperfections. The structural proteins are progressively damaged, causing collagen and elastin to lose their resiliency. The skin's water-holding proteins and sugars diminish the dermis, and the epidermis thins; the microcirculation becomes disorganized, and the subcutaneous fat cells diminish in number.

Decades of exposure to ultraviolet rays, irritants, allergens, and various environmental toxins further intensify these effects. The result is wrinkled, dry, and inelastic skin populated by unsightly lesions.

But this condition is where the copper peptides work best. This book reveals practical ways to both prevent the harmful effects of aging and to reverse skin damage once it flares up. Most of the following methods, which are based on research in this book, may seem too good to be true, however there were times when no one would even dream that antibiotics could instantly cure deadly infection or that insulin could control diabetes.

My bias is for the biological rather than the artificial, for slow, gentle, safe treatments. The only worthy products are those supported by credible, independent articles in scientific journals.

WHAT ARE REGENERATIVE COPPER PEPTIDES? Copper peptides are small protein fragments capable of binding and transporting copper ions. As of March 2017, our records indicate that at least 212 companies in the USA sell copper peptides for skin care.

Not all copper peptides have positive actions. It is important to know that not all copper peptides or copper complexes are safe and effective; many have little effect, and some are even toxic to skin. In this book, copper peptides refers to a class of copper peptides that, at a minimum, (1) speed skin repair, (2) have potent anti-inflammatory actions, and (3) increase hair follicle size. The best example of such a copper peptide is the one in your blood called **GHK-Cu (glycyl-l-histidyl-l-lysine:copper 2+)**. The second generation copper peptides are less well defined but are approximately 10-fold more effective than GHK-Cu.

The Copper Peptides mentioned in this book refer to either a human copper-binding peptide, GHK (glycyl-l-histidyl-lysine or gly-his-lys), or are based on similar small copper-peptide complexes that occur within the human body. *Basically, certain copper peptides seem to reset your genes to a younger age.*

Effects of GHK (Glycyl-l-histidyl-l-lysine)

Skin, Hair, and Many Diseases of Aging

GHK was first studied for wound healing (1983+) and later for its effects on skin and hair. In many controlled, peer-reviewed published articles, GHK was found to:

- Tighten loose skin and thicken older skin
- Repair protective skin barrier proteins
- Improve skin firmness, elasticity, and clarity
- Reduce fine lines, depth of wrinkles, and overall appearance
- Smooth rough skin
- Reduce photodamage, mottled hyperpigmentation, skin spots and lesions
- Improve overall appearance
- Protect skin cells from UV radiation
- Increase hair growth and thickness, enlarge hair follicle size

GHK Protects the Rest of Your Body

In 2010, the Broad Institute of Boston broke open GHK research when it measured the effects of GHK on 13,424 of the estimated 22,277 human genes at that time. This produced many new studies which are further detailed in Chapter 19.

The number of human genes stimulated or suppressed by GHK with a change greater than or equal to 50% is 31.2%. GHK increases gene expression in 59 % of the genes while suppressing it in 41%. Most discussions of gene expression, especially by cosmetic companies, focus on "turning genes on." Yet, *suppressing* genes may be just as important to health. Conditions such as pregnancy, acute stress, exposure to low temperatures, and so on, may activate many genes unnecessary for normal bodily functions.

When I isolated GHK from human blood, I thought it must be important for evolution to have kept it in our blood, but never expected anything like the positive effects listed below. Published reports from universities have found GHK to:

Anti-Cancer Actions

- GHK topped 1,309 genes as the best Broad Institute computer recommended bioactive for the treatment of human metastatic colon cancer.
- GHK, at 1 nanomolar, resets the programmed cell death system in human cancer cells (human neuroblastoma, leukemia, and breast cancer).
- GHK-copper plus ascorbic acid appeared to remove a sarcoma in mice.
- GHK inhibits NFKB p65 which is believed to promote cancer growth and aging.
- Repair damaged DNA at cellular level at 1 nanomolar (47 genes UP, 5 genes down).
- GHK-copper induces cell differentiation.
- Resets 84 genes to growth inhibition or cancer inhibition.

Other Positive Actions

- Topped 1,309 genes as the best Broad Institute computer recommended bioactive for treatment of Chronic Obstructive Pulmonary Disease. Restored healthy function in COPD affected cell at 10 nanomolar.
- Protect tissue in mice from acute lung injury. Increase SOD activity. Suppress p38 MAPK, IL-6, TNF alpha, and strongly suppress NFKB—a molecule, which is believed to be the primary cause of the diseases of aging.
- Cause adult stem cells to produce more growth factors, increases stem cell differentiation.
- Increase the healing of many tissues (skin, stomach, intestine lining, bony tissue).
- Induce strong anti-anxiety actions in rats within 12 minutes.
- Possess anti-pain actions.
- Strongly activate genes of the Ubiquitin Proteasome System used for cell cleansing (41 genes up, 1 gene down).
- Block cortisone's anti-regeneration effects.
- Suppress the insulin and insulin-like system that reduces lifespan in roundworms.
- Reduce fibrinogen synthesis. Fibrinogen levels are the top predictor of cardiovascular heart disease.
- Increase nerve outgrowth and strongly affect 700 nervous system genes.
- Act as a powerful anti-inflammatory.

GHK and Your Health

Can a skin cream reduce your health risks? Maybe not, but the above results indicate that GHK is very, very safe. It is estimated that a woman using cosmetics has 2.2 kilograms (4.85 lbs) of the ingredients enter her body each year.

The best evidence that GHK actual converts diseased cells to healthy cells is from:

◆ COPD studies where damaged lung cells from patients reverted to healthy cells after the addition of 1 nanomolar GHK.

◆ Cancer studies. GHK changes the gene expression of over 85 genes to cancer growth inhibition. Cells have a system to self-destruct if they make DNA incorrectly which is called the programmed cell death system. GHK, at 1 to 10 nanomolar, forces the cancer cell to reactivate the system back on and inhibit its cell growth. GHK-Cu and ascorbic acid strongly inhibit the growth of sarcoma cancer in mice.

Not all copper peptides improve skin or hair.

Gly-Lys-His is very similar to GHK but has only a fraction of GHK's activity. Note the differences in the activity of GHK and analogs on cellular DNA synthesis:

Effects of GHK and Analogs on Percentage Increase of DNA Synthesis in HTC4 Liver Cells

Peptide Concentration micrograms/liter	2	20	200	2000
Gly-His-Lys (GHK)	50	408	339	91
Gly-His-Lys-His	82	604	387	84
His-Lys-Gly	31	368	353	56
Gly-His-Orn	16	220	219	56
Gly-Lys-His	2	36	65	31
Gly-His-(e-Gly-His)-Lys	0	24	68	88
His-Gly-Lys	0	13	81	29
His-Lys	0	8	30	26
Gly-His	0	0	6	3
Gly-Lys	0	0	0	0

Plants Hate Animals

Many products emphasize plant extracts because they are "natural". Well, the natural world is pretty deadly. Plants hate animals that eat them and are often filled with poisons and carcinogens.

Any key cosmetic ingredient without data on its effects on the human genes is junk.

Yup. Changing gene expression can be good or bad. Why don't large cosmetic companies (Paint Shop Factories) publish extensive human gene data on their "discovery of the year"? Primitive science may produce sellable cosmetics, but they are not safe. Enough said.

RETUNING YOUR GENE PIANO TO HEALTH

So what does GHK do and what does this have to do with human aging? The GHK effects listed above suggest that it maintains the health of human tissue systems when it is abundant. Think of two types of aging. The first is the decline in tissue health as we age which seems to be what GHK counters. The second is a limit on the maximum lifespan. These types of aging are probably under separate controls since anything that increases total lifespan must be strongly controlled to prevent cancer.

In studies at the *University of California at San Francisco*, young (age 20–25), male medical students were found to have about 200 nanograms/mL of GHK in their blood, while the healthy, male medical school faculty (average age of 60) had 80 nanograms/mL of GHK. The medical students had 2.5 times more GHK than the oldies. One could argue that young medical students are among the healthiest humans in terms of mental, physical and social attributes.

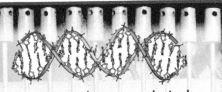

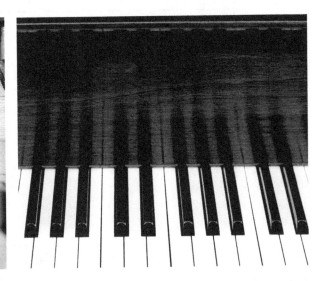

Just as a piano needs to be periodically fine-tuned to maintain melodic balance, studies suggest that GHK-Cu tunes gene expression to a healthier, younger state.

The medical school faculty is another very healthy group that tends to strongly adhere to a "health conscious lifestyle", e.g. red wine and lettuce, which may increase their lifespan about 10 years; however, the faculty still showed a sharp drop in GHK levels.

Our data on GHK suggests that the main cause of human tissue aging appears to be that the genes lose their optimal pattern of UP and DOWN (like On and Off) settings which occurs at about age 20-25. This is like piano keys. When the piano is new, it plays beautiful music, but with time, the piano keys lose their proper tuning, and the music is imperfect. Likewise, with time, human genes lose their youthful settings, and the diseases and conditions of aging set in. GHK, which was discovered during biochemical studies of human aging, appears to reset human genes to a younger and healthier condition or "tuning".

Most current theories and therapies to treat disease tend to target only one biochemical reaction or pathway. But for human aging, our data finds that we must think of simultaneously resetting hundreds or thousands of genes to protect at-risk tissues and organs. GHK may be a major step towards this resetting goal.

There Is No Quick Fix

One last item: It is important to remember that our bodies can only rebuild skin at a set pace. This is a slow process during which blemishes and damaged proteins are removed and replaced with more youthful skin. So let us now learn how to slowly and gently turn back Father Time as we reverse the signs of skin aging at a cellular level.

Throughout history, science has advanced through a mixture of astute observations and experimental studies. It is not generally realized that the successful theories of Newton, Einstein, and Darwin were built mainly on observation and thought. Like other scientific breakthroughs, the methods to reverse skin aging are accurately captured by a phrase from St. Paul: "We know in part, we prophesy in part..."

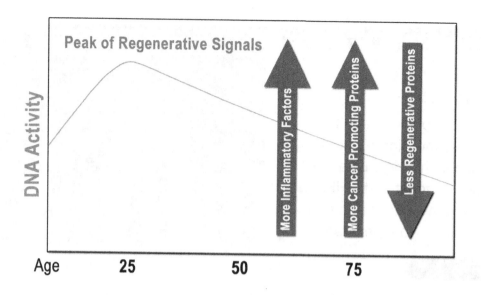

SKIN TRUTH: WHAT IS REALLY KNOWN?

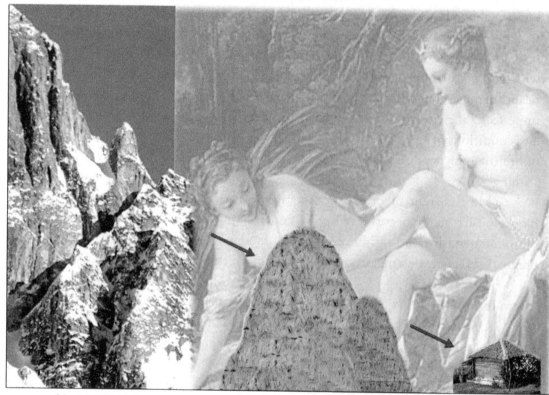

Mountain Ranges
of Ignorance

Piles and Piles
of Data

Actual
Understanding

Today, we still only
understand the skin
at a simple level.

Oily: 15% of skin lipids are squalane/squalene

Skin is smooth and blemish free

Thick acid mantle
Thick skin depth

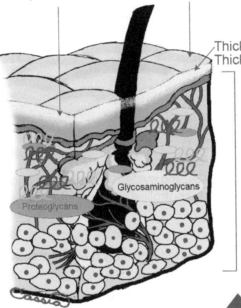

Glycosaminoglycans

Proteoglycans

Young Skin

Dense capillary beds, undamaged collagen and elastin, ample water-holding proteins, plus a thick layer of subcutaneous fat, large follicles, and stem cells converted into skin cells

ℓℓℓ : collagen and elastin

Aging

Aging Reversal

Skin is wrinkled and inelastic

Dry: 5% of skin lipids are squalane/squalene

Thin acid mantle
Thin skin depth

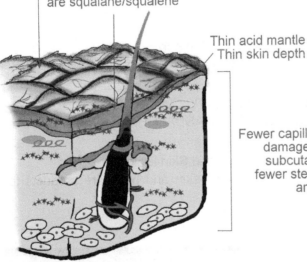

Aged Skin

Fewer capillaries, fewer water-holding proteins, damaged collagen and elastin, thinned subcutaneous fat, diminished follicles, fewer stem cells converted into skin cells, and less inflammatory GHK

⁎⁎⁎⁎⁎⁎ : damaged proteins

Biography

1938: Born in Winona, Minnesota
Ethnicity - European, Mohawk Nation, African

1956 - 1959: Navigation Equipment Specialist
U.S. Army Electronic Proving Ground, Fort Huachuca, AZ.
Worked with engineers and scientists on DECCA, the system that evolved into the Global Positioning System (GPS), computer controlled anti-aircraft artillery, and mobile aircraft landing radars.

1960 - 1962: University of Minnesota, Minneapolis, BA Chemistry & Mathematics

1963 - 1964: Graduate studies at Atherosclerosis Research Laboratory, University of Minnesota
Studied control of fibrinogen synthesis in humans and animals.

1965 - 1967: Sansum Foundation, Santa Barbara, CA. Found an impurity in blood albumin that suppressed fibrinogen synthesis.

1969 - 1973: University of California, San Francisco, PhD Biochemistry.
Isolated GHK from human blood as the active factor controlling fibrinogen synthesis and supporting replication of cultured cells.

1974 - 1978: Continued work on GHK at UCSF

1979 - 1984: Benaroya Institute, Seattle, Washington
Studied GHK's copper connection & discovered skin rejuvenation effects of GHK.

1985 - 1991: Barbara Weinstein and I started ProCyte Corporation.
Directed research on GHK. Took ProCyte to NASDAQ. ProCyte was later sold.

1994 - Present: Charlene Pickart and I founded Skin Biology.
Continued research on GHK's actions. Sold skin and hair care products to support research.

Questions? Email: ghkcopperpeptides@gmail.com

2

ARTIFICIAL & UNNATURAL SKIN TREATMENTS
WHY YOU SHOULD BEWARE OF THE "QUICK-FIX"

When I was a boy, my mother and I gazed up to the trees to hear the chirping, warbling, whistling symphony of songbirds. This feathered chorus filled the rolling hills and forests that surrounded our Minnesota farm with music. But as years went by, the birds vanished. My mother would reminisce as the thousands of birds dwindled and their music died. Then, in 1962, Rachel Carson published *Silent Spring*, which examined how chemical pesticides such as DDT endangered plants and animals and how these chemicals killed bird populations. Often, as I look at the list of ingredients in cosmetics, I reflect upon the songbirds.

After spending years in the laboratory raising skin cells, I learned just how fussy and finicky these skin cells can be about what they want. You can't just expose skin cells to any new compound. Yet chemical companies keep spewing out alien synthetic molecules for use in cosmetics, disregarding the fact that the body has difficulty handling chemicals that have never existed inside the skin before. These new chemicals are patented and then advertised as the newest "miracle" product to rejuvenate the skin.

The truth is—scientific research takes time. The most reliable and effective ingredients, which can truly improve, repair, and rejuvenate your skin, are those which are brought to you after decades of trials and errors, pondering, discussions, and experimentations.

Many consumers don't realize how difficult it is to improve upon mother nature. In order to move forward on this global journey to rejuvenation, we need to respect the spirit of nature. It took 30 years of intensive research to develop effective anti-lipid drugs, and these medications are still far from perfect. Most manufactured chemicals achieve more harm than good. For example, I've seen women lose their eyebrows by the tender age of 40, because of chemical dyes and metallic salts in makeup products.

You may ask, but why all these unnatural and artificial treatments still exist if their dangers are known? Consider this—environmental hazards associated with DDT and PCBs took decades to surface. And these alien irritants still plague our environment today.

I feel saddened to witness how toxic chemicals reduce the quality of life on earth. For years, I have spent time every summer fishing for salmon off San Juan Island, along with the local orca pod. These friendly and inquisitive whales always come over and check out the water around my boat, *Regenerate*, to see if I have found a school of big salmon. Today, these lovely creatures are plagued by toxic levels of PCBs that threaten their very survival.

QUOTABLE QUOTES: *Chuck a handful of weeds in the pot and you've got herbs – Terry Pratchett*

Speaking of survival, toxic chemicals also threaten the life of our skin. Color dyes in cosmetics such as blush, concealers and foundations, endanger the acid mantle. These products are brimming with a witch's brew of metallic salts, chemical dyes, optical diffusers, and alien synthetic chemicals. Now here's a bewitching fact. The average woman will absorb more than four pounds of this cosmetic brew into her body each year. Many of these chemicals lack a long track record of safety. I advise that you use as few color cosmetics as possible, especially when they have a list of alien ingredients which you can't even pronounce.

Plant extracts also pose risks to skin. Just because a plant is natural, that doesn't mean it cannot kill you. Rattlesnakes and poison ivy are oh so natural, and yet will sting you with their venom. Nature protects poisonous plants by filling them with toxins and carcinogens, so that they can ward off hungry animals. Safety tests demonstrate that most exotic flowers, stems, and leaves irritate the skin. Although many carcinogens enter our body from common foods, the gastrointestinal tract and liver detoxify the dangerous ingredients. The skin has no such protective system. Thus, you should only apply plant extracts and oils to your skin that are highly domesticated, and that have been used for at least a thousand years. Only a very few domesticated plants, such as Aloe Vera, have a positive effect on the skin.

Advertising Agency Science

To a true scientist, the world of cosmetic science is a strange world indeed. Being very familiar with the realm of cosmetic science, I know how easily truth, dignity and scientific facts are twisted, bent and distorted to suit marketing needs. It won't be an exaggeration to say that cosmetic companies accumulated the greatest collection of junk science on planet Earth.

Pseudo skin experts mislead with deceptive phrases like "Clinically proven". I would advise a bit of caution there. An ingredient maybe scientifically tested; however, it doesn't mean that it will have the same effect in a cosmetic product.

Materials such as retinol, squalene, and Co-Q10 need to be present at established concentrations in order to be active. However, more often a finished product contains a microscopically small percentage, yet, cosmetic companies still insist that the substance offers the same benefit.

Okay, I'm reading your mind, friends. I'll bet you're asking, "If a product is clinically proven, isn't there a study to back up its claims?" As a scientist, I have seen many flawed studies. Typically, when testing a cosmetic product, a clinician applies product to one side of a face and leaves the other side untreated. Under such circumstances, even simple oils would reduce wrinkles, just by keeping skin softer and more hydrated.

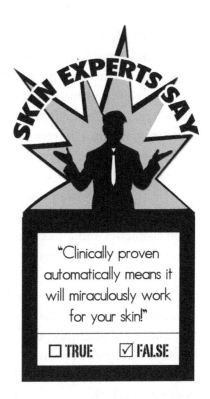

"Clinically proven automatically means it will miraculously work for your skin!"

☐ TRUE   ☑ FALSE

Extremely few of these junk science "clinical studies" ever make it into scientific journal articles.

Scientists in cosmetic companies have little influence. An executive at a very large cosmetic company once told me many years ago, "We pay our top model 20 times more than we pay our top scientist. You can guess who gets listened to the most."

If you were a fly on the wall at a cosmetic company, you would be shocked to discover how they make their wares. These companies order products from generic manufacturing plants that use standard formulas.

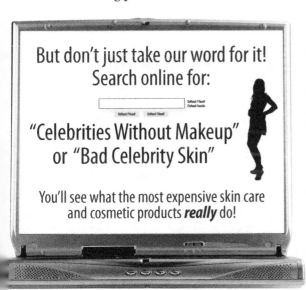

But don't just take our word for it! Search online for:

"Celebrities Without Makeup" or "Bad Celebrity Skin"

You'll see what the most expensive skin care and cosmetic products *really* do!

Products with similar ingredients are given different fancy names such as Night Active Defense Cream, Anti-Gravity Skincare Lotion (this could save a fortune on airline fares if it worked), Cucumber Regenerative Tightening Gel, Natural Environmental Conditioner, Stress-Reducing Lymphatic Drainage System, and so on.

What links all of these products together is a lack of credible evidence that they do anything positive for the skin.

Beware of "Quick Fix"

Most modern cosmetic products are designed to produce an immediate and visible effect. There are plenty of ingredients, developed with only one goal—make you look dewy and youthful at the cosmetic counter, so you will buy products. Wetting agents puff up the skin so that wrinkles and lines appear less noticeable. Then dyes and optical diffusers give skin a better color and "glow" and hide blemishes. There is nothing wrong with this approach. After all, we all want to look younger and more radiant. However, there are products, which achieve this noble goal by literally destroying your skin.

The fact that a product feels smooth and sensuous, does not necessarily relate to improving skin health. Cosmetic companies created the legend that skin "adapts" to good cosmetics and looks bad when you stop using them. But the truth is that so often these smooth and sensuous creams and serums are quite rough on your skin's delicate structures.

For example, some moisturizers may damage the skin barrier by breaking the water-resistant layer of proteins and oils of the upper skin. This allows water to go into the epidermis, plumping skin and smoothing out wrinkles. However, this also weakens the skin barrier and lets in more bacteria, viruses and allergens.

Another issue is stabilizers and preservatives, which extend the shelf life of a cosmetic product, but can be toxic for skin cells. The majority of cosmetic skin products are designed for long-term stability, that is, they can be frozen or thawed without change and have a long shelf-life, preferably years. But skin is a living tissue. Thus, effective products should be more akin to perishable foods than perfectly stable creams or clear solutions.

Truth…or Fiction?

By now, you may wonder why the cosmetic industry is selling treatments that are useless or even harmful for our skin. Sure, the big cosmetic corporations have enough resources to develop effective products based on real science. Unfortunately, it is much easier and safer to sell deception.

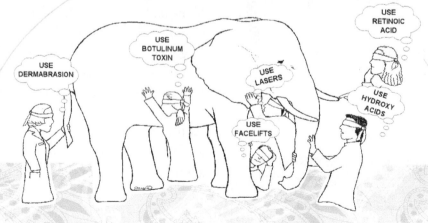

Based on the Indian fable: "Six Blind Men and An Elephant"

Consider for a moment how many products claim to reduce wrinkles. Based on TV advertising and magazine ads, it would be easy to believe that every product on the market achieves a miraculous anti-wrinkle effect. The truth is that the cosmetic industry's main objective is to manufacture innocuous products that do not in any way irritate the skin. This is a good goal; however, this often means that it is much safer and more profitable to invest money and resources into technologies that create illusion of improvement, than it is to search for truth. Real scientific research takes time and results are uncertain. Fake science is quick and impressive.

This is why so many cosmetic companies depend on advertising to create the illusion that their products benefit the skin. This is why these products often have to employ unnatural and artificial methods to cause a sort of "skin renewal" or the appearance of skin renewal. This is why it is so rare to find a product, which works by activating the skin's natural repair systems.

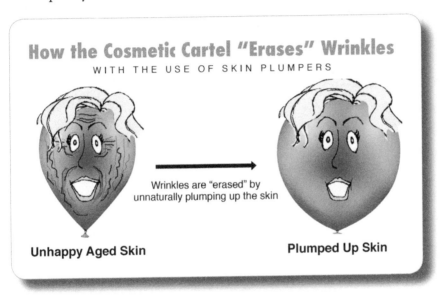

How the Cosmetic Cartel "Erases" Wrinkles
WITH THE USE OF SKIN PLUMPERS

Wrinkles are "erased" by unnaturally plumping up the skin

Unhappy Aged Skin

Plumped Up Skin

Beauty Takes Time

We live in a very exciting time, when so much is available to us to beautify, renew and rejuvenate our skin. Advanced technologies such as lasers, microwaves, heating lights, and other popular methods of skin care induce collagen formation and, in turn, younger skin. However, there is no quick fix without risk.

The idea behind many of these methods is that often controlled skin damage will stimulate a vigorous regenerative response. Another common approach is creating temporal collagen tightening, which takes care of wrinkles. When used with care and by a trained skin care specialist, they can make your skin look younger. They also can lead to scarring, skin sagging, discoloration, and further damage.

Some other methods such as nerve toxins and skin fillers can reduce wrinkles, and they can also produce an expressionless or a hardened "mask-like" face.

Surgical procedures, such as face lifts and implants, are followed by a long recovery period as scar lines fade, and the skin adjusts to its new position. In addition, no one is sure what the future impact of such procedures will be.

Today you may be surprised to hear that in the past X-ray machines were used to treat acne. A few decades later, these patients are developing cancer from the treatment. And in the past, silicone injections were applied directly into women's faces and breasts, and later, many of these women found that the silicone slowly slid down inside their skin, necessitating surgical removal to avoid the consequence of disfigurement. The secret to beautiful skin cannot be found in any of the multitudes of products or procedures you see in advertisements. Rather, true beauty emerges from the idea that slower is better.

Our bodies can only rebuild skin at a set pace. This is a slow process during which blemishes and damaged proteins are removed and replaced with more youthful skin. So let us now learn how to slowly and gently turn back Mother Time as we reverse the signs of skin aging at a cellular level.

Unnatural and Artificial Methods of Skin Renewal

METHOD	MECHANISM OF ACTION	RESULT	SIDE EFFECTS
Laser Resurfacing	CO2 Lasers evaporate (ablate) the epidermis and cause heat damage to the dermal proteins. Deep damage brutally forces the skin into reparative response.	Immediate tightening of the skin due to skin protein denaturation. Works well for removing local skin lesions. Using lasers for larger areas increases the risk of side effects. If reparative process goes well, skin will look better with fewer wrinkles.	Redness and inflammation in post-treatment period, possibility of scarring, discoloration, hyperpigmentation, prolonged redness and a possibility of damage to skin's stem cells. Use SRCPs to promote healing and reduce side effects.
Deep Chemical Peels (phenol)	Chemical burning of the epidermis, possible damage to the dermis. Deep damage brutally forces the skin into reparative response.	If regenerative response goes well - improvement of wrinkles and skin elasticity, removal of pigmented spots.	Painful procedure (requires anesthesia), risk of heart failure (needs to be performed with heart monitor), redness, swelling and inflammation in post-treatment period, high risk of permanent skin discoloration and scarring, poisoning of skin cells. Permanent sensitivity to the UV-rays – no tanning allowed. Sharp contrast with the untreated skin may create an effect of a "clown mask".
Medium Chemical Peels (20-35% TCA, Jessner Chemical Peel)	Chemical burning of the epidermis with trichloroacetic acid. The skin is damaged and pushed into reparative response.	Reduces the depth of wrinkles, lightens pigmented spots.	Redness, swelling, possibility of hyper-pigmentation. Use SRCPs to promote healing and reduce side effects.
Deep Dermabrasion	Mechanical removal of epidermis. The skin is brutally forced into reparative response.	Improvement of wrinkles due to reparative process.	Infection, scarring, long-lasting redness, inflammation. Use SRCPs to promote healing and reduce side effects.
Fillers (Collagen, Hyaluronic Acids, Synthetic Gels)	The skin is injected with various alien substances – dissolvable such as bovine collagen, fat or hyaluronic acid, or permanent (various synthetic gels and combination of collagen with synthetic gels).	Typical fillers plump the skin, masking wrinkles or age-related degeneration of tissue. In some instances, skin develops inflammation and surrounds the filling material with connective tissue, which produces tightening effect. No real rejuvenation is produced.	Can produce local hardening of skin. Some permanent fillers (synthetic gel) can produce disfigurement (bumps, depressions etc) if done incorrectly. Can cause chronic inflammation, speeding up aging.
Nerve Toxins	Block nerve stimulation of the skin's muscles, relaxing mimic wrinkles. Poison skin nerves and disturb their function.	Relaxation of "frown and smile" lines on your face. Does not stimulate skin remodeling.	Can travel in your brain, causing long lasting headache or weird taste in your mouth, damage skin nerves, can get to the surrounding muscles, producing drooling mouth, drooped eyelids etc. May create unnatural, emotionless expression.
Radiofrequency (RF) Non-ablative Technology (microwave)	Often promoted as safer alternative to lasers (does not evaporate upper layers of skin). In reality, they just contract skin collagen like bacon in the microwave.	Immediate contraction of collagen creates an illusion of skin tightening. Does not make the skin younger, but on the contrary, adds more damage to its proteins.	May accelerate skin aging.
Infra-red (IF) Light Technology	Often promoted as safer alternative to lasers (does not evaporate upper layers of skin). Infra-red radiation passes into the dermis, causing heat damage.	Immediate contraction of skin proteins creates an effect of skin tightening. May stimulate mild skin repair in response to heat damage, but does not promote removal of damaged proteins.	May accelerate skin aging, causing more damage.
Surgical Facelift	Surgical removal of loose skin, tightening of skin.	Gives good result with extensive sagging or loose skin. The skin doesn't get younger; it just gets tighter.	Painful, costly, with long healing period. Often create unnatural (tightened) look of the skin. Possibility of keloid formation. Use SRCPs to promote healing and reduce side effects.
Biologically Active Peptides	Claim to stimulate skin renewal and collagen synthesis. But most of them never get below skin surface.	Only a few of them were tested in clinical studies.	Certain growth factors, such as TGF-beta produced scarring in wound healing studies.
Stem Cells (frozen or extracts)	Claim to stimulate skin renewal.	No published studies on the efficiency of any cosmetic treatment with frozen stem cells.	
"Miracle" Ingredients	New miracle ingredients are launched and heavily promoted every several months. Claims are usually carefully formulated such as "visibly reduces appearance of wrinkles", "makes skin look younger" etc.	In most cases, an effect is produced by other ingredients in the formulation that create temporary tightening or swelling of the skin (synthetic polymers, silicones, mild irritants etc). The effect is usually gone the next morning or when you stop using the product. Always ask for independent studies published in scientific journals.	

3

UNDERSTANDING YOUR BEAUTIFUL SKIN
How to Baby the Skin You Were Born With

When it comes to skin care, especially anti-aging skin care, accurate and unbiased information is invaluable. Not only will it save you money, but it also can protect your skin.

Knowledge is power. Knowledge about your skin gives you power not only to preserve its youth and beauty but also to reverse many signs of aging, restoring a smooth and bright appearance. In this chapter, we will take a closer look at your skin's structure. Knowing how your skin functions can save you thousands of dollars spent on cosmetic products, which are useless or even harmful.

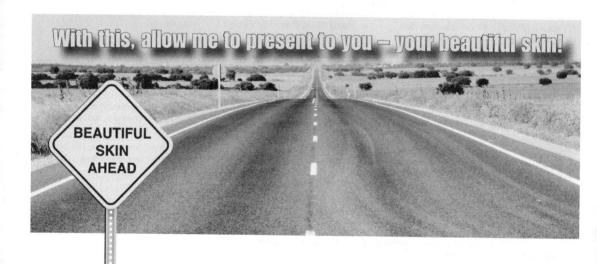

With this, allow me to present to you – your beautiful skin!

BEAUTIFUL
SKIN
AHEAD

The First Frontier

When you think about your skin, think—layers. Your skin has layers, which have different functions and structure. Why is this important to understand? Because when you look at yourself in the mirror, what you see is the outer layer of your skin. And most cosmetic products work on the surface only, affecting appearance of this very first layer.

However, the overall appearance of your skin is determined by health and functionality of all layers. When you understand layers of skin, you can start distinguishing between products which only temporarily improve your skin's appearance and those which can have more lasting effect.

The primary goal of our skin is to be a strong barrier that protects our tender inner organs from the harsh environment. It is not just an attractive façade, a pretty covering for our bodies. It is the first frontier that keeps away harmful microorganisms and toxins, shields us from UV-rays, and prevents our body from drying out in the dry air or, on the contrary, from swelling with water like a sponge.

It also allows one to experience and interact with the world through the many senses. Finally, it allows us to interact with each other. It may even make other people fall in love with you.

THE LAYERS OF OUR SKIN

Labels: Hairs, Collagen Strands, Elastic Fibers, Keratinocytes, Fibroblasts, Hair Follicle, Epidermis, SKIN, Nerves, Dermis, Hypodermis (subcutaneous tissue), Fat Cells, Macrophages, Sebaceous Gland, Blood Vessel, Water Holding Proteins and Sugars:

Surprisingly, this vital barrier is very thin—from 0.03 mm on the eyelids to 1.3 mm on palms and soles. The secret to why the skin can serve its protective function so well lies in its highly sophisticated structure, which is one of Nature's wonders. Every wrinkle and spot on our face that mars our beauty is not just a superficial lesion, but corresponds to the inner damage of the skin structure.

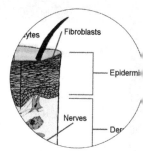

Human skin can be divided into three distinctive layers—epidermis, dermis and subcutaneous fat (see the picture). Each layer is important, and each contributes to both the skin's appearance and protective function.

The Epidermis

Just like all living cells, the cells in your skin require a comfortable, stable environment in order to function well. You may think of your body as a warm, secure, comfortable house, where all the residents can feel happy and protected. Imagine yourself in that house—warm and secure. Now imagine what would happen if the roof started leaking, and holes appeared in the walls. Would you still feel comfortable? I think not.

In the same way, your skin's cells and your entire body won't feel comfortable or be able to function properly if the skin's upper layer is damaged.

The outermost layer of skin is called the **epidermis**. Its thickness is only 0.03 mm in the eyelids and 1.3 mm in palms and soles. Since this layer has to withstand a significant amount of wear and tear, one may wonder how it manages this without getting worn out within a few months. In order to achieve this, Mother Nature devised a unique multilayered structure that continuously repairs and renovates itself.

Skin renewal is made possible by **stem cells**—very special cells, which possess almost unlimited renovating power. If stem cells remained active through our entire life, we would never have any problem with wrinkles. Unfortunately, as we age, our stem cells start losing their ability to renew skin. One of the most fascinating qualities of GHK is its ability to invigorate stem cells, bringing them back to a much more youthful state.

The outmost layer of the epidermis is called the stratum corneum—a layer of tough, hard and quite dead keratinous scales, which can withstand all those insults coming from the hostile environment.

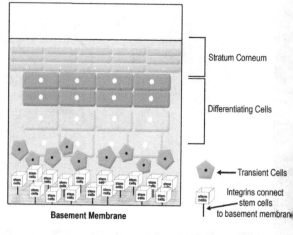

The stratum corneum is often compared to a brick and mortar wall because its hard, protein-rich scales (bricks) are held together with fatty substance (mortar).

This brick-and-mortar layer is called the **epidermal barrier**. A damaged barrier leaves skin unprotected against swarms of invaders (viruses, bacteria and harmful chemicals) as well as moisture loss. This is why our skin constantly renews its stratum corneum—when keratinous scales get worn out and damaged, they are sloughed from the surface and promptly replaced.

As we age, the rate of skin turnover goes down. At the age of 50, it usually takes 6-7 weeks to renew the epidermis. This leads to thinning out of the epidermis, thickening of the stratum corneum, roughening of the skin surface, and dry skin.

MY SKIN WILL LOOK BEAUTIFUL IF:

1. Its epidermis is well developed and supple with fully functional stem cells that ensure its repair and renewal.

2. Its stratum corneum is relatively thin and transparent with enough NMF to keep it moist.

3. The epidermal barrier is intact and well functioning.

4. The epidermis goes through complete renewal cycle every 2-4 weeks.

The Dermis

The dermis is a layer that cushions the epidermis, supplies it with water and nutrients, as well as gives our skin its nice plump appearance and wonderful resilience. The dermis is only slightly thicker than the epidermis—0.03 mm on the eyelids and up to 3 mm on the back. The dermis can be compared to a mattress. Its "springs" are fibrous proteins that give it resilience and elasticity (they are called **collagen and elastin**), and its "stuffing" is formed by water-binding gel made of large sugar based molecules (**proteoglycans and glycosaminoglycans**).

The components of the dermis are produced by special cells—fibroblasts. These cells also play a key role in skin repair and renewal. Its main function is to produce skin's protein, including collagen and elastin.

When we age, fibroblasts start losing their ability to make good collagen, which leads to wrinkles and sagging. As you will learn in the following chapters, GHK plays a key role in maintaining health and youth of skin fibroblasts, ensuring proper collagen synthesis.

MY SKIN WILL LOOK BEAUTIFUL IF:

1. Dermal fibroblasts are fully functional and active.

2. The dermis is thick and has enough collagen, elastin and glycosaminoglycans.

3. Dermal proteins have proper structure.

4. The dermis renews itself at a proper rate.

The Subcutaneous Fat

The **subcutaneous fat** insulates the body and gives it additional cushioning. It also gives our faces and bodies their pleasant and alluring shape. As we enter old age, fat cells start to deplete, and it has a devastating effect on our appearance.

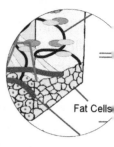

Fat Cells

So when all those slimming ads in fashion magazines urge you to declare a war on your fat, just think what would happen if it went away completely. The truth is that your skin needs subcutaneous fat—it is nothing less than a foundation of your beauty.

Today it is known that fat cells can produce female hormones, such as estrogens, supporting hormonal health of the skin during pre-menopause.

Subcutaneous fat also contains stem cells that produce cytokines and growth factors activating wound healing and fibroblast function. Therefore, skin fat appears to be even more important than just a soft cushion underneath our skin.

Oil Glands and Hair Follicles

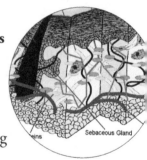

Sebaceous Gland

The entire surface of our skin is covered with **hair follicles** (except eyelids, palms, and soles). Hair follicles harbor stem cells, which play a key role in skin repair.

Closely associated with hair follicles are the **oil glands** that produce sebum or skin oil. Too much sebum can make your skin look oily and yet, it plays an important protective role, smoothening the skin surface and reducing water loss.

If you look at your skin's surface, you will notice that it has **pores**. In some areas, they are more visible and in others—very hard to see. They are simply the openings of the oil glands. When the skin produces too much oil, pores may get clogged with sebum and dead skin cells, eventually forming comedones—whiteheads and blackheads.

The activity of oil glands is governed by hormones—male hormones (androgens) increase it, and female hormones (estrogens) reduce it. GHK has an ability to naturally reduce excessive sebum production, preventing pore blockage.

Protective Systems of the Skin

Do you like gardening? How about playing outdoor sports? Going to a petting zoo? How often do you shake hands? All those activities shower your skin with myriads of microorganisms—viruses, bacteria, and fungi. And yet, most of the time we are just fine, even when we forget to wash our hands.

You also know that the sun can be damaging to your skin. But how many hours did you spend in the sun when you were a kid? And yet, your skin remained smooth, rosy, and beautiful for many years.

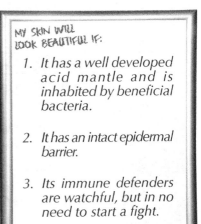

All of this is possible because our skin has such powerful reparative and protective systems. Without them, we would be doomed. We would have to live in sterilized, protective cocoons and could never touch the beach sand or the garden soil. Shaking hands would be suicide.

First of all, our skin is protected by the **acid mantle**—an emulsified mixture of sweat and skin oil. It contains a noticeable amount of lactic acid and has an acidic pH of about 4.7-5.5 (neutral pH is 7.0, and above it is alkaline). In addition, the acid mantle contains **antimicrobial peptides** that kill bacteria and fungi. The skin oil repels water and softens our skin. It is also rich in antioxidants, protecting skin from UV-radiation. Frequent washing with harsh alkaline soaps can strip the acid mantle from the skin and increase a chance of drying and bacterial invasion. The stratum corneum provides a mechanical barrier—if it is damaged, skin can get infected.

When the acid mantle and the epidermal barrier function well, all alien chemicals and pathogenic bacteria are stopped before entering the skin.

KEEPING YOUR SKIN YOUNG Now you can see that healthy skin structure means a younger-looking and more radiantly beautiful you. Yet, due to a number of internal and environmental factors, all structures of our skin slowly accumulate damage.

Damage to your skin's barrier opens the gate to toxins, water loss, germs, and allergens. Damage to the epidermis leads to slower skin renewal and skin repair rates, resulting in a dull and lifeless appearance. Damage to the dermis causes wrinkles, skin sagging, uneven skin tone, and the loss of elasticity. Even when we smile and cry, we cause damage to our skin by stretching it with muscle movements!

But can you battle skin damage by trying to avoid it? Not if you want to win the war on aging! While taking steps to protect your skin from ultraviolet light, allergens, detergents, damaging soaps, irritants, acne scars, airborne pollutants, chemical sunscreens, and so on will reduce certain types of damage, this is only a small piece of a much larger puzzle. You can hide from the sun until you evolve into a mole, but this will not keep your skin young.

In the next chapter, you will discover the Holy Grail of skin care—a method that can bring, not illusionary, but real changes to your skin.

WHY WE LOOK OLDER?

A number of changes sabotage skin as it ages. These include:

	Effect of Aging	Effect of Skin Remodeling
SKIN	Thinner, more fragile skin	Thickened skin dermis and epidermis
	Less elastic skin	Rebuilt new collagen and elastin
	Less keratinocyte replacement for skin's surface	Increases keratinocyte flow to surface and replaces damaged old skin components with new material
	Less subcutaneous fat ("baby fat")	Increased subcutaneous fat
	More skin lesions, imperfections, blotchiness	Activate scar removal system that removes lesions and scars
	Poor blood capillary networks	Rebuilt capillary networks for better tissue nutrition
	Flabby, less firm skin	Increased synthesis of water-holding proteins
	Inflammation	Anti-Inflammation
HAIR	Less hair growth	Increased hair growth
	Smaller hair follicle size	Increased follicle size
	Thinner hair shafts	Thicker hair shafts
	More breakage of hair shafts and split ends	Thicker, more break resistant hair shafts

1. Cells replace themselves at a reduced rate, producing a thinner, more fragile skin. Skin replaces itself every three weeks at age 20 but only every nine weeks by age 70.

2. Antioxidants lose their ability to protect the skin by 80 percent between ages 15 and 60.

3. Protein damage accumulates and ages the skin as a result of scars, sun damage, oxidative damage, or the cross-linking of skin proteins by sugars.

4. The skin's oil producing sebaceous glands produce less sebum or "oil." Thus, although we develop less acne, our skin grows drier. This drop in oil emerges at around age 25 and dramatically slows down after age 45.

5. Collagen and elastin break down causing our skin to wrinkle and sag. At the same time, water-holding proteins decrease, resulting in drier skin. We begin to form wrinkles and lose elasticity by age 25. The problem intensifies with passing years.

6. Vellus hair follicles diminish in size and efficiency. This colorless fine hair covers most of our body. Since these follicles supply new stem cells for skin repair, a loss of follicles damages the skin.

Questions? Email: ghkcopperpeptides@gmail.com

4

THE HOLY GRAIL OF SKIN CARE
A SAFE AND NATURAL APPROACH TO SKIN AGING REVERSAL

So far, we have been talking a lot about the aging process. But have you heard about the "anti-aging process"? Yes, such a process actually exists! It is the natural process that takes place in every cell and every tissue of your body every day of your life.

Old cells die and new cells emerge. Old structures fall apart, and new ones are created. Wounds heal, and then scar tissue is slowly dissolved over the course of many years. In skin, this process is called skin remodeling.

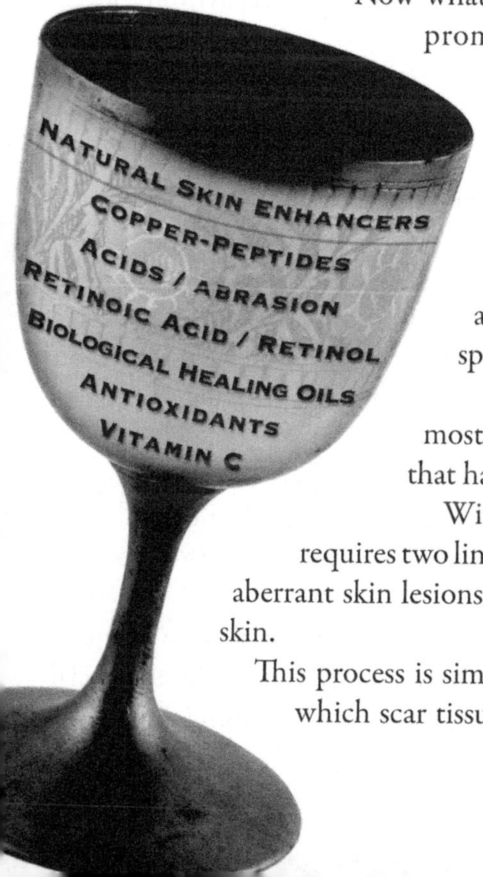

Now what do you think would happen if all damage were promptly removed all at once? What if every time an aberrant cell popped up in your skin, it was immediately destroyed and replaced by a new one? Or what if every time collagen fibers were damaged, your skin took them apart and created new ones instead? Sounds great, doesn't it? If that were the case, there would be no damage accumulation, no wrinkles, no sagging, and no age spots. That is what we ALL want!

So wouldn't you agree that the safest and the most natural approach to skin aging reversal is the one that harnesses the power of skin remodeling?

Without a doubt. Restoration of younger skin structure requires two linked processes: the removal of damaged proteins and aberrant skin lesions, and their replacement with normal, blemish-free skin.

This process is similar to the remodeling phase of wound healing in which scar tissue is removed over the course of several years, and

NATURAL SKIN ENHANCERS
COPPER-PEPTIDES
ACIDS / ABRASION
RETINOIC ACID / RETINOL
BIOLOGICAL HEALING OILS
ANTIOXIDANTS
VITAMIN C

the skin is slowly restored to its original state. In young children, this process functions efficiently, and skin damage is rapidly removed. But in adults, this process slows drastically, and various skin lesions may persist for years or decades. As skin remodeling becomes less and less efficient, skin damage accumulates, resulting in wrinkled, sagging, uneven skin.

The Holy Grail of Skin Care

How would you like to baby your skin back into the soft, supple, luscious skin you were born with? What if, like a child, your skin could repair itself from scars and other damage within a week or two?

The good news is that young glowing skin is within reach. You can flash skin "soft as a baby's bottom" if you learn methods to remodel and rejuvenate this largest organ in your body. When we remodel our skin, we repair and replace old skin. So it's out with the old and in with the new. The remodeling process, which removes children's scars and damaged skin, also repairs adult wounds. Thus wound healing, like skin remodeling, repairs and rejuvenates skin. When our skin repairs itself, we emerge with a new blemish-free complexion. This restoration works beautifully for children. However, as we age, adult skin remodels far more slowly.

When children get sunburned or injure their skin, they do not develop wrinkles or blemishes. Their skin repairs quickly. So in order to win the war against wrinkles, it makes sense to arm ourselves with the secret to youthful adult skin. Our victory lies in enhancing the skin remodeling process.

When cosmetic products produce skin remodeling, they triumph as the Holy Grail of skin care. According to legend, the Holy Grail possessed the magical power to heal all wounds. And when we remodel skin with potent potions that heal us from wicked wrinkles, the result is pure magic.

The Skin Remodeling Process

Let us look at the skin remodeling process more closely. What actually happens in the skin when it is undergoing remodeling, and how can this process be used to rejuvenate your skin?

In a way, skin remodeling is very similar to remodeling your home. If, for example, you want your freshly painted wall to look nice and last longer, you should first power wash the surface to remove all the old peeling paint. If you want to install new carpet, you always remove the old one first. Similarly, the first stage of the skin remodeling process includes removal of damaged structures.

In the case of wound healing, your skin uses special enzymes to dissolve damaged tissue. If you want to mimic this process for the purpose of skin rejuvenation, you may want to dissolve the damaged area with hydroxy acids or remove it manually (for example, by using skin abrasion).

Now the question for you to consider is: Should we try to remove as much damage as possible at once, or should we go slowly? The answer is: It is absolutely crucial to remove the lesion slowly to avoid triggering skin inflammation or scar formation. Many methods of skin exfoliation produce way too much damage. As a result, they often leave redness, scars, and unwanted pigmentation. You will read more about this in the following chapters.

As soon as you start removing upper skin layers, your skin will activate its repair mechanisms. Unfortunately, this process often involves inflammation. If you use gentle methods of exfoliation and your skin is healthy, this inflammation will soon subside. You may notice some redness or feel a slight burning sensation, but there won't be any lasting discomfort or side effects.

However, if your skin is already damaged and has a disrupted barrier, it may respond with too much inflammation. Therefore, it is very important to baby your skin back to health before attempting remodeling.

You may think of it this way: Imagine a strong fortress guarded by well-trained and well-nourished, healthy soldiers. If there is a slight breach in the fortress's walls, it will be quickly and efficiently repaired. However, if the walls have numerous weak spots, and the defenders are under-nourished and exhausted, any breach in defense may open the way to invaders, bringing war and destruction upon the fortress's residents.

Your skin is your fortress. It is necessary to make sure that your skin is in top regenerative condition, before removing damage. In the next chapters, you will learn how to guide your skin through the skin remodeling process without any risk of further damage.

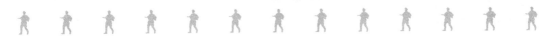

After damage is removed from skin, the repair process is triggered. As a part of this process, your skin releases and activates a special kind of enzyme called a matrix metalloproteinase. These enzymes dissolve damaged collagen, elastin, and glycosaminoglycans in your skin. Even though this stage is essential for skin rejuvenation, it may potentially lead to more damage, since over-activation of metalloproteinases may cause too much destruction.

Therefore, regulation of metalloproteinases is another important part of a well-balanced skin remodeling process. Many methods can activate skin repair, but they do not provide any means of controlling it and preventing it from wreaking havoc on your skin.

In the final stage, skin cells produce new skin proteins and glycosaminoglycans to complete the repair process. If too much collagen is produced, if the collagen types are not present in the correct ratio, or if the skin fails to assemble collagen and elastin into their proper structures, your skin may develop scars and an uneven, dimpled appearance.

Therefore, even if some methods can stimulate collagen production, it is still not enough to correctly rejuvenate skin. More collagen is not necessarily a good thing. In fact, the difference between disorganized collagen and properly assembled collagen fibers is the same as between a pile of bricks and a brick wall. Just look at keloid scars—they have plenty of collagen, but this collagen does not have proper structure. The result is a disaster.

Another part of skin remodeling is the formation of a smooth and even epidermal layer. This is another instance where you need a precise balance to achieve a glowing, supple, even skin appearance.

Your method of skin remodeling should ensure proper formation of the skin barrier, otherwise you'll end up with sensitive, dry, inflamed skin. Having an impaired skin barrier is just like having a leaky roof in your house. Even if the walls are freshly painted, and the floors are covered with luxurious soft carpet, you won't be comfortable until you fix that roof.

As you can see, the skin remodeling process needs to be precisely balanced and well-coordinated. This is why it is so important to select the right method of skin remodeling.

The Ideal Skin Remodeling Solution

The ideal skin remodeling technique should possess the following characteristics:

It should be SAFE. As it enhances the skin remodeling process, there should be no excessive irritation or inflammation.

It should work alongside the NATURAL skin remodeling process.

It should STIMULATE not only collagen, but also elastin and glycosaminoglycans.

It should STIMULATE removal of old proteins in a precisely balanced way without any risk of degrading skin structure.

It should result in a smooth, clear, elastic, resilient skin with HEALTHY structure and youthful glow.

THE SKIN'S NATURAL RENEWAL SYSTEMS AND PROTECTANTS

230 Million Years of Skin Renewal

Over the past 230 million years, skin renewal has depended on only a small number of biological compounds. Dinosaurs and reptiles used similar molecules to heal their skin. Although their ancestors diverged during the Triassic Period, the wound healing process has evolved minimally over time. In essence, skin has not changed much over 230 million years.

Our skin has reemerged with the power and resilience to renew itself, to remove blemishes, scars, and tighten the skin. The goal of skin remodeling is to tap the natural activators within us. In the next chapter, we will explore natural renewal molecules that I like to call the magic tools of skin renewal.

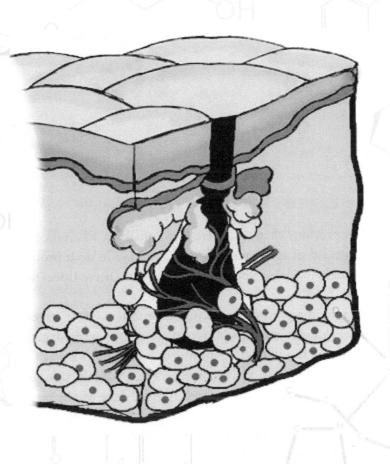

Questions? Email: ghkcopperpeptides@gmail.com

6 MAGIC HELPMATES TO BEAUTIFY YOUR SKIN
AND THE 3 R's OF SKIN RENEWAL—REBUILD, REMODEL, AND RENEW

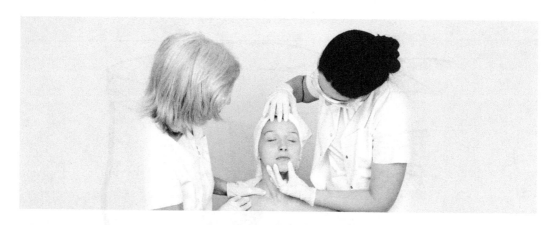

As discussed in previous chapters, there is no quick fix when it comes to skin aging reversal. To get rid of age-related damage, we have to do it properly. Step by step, your skin has to be remodeled, rebuilt, and renewed. These three "Rs" are absolutely essential.

For example, many modern cosmetic products claim to stimulate collagen synthesis. But if we just stimulate synthesis of new collagen without getting rid of the old and worn out proteins, the skin will continue to accumulate damage, such as wrinkles, spots, and other imperfections. Other products may contain substances that remove damaged skin layers. But without proper rebuilding, there will be no rejuvenation.

Only by diligently following the path of Mother Nature (by remodeling, rebuilding, and renewing the skin at the same time) can we win the battle against aging and restore our beautiful skin to its youthful glory. It may not be as fast as we want it, but trust me—there is no shortcut.

We shall now explore six magic tools that you can use to repair, renew, and rebuild your skin.

1. Skin Remodeling Copper Peptides (SRCPs) are key players in dermal restoration. SRCPs work by using the human body's systems to get rid of damaged and worn out proteins, while orchestrating and facilitating skin repair and renewal. They are clinically proven to reduce wrinkles, increase skin thickness, lessen sagging, and produce other anti-aging effects.

2. Exfoliating Hydroxy Acids such as alpha hydroxy acids (AHAs) and beta hydroxy acids (BHAs). These molecules increase the effects of copper peptides by loosening and exfoliating old and worn out layers of skin so that newer layers rebuild more quickly and completely. Also, physical methods of **Abrasion** and skin needling further break up scar tissue and damaged skin to aid in remodeling.

3. Biological Healing Oils (such as emu oil) compensate the age-related depletion of natural skin oil, moisturizing the skin, helping it to rebuild a protective barrier, and speeding up the repair process.

4. Retinoids —members of vitamin A family. Just like AHAs and BHAs, retinoids work with SRCPs to rebuild the skin. Trans-retinoic acid (tretinoin, Retin-A) and cis-retinoic acid (isotretinoin) are prescription drugs that are used to treat acne and sun-damaged skin, while retinaldehyde, retinol, and retinyl esters are used in cosmetics for the same purpose.

5. Vitamin C (ascorbic acid)—an antioxidant vitamin that works together with vitamin E to protect your skin from damaging free radicals. When taken internally, it works with copper to help new collagen synthesis. However, to achieve the effect of aging reversal, vitamin C has to be combined with SRCPs to ensure skin remodeling.

6. Protective Antioxidants are natural compounds that scavenge and remove skin-damaging free radicals.

SKIN REMODELING COPPER PEPTIDES (SRCPS) TARGET SKIN REPAIR

How do SRCPs hit their magic mark? These miraculous molecules are the number one remodelers essential for renewing and restoring youthful skin. Exceptionally safe and exceptionally gentle, there is nothing else quite like SRCPs in the human body. However, be aware that not all copper peptides are created equal. Not all are SRCPs. I have analyzed and tested several other types of copper peptides and found little or no activity. And some copper peptides can even be toxic to the skin.

As I described in Chapter 1, SRCPs help trigger the natural mechanism of renewal and restore the skin to a biologically younger and healthier condition. We have learned a great deal about SRCPs in the past three decades. The first SRCP that I discovered and used for remodeling consisted of a small copper peptide complex present in human blood, saliva, and urine. This blue-colored molecule, technically called GHK-Cu (glycyl-l-histidyl-l-lysine:copper(II)), reversed certain effects of aging in human and animal experiments. In 1984, a few colleagues and I created a company, Procyte (Latin "for the cell"), to develop GHK-Cu into useful products.

It is now used in cosmetics and hair-care and applied after clinical skin renewal procedures, such as chemical peels, laser resurfacing, and dermabrasion, to improve post-treatment skin recovery.

The GHK-Cu Breakthrough: Call Me Mr. Blue

As discussed, many copper peptide products on the market are inept at renewal. So, as with all cosmetics, it's consumer beware. However, years ago, as I began my skin renewal journey, I discovered the uniqueness of GHK-Cu, this blue jewel of a molecule with the power to heal.

Thus, I embarked upon my pilot study with 20 women in 1989. I investigated the wound healing and anti-inflammatory actions of GHK-Cu. To my delight, I discovered that skin creams containing GHK-Cu increased the thickness of the dermis and epidermis, enhanced elasticity, reduced wrinkles, and resulted in the removal of imperfections, such as blotchiness and sun damage, while producing a significant increase in subcutaneous fat cells.

I used my discovery to obtain patents on the cosmetic uses of GHK-Cu. Unfortunately, these observations languished for another 10 years. Most skin-care researchers found it difficult to accept that a single biochemical compound could both heal and beautify the skin.

Today the situation has changed significantly. First of all, numerous studies have established GHK-Cu's capacity to heal wounds and remodel the skin in experimental animals. We also learned a great deal about molecular actions of GHK-Cu, such as its ability to stimulate production of skin's proteins, increase the level of antioxidants and other natural protectors (such as decorin), restore function of damaged skin cells, and revive skin's stem cells.

Finally, between 2002 and 2005, leading dermatologists published nine placebo-controlled studies confirming GHK-Cu's ability to reverse human skin aging. At long last, an increasing number of researchers are beginning to see the light at the end of the blue GHK-Cu tunnel. They now realize that one SRCP can both heal broken and damaged skin and improve the quality of intact, undamaged dermis. (See references in Chapter 23).

Proof in the Cosmetic Pudding

GHK-Cu clinical studies have demonstrated that SRCPs produce the following cosmetic actions on human skin as shown in the graphic:

Reducing fine lines
Smoothing rough skin
Improving skin firmness
Improving overall appearance
Improving skin clarity and "glow"
Calming irritated and reddened skin
Reducing the depth of deep wrinkles
Tightening loose skin and improving elasticity
Tightening the protective skin barrier proteins
Reducing spots, photodamage, and hyperpigmentation

Second-Generation SRCPs Cosmetic Breakthrough

Just when it appears that we have developed the perfect cosmetic, it gets even better with the advent of a second generation of copper products. Although the original GHK-Cu performed well in many studies, especially around the eyes, its mildness makes it best suited for sensitive skin. GHK is a gentle molecule that feels both soothing and elegant. However, for those who seek stronger products, my search continued.

GHK and other peptides are now present in the formulations of many cosmetic products worldwide.

Therefore, in 1994, I started Skin Biology to develop improved, second-generation SRCPs with enhanced potency, breakdown resistance against bacteria, and high adherence to the skin. GHK is quickly destroyed by certain types of enzymes that breakdown peptides (carboxypeptidases), so I isolated peptide fragments from soy protein digests that possessed the desired qualities when bound to copper(II). Such peptides do not cause allergic reactions and have a long history of safe use in cosmetic products.

These new copper peptides outperform prior SRCPs in their ability to heal wounds. In my tests, the second-generation SRCPs have proven to be even more effective than the first. In veterinary studies, creams made from the new SRCPs produced rapid and scar-free healing in dogs and horses. At the *University of California, San Francisco*, Howard Maibach and colleagues tested these new copper peptides in four small, placebo-controlled human studies. They found that creams made from the new complexes produced significantly faster healing and reduced redness and inflammation after mild skin injuries.

This truly is a cosmetic breakthrough. Our work on the new SRCPs had an unexpected result. Somewhat accidentally, women and men began using these products for cosmetic purposes and reported improved skin condition and hair vitality. They found that when they combined breakdown-resistant SRCPs with hydroxy acids, the two products removed many types of blemishes and scars from the skin. Soon thereafter, many reported that the products reduced wrinkles, tightened skin, and improved their hair growth and condition.

Recent studies by Lipotec, the *Barcelona Bioinorganic Chemistry Institute*, and the *University of Milan* examined the mixed soy peptides that I first used at Skin Biology. They found that such peptides increased the synthesis of collagen-3 by 300% in fibroblasts. At age four, 90% of human skin collagen is collagen-3. This declines to less than 10% at age 50. So if more collagen-3 is produced in the skin, then our adult collagen should become more like the collagen in children (See Chapter 19). And we would all love to travel back to our young, lush, collagen-rich skin.

Damaged Skin Must Be Babied Back To Health

As your skin barrier repairs and rebuilds, it will strengthen and grow to shield itself. As a result, fewer materials, including SRCPs, will be able to penetrate it. The area surrounding our eyes is especially thin and delicate. You need to baby it back to health.

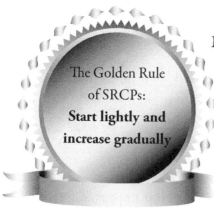

The Golden Rule of SRCPs:

Start lightly and increase gradually

Many women have wreaked havoc on this fragile skin over years by applying harsh color cosmetics and make-up removers.

So as you start with milder SRCPs, your skin will have an opportunity to adjust. You can then transition to stronger products if this sensitive area needs a more intensive rebuilding. So remember the Golden Rule, and baby your skin.

SRCPs and Wound Healing

As we've discussed earlier, baby skin remodels its rosy glow in one to two weeks. However, that rejuvenation halts to a snail's pace over time. So here's where the SRCP magic bullet hits its mark. SRCPs accelerate the pace of wound healing. And the process of remodeling uninjured skin appears similar to how skin remodels itself after wounding. Numerous studies have demonstrated that SRCPs accelerate the healing of wounds and damaged skin and also cause strong remodeling of intact, undamaged skin (For more details see Chapter 19).

Our bodies use the same biochemical mechanisms for closely related purposes. Many dermatological techniques used for skin remodeling (such as lasers, dermabrasion, and chemical peels) actually induce a mild wounding to trigger the remodeling process.

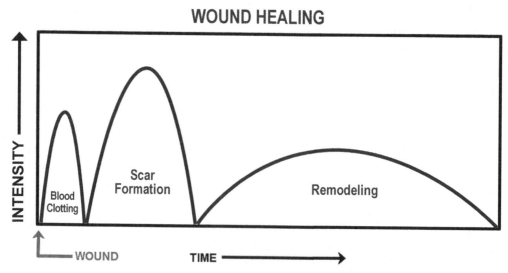

WOUND HEALING

INTENSITY

Blood Clotting

Scar Formation

Remodeling

WOUND   TIME

SRCPs: • **Stimulating Wound Healing**
• **Activating Remodeling of Intact Skin**
(Not all copper peptides and copper complexes are SRCPs, some used in cosmetics actually inhibit skin repair)

EXCITINGLY, RESEARCH SHOWS THAT THIS SAME MECHANISM CAN BE USED TO REDUCE WRINKLES

Example of Reversing Skin Aging by Skin Remodeling

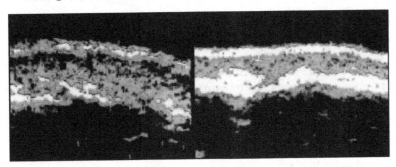

SRCPs REALLY WORK! When we apply SRCP complexes to our skin, these wondrous blue molecules create an environment that helps the skin tighten its barrier and increase its collagen production and elastin density. The above photos show ultrasound scans of a 59-year-old woman before (left) and after (right) one month of treatment with SRCPs. Notice how the scan also illustrates the ultrasonic reflection in tighter, denser areas resulting from closer cellular binding and increased amounts of collagen and elastin. This creates the opposite effect from the usual thinning and loosening of skin produced by aging.

" I have studied methods of reversing human aging for my entire career, and I found a special fraction of peptides from soy proteins that possess remarkable skin regeneration properties ...I'm lucky; I enjoy what I do."

Loren Pickart, PhD

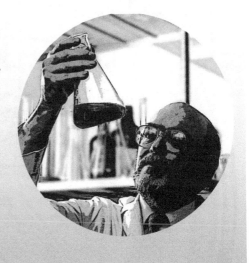

WHAT IS THE SKIN RENEWAL CYCLE? Why is it important? For the first time in the history of skin renewal and wound healing, the Skin Renewal Cycle offers a scientific explanation for how skin repairs itself. This cycle illustrates the biochemistry and cell biology involved with skin repair and remodeling. These mechanisms are based on the many reported actions of the human tripeptides GHK and GHK-Cu from stem cells that lead to the replacement of damaged skin. From these behaviors, we can predict practical actions that will help skin building. For a more detailed explanation, see Chapter 19.

The Skin Renewal Cycle Suggests That...

1 A certain amount of skin damage is needed to activate the early stages of rebuilding. Such damage could be induced by physical abrasion or by acid peels. Even mildly destructive actions, like those caused by lasers or heating devices, can trigger some of these early stages of renewal.

2 An oxidation always accompanies tissue damage as neutrophils (white cells that arrive after injury and help kill bacteria) and macrophages (white cells that remove cellular debris and pathogens, and then secrete various growth factors) plus toxic oxygen radicals kill bacteria after wounding. This explains some of the skin healing actions of mild hydrogen peroxide.

3 SRCPs (Skin Remodeling Copper Peptides) are essential for the later stage of repair where inflammation is suppressed and skin remodeling begins. This requires adequate copper in the tissue.

4 Abnormal skin conditions such as psoriasis and the slow removal of skin scars and lesions may result from inadequate amounts of SRCPs in the skin.

5 SRCPs have multiple and powerful anti-inflammatory actions that protect skin.

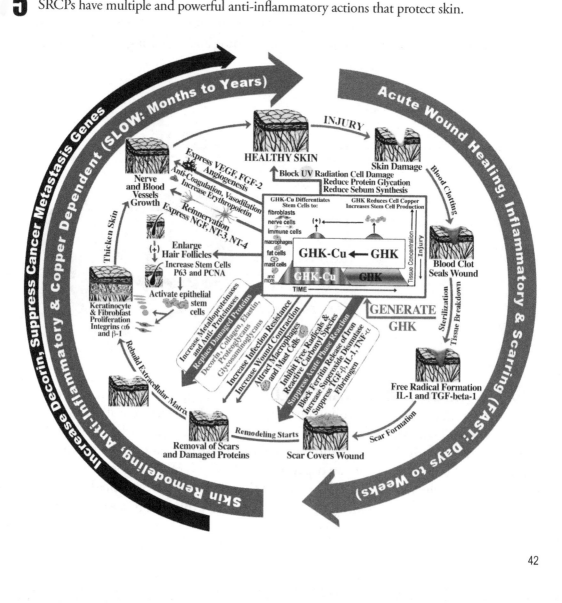

	NATURAL ACTIVATORS	CELL BIOLOGY AND BIOCHEMISTRY	COMMENTS
1.	**Skin Remodeling Copper Peptides (SRCPs)** **Used in human body** **Exist in tissues, plasma and saliva**	1. Anti-inflammatory: Increases Super-oxide Dismutase. Blocks Interleukin-1, TGF-beta-1, and release of oxidizing iron. Detoxifies free radicals and reactive carbonyl species. 2. Activates removal of damaged proteins, scars, and blemishes. 3. Helps synthesis of new collagen, elastin, and water-holding molecules for firmer, more elastic skin. 4. Helps rebuild microcirculation for better skin nutrition and youthful "glow". 5. Helps tighten collagen strands and loose skin. 6. Repairs skin barrier to be more protective against viruses and bacteria, and lose less moisture. 7. May increase production of stem cells for the skin. 8. SRCPs without copper increase stem cell production / SRCPs with copper differentiate stem cells into cells used for rebuilding skin. 9. Increases proliferation of fibroblasts and keratinocytes. 10. Protects keratinocytes from UV radiation. 11. Reduces protein glycation. 12. Activates epithelial (adult) stem cells and slows aging throughout the body by increasing p63. 13. Suppresses cancer metastasis genes.	Very safe.
2.	**Exfoliating Hydroxy Acids**	Normally on and in skin. Lactic acid and salicylic acid are normally on the skin.	Irritating if used excessively.
3.	**Biological Healing Oils**	Emu oil is similar to human skin oils. Squalane is normally in the skin.	Emu oil and squalane have proven healing effects.
4.	**Retinoic Acid**	Normally in skin. Proven to remodel skin but may act by irritation and exfoliation. Role in skin appears to help differentiate stem cells into skin cells.	Often used with SRCPs for better effects with less irritation.
5.	**Vitamin C**	Normally in skin. Acts with copper(II) to tighten collagen strands.	Best if taken as a supplement (500 mg - 1 g daily)
6.	**Protective Antioxidants**	Naturally occur in our skin, but are depleted as we age. Prevent free radical damage to skin proteins and skin barrier.	Only natural antioxidants are protective. Avoid artificial and exotic antioxidants.

ALPHA HYDROXY ACIDS (AHAs) FOR SKIN RENEWAL

The origin of alpha hydroxy acids traces back thousands of years to the days of Cleopatra. In the ancient book *Beautification*, Cleopatra described how she applied fruit acids, sour wine, and sour milk (all of which contain AHAs) to renew and beautify the skin. The book was on the Egyptian "best-seller" list for 200 years.

In 1974, Doctors Ruey Yu and Eugene Van Scott investigated the effects of alpha hydroxy acids (AHAs) on skin. It took another 15 years of research until these compounds made their way in cosmetic products. Today, AHAs are proven to speed up skin turnover, remove skin lesions, and restore the skin's firmness, elasticity, and internal moisture-holding properties.

AHAs work by loosening dead cells in the skin's outer layers, helping to remove old and worn out layers. They also create an acidic environment that stimulates the skin's own exfoliating enzymes, speeding up natural skin renewal processes. As a result, the newer skin rebuilds more quickly and completely. However, a word of caution before you rush to buy AHA products—just as any truly active ingredients, they have to be present in certain concentration in order to produce an effect. Consumer cosmetic products should contain at least 10% AHA, while estheticians in beauty salons carefully use 20-30% solutions. Up to 50-70% concentrations are sometimes used by expert dermatologists; however, at such concentrations, AHAs lose their gentleness and may inflict too much damage to the skin.

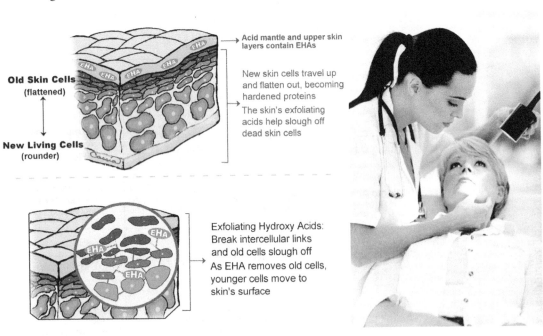

Since AHAs may be irritating at working concentrations, many cosmetic products contain minute amounts of these acids and consequently offer no benefit to skin.

Similar to AHAs are BHAs (beta-hydroxy acids) such as salicylic acid. Initially, they were used by medical doctors in high concentration for removal of pigmented spots and in low concentration for their anti-inflammatory and antibacterial action in acne treatment. In today's cosmetic products, BHAs are used for gentle exfoliation of oily and acne prone skin.

AHAs work best on the skin surface, while BHAs can travel into the oil glands, which makes them really helpful for people with oily skin and acne. The most natural AHA is lactic acid, which is naturally present in skin. Salicylic acid (BHA) is present in skin and in certain plants (e.g. raspberry and willow tree bark).

AHAs and BHAs work synergistically with SRCPs, removing upper layers of worn and damaged cells, speeding up skin renewal, and improving intake of SRCPs into the skin.

Peel Away Mother Time

How about a rub-a-dub-dub when you get out of the tub? We can mildly abrade our skin by gently rubbing or scrubbing with a Loofah brush, sponge or wash cloth.

With gentle abrasion, we remove older skin and blemishes while helping our skin to rebuild. Animals will often rub against a tree or fence post to help heal damaged areas of their body. Our skin adapts well to abrasion and slight damage by launching a strong regenerative skin-repair response. Methods such as micro-dermabrasion, a mild abrasion of the skin's upper surface, have proven very effective.

BIOLOGICAL HEALING OILS (BHOs) BABY YOUR SKIN

Biological healing oils contain fats or lipids that exist naturally in the epidermis and on the skin's surface. The surface of the skin is covered with sebum, which is a special mixture of neutral fat and fatty acids (60%), waxes (25%), cholesterol and its esters (3%), and squalene (12%). The stratum corneum contains so called epidermal lipids, which are a mixture of ceramides (approximately 40%), palmitic acid (approximately 25%), cholesterol (25%), and cholesteryl sulfate (10%).

Today we know that skin needs good oils to stay moist and supple, but for quite a long time, there was a discussion on whether the skin needs oil or just more water to be soft, plump, and smooth. The first scientist who proposed using oils to heal skin was Albert Kligman in the 1960's. He also coined the term "corneotherapy"—a method to correct skin's disorders by treating its stratum corneum.

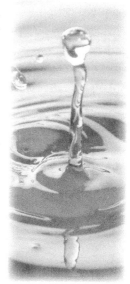

It has been established that oils which are similar to the skin's oils help beautify our skin by protecting its barrier. They waterproof the skin. The oils also help repair the skin barrier by acting as glue that binds the outer proteins together, keeping them relatively dry, hard and protective. If you were to visualize these proteins as bricks in a wall, the BHOs would act as mortar holding them together. BHOs also moisturize the skin by blocking excessive water loss. Unfortunately, these naturally occurring oils lessen as we age.

We can apply these oils to our skin to modify the level of SRCP absorption. Depending on how we layer these oils with SRCPs, BHOs will either increase or reduce SRCP effects. For example, if we apply BHOs over a milder SRCP product, the oil then pushes more SRCPs into the skin or hair follicle, thus increasing its effects. However, to reduce SRCP effects on irritated skin, we can apply BHOs before SRCPs. This reduces the uptake of SRCPs and thereby produces a milder reaction. Emu oil contains a molecular structure similar to natural skin oils. Indigenous people of Australia have used this amazing oil to moisturize and heal for thousands of years.

A word of warning, since natural oils may feel a bit greasy on your skin and not so easily incorporated into cosmetic formulations, many modern cosmetic products that claim to soften and moisturize your skin contain no natural oils whatsoever or very little of them. Instead, they achieve the illusion of nourishment and moisturization by adding artificial oil-like substances such as silicones and fatty acid esters. These ingredients are very different from natural skin lipids and may damage your barrier structures. They also can be comedogenic—that is, they can clog the pores, creating blackheads.

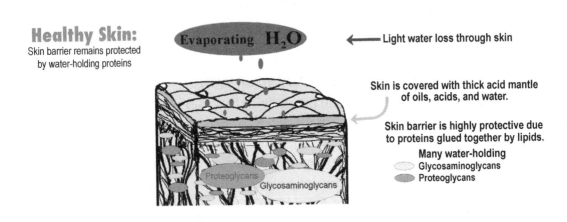

Healthy Skin:
Skin barrier remains protected by water-holding proteins

Evaporating H_2O

Light water loss through skin

Skin is covered with thick acid mantle of oils, acids, and water.

Skin barrier is highly protective due to proteins glued together by lipids.

Many water-holding
Glycosaminoglycans
Proteoglycans

Proteoglycans

Glycosaminoglycans

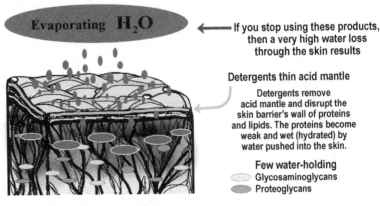

False Cosmetic Moisturizers:
Product quickly makes skin attractive at cosmetic sales counter, but slowly damages the skin, inhibiting normal skin renewal and producing a daily moisturizer need somewhat like a drug addiction

Evaporating H_2O

If you stop using these products, then a very high water loss through the skin results

Detergents thin acid mantle

Detergents remove acid mantle and disrupt the skin barrier's wall of proteins and lipids. The proteins become weak and wet (hydrated) by water pushed into the skin.

Few water-holding
Glycosaminoglycans
Proteoglycans

The wetness of the upper skin layers stops the signals to the lower layers to produce more skin cells to move to the surface and reduces the production of water holding molecules in the skin.

RETINOIDS—MAGNIFY THE POWER OF SRCPs

Even before its official discovery, vitamin A was used for centuries for its skin benefits. In ancient Greece, doctors used raw liver (rich in vitamin A) to cure certain skin diseases.

During World War I, it was observed that a deficiency of vitamin A leads to extreme skin dryness (xerosis) and thickening of the stratum corneum (hyperkeratosis). Initially, cod liver oil was used in cosmetics as a source of vitamin A; however, not everybody appreciated its strong fishy smell.

In the 1830's, H.W.F. Wackenroder isolated beta-carotene—a plant precursor of vitamin A. In the 1930's, a highly active, but still impure, form of vitamin A was isolated. In 1942, J.G. Baxter isolated pure vitamin A, and in 1947, A. van Dorp succeeded at synthesizing vitamin A.

In 1968, the pharmaceutical company Hoffmann-La-Roche began research on retinoids—chemical compounds that have structures and effects similar to vitamin A. In 1979, they were able to develop the first anti-acne products with retinoids.

Today's retinoid family includes vitamin A (retinol), retinoic acid, retinaldehyde, retinyl esters, as well as their synthetic derivatives. Today, it is known that vitamin A is a natural gene regulator which is closely involved in cell growth and differentiation as well as in many other biological processes. In the skin, retinoids increase skin thickness, speed up cell turnover, stimulate glycosaminoglycan synthesis, and reduce oiliness and inflammation.

Vitamin A derivatives (retinoids) include prescription retinoids (such as retinoic acid, also known as tretinoin) and OTC retinoids (such as adapalene and retinol). Retinoic acid is approved by the U.S. Food and Drug Administration for treatment of aged skin.

In 2016, FDA also approved another retinoid, adapalene (brand name Differin) as a once-daily topical gel for the over-the-counter (OTC) treatment of acne. The main problem with retinoids is skin irritation, which discourages many people from using them.

Many people use SRCPs and retinoic acid products together and report better results with less irritation. Retinoic acid can function in a similar manner to AHAs by helping SRCPs speed up skin renewal. Cosmetic products may contain retinol, retinaldehyde, or retinyl esters.

Retinol has to be present in high concentration (about 1-2%), to produce an anti-aging effect. Unfortunately, this high level can be irritating. Many people use SRCPs and retinoic acid products together and report better results with less irritation.

Retinoic acid can function in a similar manner to AHAs by helping SRCPs speed up skin renewal. For women with mature dry skin, retinol in low concentrations adds skin oil, which moisturizes the skin.

However, retinol can increase acne for those between 18 and 30 years of age. Paradoxically, persons between ages 25 and 40 often report that these creams help with chronic cystic acne.

When using retinol cream, it is best to start slowly and work up to a higher dose. Many women have asked me to clarify how the effects of retinoic acid and retinol differ. Cosmetic companies often foster confusion regarding these two products in order to promote their merchandise.

Retinoic acid, contained in various commercial products, helps remodel skin. Retinoic acid requires a prescription. Retinol, a weaker form of vitamin A sold by cosmetic companies, does not require a prescription. Although retinol offers many benefits, it does not remodel skin.

The following chart highlights the differences between the two:

	Retinoic Acid	Retinol
Chemical Name	Retinoic Acid	Retinyl alcohol
Common Name	Vitamin A acid	Vitamin A
Prescription Drugs	Retin-A	Not a drug
Effect on skin oil	Reduces skin oil	Increases skin oil
Effect on wrinkles	Strong wrinkle reduction	Mild effect on reduction of fine lines

VITAMIN C (ASCORBIC ACID) TIGHTENS YOUR SKIN

Vitamin C was discovered in 1932 as a factor in lemon juice that prevents scurvy—a potentially fatal disease which manifested with bleeding gums, loose teeth, hemorrhages, and connective tissue fragility. Today it is known that scurvy is not the first but the last and final symptom of vitamin C deficiency, since many more less noticeable but important deleterious changes occur in earlier stages of vitamin C deficiency. Many of them involve skin.

Our tissue cells use vitamin C and a copper enzyme called lysyl oxidase to cross-link and tighten collagen. It also serves as a powerful antioxidant that, together with vitamin E, scavenges and detoxifies harmful free radicals. In order to reap the skin tightening benefits of vitamin C, your system requires adequate amounts of both copper(II) and vitamin C. Since ascorbic acid is very unstable in cosmetic formulations and cannot penetrate the skin well enough, it is best to put copper products on the skin and raise your vitamin C levels with oral supplements. You can take 500 mg to 1 gram daily since increased vitamin C is easily tolerated.

We need about 20 milligrams of vitamin C daily to stay alive. However, based on natural diets of other primates, studies suggest that 5 grams per day would be a better dosage for humans. Our ancestors evolved on a diet very high in vitamin C. The diet of primates, such as gorillas, chimpanzees, and monkeys, contains high levels of vitamin C that would be comparable to ingesting 5 grams daily in humans.

Protective Antioxidants

In 1937, after several years of research, Olcott and Emerson established that vitamin E (alpha, beta, and gamma tocopherols and other related substances) is an effective antioxidant in fatty liquids such as milk. But although it was known that the human body contains many fatty substances, for a long time many researchers would not accept the idea that the same oxidative reactions that occur in milk and fatty solutions may be important in biological systems as well.

It took decades of research before the physiological role of natural antioxidants was established, and their part as protectors against aging was proven.

Now it is known that the human body and, in particular, the skin have an elaborate antioxidant system that includes vitamins such as vitamins A, E, and C, low-weight molecular substances such as co-enzyme Q10 and alpha-lipoic acid, and antioxidant enzymes such as superoxide dismutase (SOD), catalase, and glutathione peroxidase.

Also, our body makes use of many antioxidants present in food such as lycopene, lutein, flavonoids, and others. Taken together, all those antioxidants control free radicals in our body, protecting it from aging. Unfortunately, antioxidant defense weakens as we age. SRCPs were proven to increase the level of natural antioxidants in our skin, prolonging skin youth.

Antioxidants are often added to cosmetics to protect skin against free radicals caused by excessive UV-radiation and environmental pollutants. However, it is important to stick with ingredients normally used in the body which include the vitamin E family, tocotrienols, lutein, lycopene, CoQ-10, and alpha-lipoic acid. Our body has learned what it needs over several hundred million years.

Exotic antioxidants that the body chose not to use in the past can harm us today. So just say "no" to artificial compounds advertised as more potent than the body's natural antioxidants. Remember also that many heavily advertised natural antioxidants are present in fruits and vegetables and work better when taken internally.

For example, instead of buying an expensive cream with grape seed extract containing a potent antioxidant resveratrol, just indulge in a glass of red wine.

While free radicals can damage skin and other tissues, we need a certain amount of them for many key reactions within the body. For example, immune cells require free radicals in order to kill bacteria, viruses, and cancer cells. Mitochondria use free radicals to produce energy. Artificial antioxidants are so powerful that they cause tissue damage by shutting down key reactions. Some have even produced cancer.

It's all about maintaining a delicate balance. Too much or too little of a good thing can create ill health. Artificial antioxidants cause havoc. Only when we nourish the body with what it needs can we renew and revitalize our largest organ—the skin.

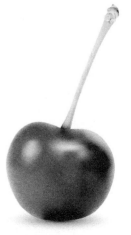

Tips for Natural Skin Renewal

The following methods will help optimize your results.

If you have sensitive skin and want to decrease the activity of SRCPs, start by applying a biological healing oil (BHO). When you apply a BHO supplemented with the skin's natural antioxidants *before* applying SRCPs, you reduce the effect. These healing oils penetrate the skin and form an oil barrier that slows the SRCP uptake into your skin. Women often use this method for irritated or sensitive skin, such as after laser burns or deep peels.

After you have used copper peptide topicals for a while, you may want to step up the remodeling. To increase the activity of SRCPs, follow the product application with a biological healing oil. When you apply a BHO *after* SRCPs, you increase the effect because the oil pushes more SRCPs into the skin. These biological oils not only enhance SRCPs, they also make great eye make-up removers, because they are much kinder to your skin than the make-up removers manufactured by cosmetic companies. Women often use this method to gently cleanse the skin around the delicate eye area.

In addition to biological oils, exfoliating hydroxy acids (EHAs) increase remodeling. EHAs can help rebuild and loosen older skin and scar tissue. Hydroxy acids exist naturally on the skin's surface and work synergistically with SRCPs. Lactic and salicylic acids are the most natural exfoliators. Normally, a person can use one product in the morning and the other at night. Stronger hydroxy acids work faster, but overuse can irritate the skin. Some people use SRCPs and hydroxy acids on alternate days.

Now how about an additional way to remodel our skin? When we scrub our skin with a loofah, the abrasion can help remove lesions. Various types of abrasion inflict mild damage that stimulate removal of scars and older skin. Abrasive methods, whether applied at the doctor's office or at home, remove damaged skin.

Dermatologists offer dermabrasion, which helps remove elevated and flat scars and lesions, and needling (subcision), which removes and loosens scar tissue in depressed scars and pitted acne. At-home abrasion methods include microdermabrasion units, files, pumice stones, and good old loofahs and brushes.

IN CONCLUSION The six magic tools of skin rejuvenation—SRCPs, exfoliating hydroxy acids, healing bio-oils, retinoids, vitamin C, and protective antioxidants—have earned their badges of honor. It took decades of research in many scientific laboratories before their molecular actions were elucidated, their skin effects proven, and their safety well established. From these examples, you can see what it really takes to develop a genuinely science-based cosmetic ingredient—one that truly works without hurting the skin. I hope it will make you a bit suspicious when you are offered a new miracle anti-aging cure that no one has heard about just a month or so ago.

However, out of these six powerful tools of skin rejuvenation, only SRCPs provide the most complete spectrum of skin age reversal activity, remodeling, rebuilding, and renewal (the three "Rs" of skin rejuvenation). All of the remaining five tools work as the trusty side-kicks, intensifying and enhancing SRCP action. In the following chapters, you will learn how to use the synergistic action of SRCPs and other scientifically proven age reversal agents to solve various skin problems.

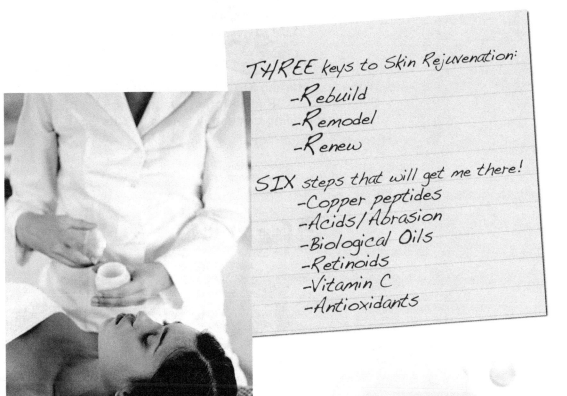

THREE keys to Skin Rejuvenation:
- Rebuild
- Remodel
- Renew

SIX steps that will get me there!
- Copper peptides
- Acids/Abrasion
- Biological Oils
- Retinoids
- Vitamin C
- Antioxidants

My Personal Tips Page

Figure 1: Milder Effect
Apply Oil First
Apply SRCPs on Top

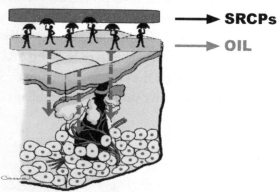

When first starting SRCPs for skin renewal:
Slow down SRCP penetration by applying
biological healing oils lightly before SRCPs

Figure 2: Stronger Effect
Apply SRCPs First
Apply Oil on Top

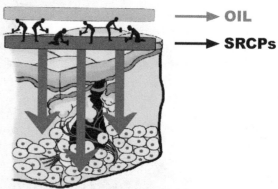

After a period of time for enhanced results:
Apply biological healing oils after applying
SRCPs to skin to increase SRCP uptake

Questions? Email: ghkcopperpeptides@gmail.com

6

SAY GOODBYE TO FINE LINES & WRINKLES
ACTIVATING YOUR BODY'S OWN WRINKLE REMOVAL SYSTEM

 QUOTABLE QUOTES: *Skin should be like fine wine… Getting better with age!*
– Submitted Comment

The good news is that copper peptides really do work without taking you to the poor house. The key to younger-looking, healthier skin is skin remodeling. In this chapter, you will discover the most effective methods for natural skin renewal. Let us now embark upon a journey to turn back the wrinkled hands of time. To understand how to battle wrinkles, it helps to know how a wrinkle develops.

Fine Lines

Fine lines are superficial wrinkles that first appear in areas with thin, drier skin, such as around the eye. These wrinkles are the easiest to remove. Practically anything that creates mild skin swelling will work for fine lines. Some "anti-aging" products contain mild irritants, which increase blood flow and cause low-grade inflammation. Another common approach is to use detergents, which damage skin barrier and cause temporary swelling of the upper layer. Many products contain polymeric substances, which mechanically tighten skin. The result is fast and amazing—it pleases our hearts to see that just a few seconds after we apply this seductive smelling and soft-to-the-touch cream to our face, our skin becomes noticeably younger. Unfortunately, such products do not rejuvenate skin and can even accelerate aging.

To truly get rid of this type of wrinkle, you need to gradually restore your skin barrier and increase the amount of water-holding molecules in your dermis. SRCPs have been clinically proven to strengthen the skin's barrier and to increase the production of glycosaminoglycans and proteoglycans in the skin. Therefore, they are able to restore skin's natural capacity to bind and hold moisture, eliminating those fine lines without inflicting any damage to your skin.

Expression Wrinkles

Expression wrinkles are caused by facial muscles stretching skin. They appear on our forehead, around the eyes, and at the sides of the mouth (often called smile and frown lines). Although they are called expression wrinkles and develop in places where our facial muscles stretch our skin, their primary cause is actually loss of skin elasticity.

When you stroke a child's skin, you will notice that it feels tight and elastic, like the surface of a balloon. This is why children can laugh, cry, and make faces and still have smooth and beautiful skin.

Unfortunately, as we age, our skin thins and becomes loose and inelastic. Over time, muscle tension in the face becomes stronger than the skin's elasticity, and muscle contractions begin to create wrinkles.

Wrinkles: Skin Elasticity vs. Muscle Tension

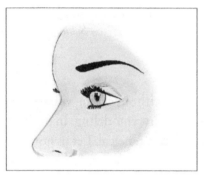

Skin elasticity pulls in
all directions
(like surface of a balloon)

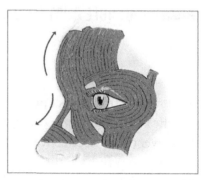

Muscle fibers pull along
axis of muscle fibers

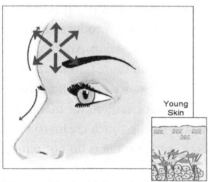

Young skin is thick and elastic,
resists muscle tension,
and is wrinkle free

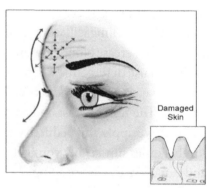

Older skin is less elastic
and cannot resist muscle wrinkling,
producing brow lines & "crows feet"

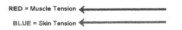

RED = Muscle Tension
BLUE = Skin Tension

© Loren Pickart PhD

54

Fortunately, there is a way to reduce mimic wrinkles, and this is by restoring the skin's natural elasticity with the help of SRCPs. The wonderful thing about this method is that you can get rid of your wrinkles and still retain your ability to smile, laugh, and even make faces if you wish.

Sagging and Loose Skin

There is one law that everybody has to obey—the law of gravity. Every living moment of our life, Earth's gravity pulls us down. That is why it is much easier to lie down than it is to stand up. Our skin feels this pull too. When we are young, our strong facial muscles and elastic, resilient dermal proteins manage to defy gravity, keeping our skin from sagging. But as we age, muscle tension and collagen elasticity decrease. This is where our skin's ability to stretch plays a bad trick on us, because we develop folds and flaps under our checks, eyes, and chin.

Surgeons solve this problem by cutting off excess skin and tightening up the remaining part. This is called a surgical facelift, and it is a very efficient method of removing flaps and folds. However, a facelift does not change the structure of the skin because it does not remove old skin proteins, nor does it facilitate the production of new ones.

Loss of Collagen Elasticity

The most difficult wrinkles are those that develop due to accumulating damage of the skin's collagen and elastin. This should be a very slow process, but it is greatly accelerated by excessive UV-radiation. When collagen and elastin are damaged, the skin's surface becomes uneven with dimpled, bumpy areas. A combination of collagen damage and mimic wrinkles, along with the pull of gravity, produces deep creases such as nasolabial folds.

Just as in the case of fine lines developed due to lack of moisture, if you swell skin with water, its surface will temporarily look smoother and firmer. However, under this seemingly younger skin, there will still be vast areas of broken, damaged, and inelastic collagen. So as soon as you stop applying the anti-aging cream, the damage becomes visible again!

In contrast, the natural wrinkle-reduction methods described in this book restore skin thickness and elasticity, essentially transforming it to act more like biologically younger skin. The key goal here is to firm and moisturize, thereby bringing you back the skin you were born with. The remodeling process tightens skin by replacing damaged proteins with new elastin and collagen, and it moisturizes by increasing the water-holding proteoglycans and glycosaminoglycans.

Remember, the power of copper peptides was first discovered in the field of wound healing. Since the process of healing wounds works similarly to repairing skin, this makes SRCPs extremely effective.

This repair process is just what the doctor ordered to naturally decrease the appearance of wrinkles. SRCPs in creams or serums have been shown in many studies to firm, moisturize, and reduce wrinkles. And as previously noted, copper peptide products may work even better when combined with hydroxy acids, which enhance the remodeling process.

TREATING DIFFERENT TYPES OF WRINKLES
As you can see, not all wrinkles are created equal. We all have them, and each and every one of us wants to get rid of our wretched wrinkles—yes, that includes you and me!

Unfortunately, there is no one simple method for removing those time-telling lines. You should use a different approach to remove lines on the forehead, around the mouth, on the cheeks, and at the edge of the eyes (known as crow's feet) than the approach you would use on lines around and under the eyes. The latter type requires special care because the thin skin surrounding the eye is prone to damage.

Nasolabial folds, those unflattering furrows that frame our sweet smiles, often concern clients more than any other wrinkles. These deep lines lie between the nose and corners of the mouth. They may run side to side, but they most often appear vertically. They are associated with hanging skin. These furrows or folds tend to make a person seem sad or much older than their actual age.

Treating Facial Wrinkles
In the days of Cleopatra, ladies pampered their bodies with wine baths to have smooth silky skin. And guess what? We can reduce wrinkles by alternating the application of hydroxy acids with SRCPs. Hydroxy acids remove upper layers of skin, while SRCPs stimulate repair.

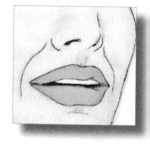

SRCPs can be used to help remodel and rebuild the skin. While stronger hydroxy acids work better in the short term, they have a tendency to irritate.

Heavy-duty hydroxy acids can lead to a rash or peeling when skin is removed due to the strong acid concentrate. Overall, I recommend you take a slower approach to obtain the same result without irritation. Just apply lighter, less concentrated hydroxy acids for a longer period of time.

As your skin adjusts to the SRCPs (particularly when combined with hydroxy acids), you may experience a brief two-week period of skin loosening before it tightens. Damaged skin can behave somewhat like hardened scar tissue, since its toughness holds everything in place.

As SRCPs help remove this damage, your skin may briefly slacken. Skin fibroblasts then begin the rebuilding process by first producing collagen and elastin, after which they slowly pull the protein strands together and tighten the skin.

You might also notice the exposure of deeply buried scar tissue. Normal scar tissue often covers old wounds and blemishes, thereby concealing them. As an example, cystic acne can form hard blemishes under the skin, which are later covered by superficial skin cells.

As the skin exfoliates, these old lesions may become visible. When you apply SRCPs and hydroxy acids to problem areas, this helps to remove the buried damage.

Treating Wrinkles Around the Eyes

As the thinnest skin on our body, the delicate eye area presents us with one of the most difficult regions to repair, keep healthy, and keep youthful in appearance.

This fragile skin tends to get irritated and may stay in a condition of sub-clinical inflammation. Years of applying color cosmetics and other make-up, which contain a high concentration of dyes and metal salts, can produce extensive damage and sagging. In addition, the cleansers we use to remove make-up can cause further irritation by stripping away protective lipids from the skin.

To ensure that your delicate skin around the eye does not become damaged or irritated, start with restoring its protective barrier by applying biological healing oils. Then you may start using gentle cosmetic products that contain low concentrations of copper peptides, gradually working up to higher concentrations. When it comes to eye skin care, patience is the key.

I have discovered that using a progressively stronger remodeling system to treat the skin around the eyes leads to better results.

Many start with a relatively weak cream. Then as the skin adjusts to the SRCPs and becomes somewhat thicker and more protective, they move on to stronger products. So I advise that you begin by using the milder products gradually and at low concentrations.

If a product should irritate your eye area, I suggest that you apply a biological healing oil to slow the uptake of the product as was mentioned earlier in the book. Applying a biological healing oil (BHO) before the SRCP product will result in a much milder response.

You will recall that if you apply a BHO after a SRCP product instead, the oil will push more of the SRCPs into the skin and intensify their effect. In this manner, it is possible to adjust the SRCP action to receive maximum results. In general, hydroxy acids, even at a very low concentration, should not be used around the eyes.

When you first begin to treat the delicate eye area, I suggest you follow these tips in order to help adjust to your new regimen:

My Steps to **BEAUTIFUL EYES**

1 Start by cleansing around the eye area to remove make-up. Use a very mild make-up remover, such as a biological healing oil. Rinse with clear water. Apply a mild copper peptide product designed specifically for use around the eye area while the skin is still wet.

2 Because the skin may be badly damaged, start with a very gentle copper peptide topical, perhaps a product containing GHK-Cu, and then gradually increase the amount you apply over time. If you experience irritation, that means you have applied too much copper peptide through a very damaged skin barrier. In this case, you might try a gentler approach of alternating with a biological oil one night to replenish skin lipids and a SRCP product every second night.

As your skin barrier repairs itself, you will grow less sensitive to products. With time, the area around your eyes should tighten and firm, and you can progress to more powerful products.

3 If you experience excessive dryness, use a little less of the SRCP product and cover it with a light amount of a biological healing oil.

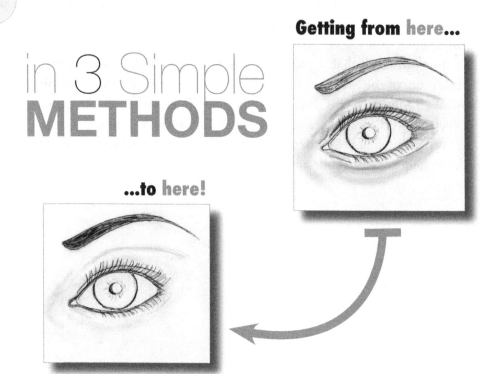

in 3 Simple **METHODS**

Getting from here...

...to here!

SKIN CARE GUIDE

How to Tighten the Delicate Area Around the Eyes

The key to remodeling this delicate area is to go slow by applying a thin layer of mild copper peptides underneath the eye, on the outside areas, or under the brow bone to affect a lift of the upper lid area before slowly graduating to stronger products.

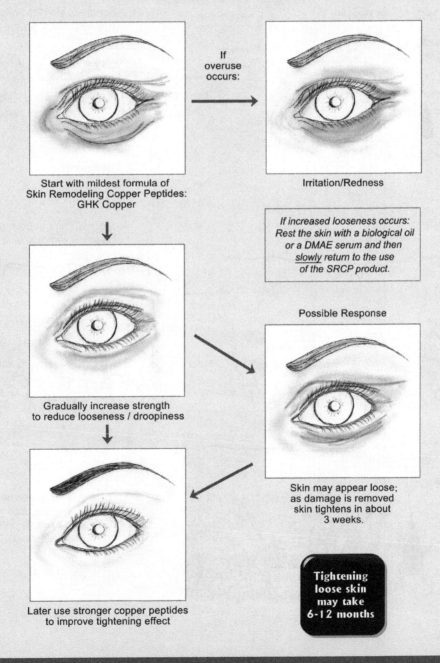

If overuse occurs:

Start with mildest formula of Skin Remodeling Copper Peptides: GHK Copper

Irritation/Redness

If increased looseness occurs: Rest the skin with a biological oil or a DMAE serum and then <u>slowly</u> return to the use of the SRCP product.

Possible Response

Gradually increase strength to reduce looseness / droopiness

Skin may appear loose; as damage is removed skin tightens in about 3 weeks.

Later use stronger copper peptides to improve tightening effect

Tightening loose skin may take 6-12 months

A PERSONALIZED HOW TO GUIDE · DESIGNED FOR MY SKIN

SKIN CARE GUIDE

How to Reduce the Appearance of Wrinkles with Hydroxy Acids and SRCPs (Natural Method)

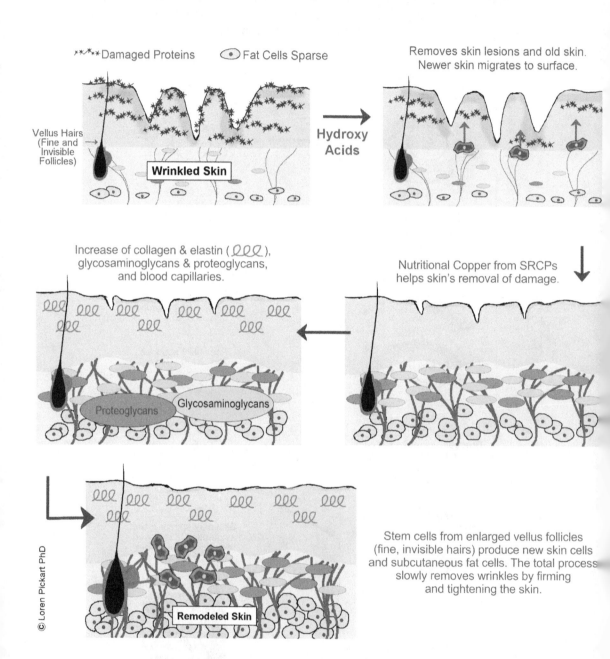

*✗** Damaged Proteins   ⊙ Fat Cells Sparse

Removes skin lesions and old skin. Newer skin migrates to surface.

Vellus Hairs (Fine and Invisible Follicles)

Wrinkled Skin

Hydroxy Acids

Increase of collagen & elastin (ℓℓℓ), glycosaminoglycans & proteoglycans, and blood capillaries.

Nutritional Copper from SRCPs helps skin's removal of damage.

Proteoglycans   Glycosaminoglycans

© Loren Pickart PhD

Remodeled Skin

Stem cells from enlarged vellus follicles (fine, invisible hairs) produce new skin cells and subcutaneous fat cells. The total process slowly removes wrinkles by firming and tightening the skin.

SKIN CARE GUIDE

How to Reduce the Appearance of Nasolabial Lines

Laugh lines are definitely nothing to smile about...

The strongest form of copper peptides should always be started slowly:

1. In the morning after cleansing, apply a hydroxy acid into the crease area.

2. At night, work in an effective copper peptide cream very lightly directly into wrinkle.

3. REPEAT CONSISTENTLY...

You can expect a significant reduction in fine lines after 3 to 4 months of applying this method. An eyebrow brush can be used to add a little abrasion while working products deep into the skin.

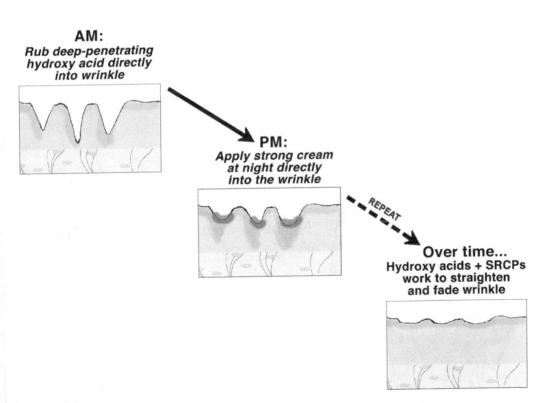

AM:
Rub deep-penetrating hydroxy acid directly into wrinkle

PM:
Apply strong cream at night directly into the wrinkle

REPEAT

Over time...
Hydroxy acids + SRCPs work to straighten and fade wrinkle

SKIN CARE GUIDE

Other Methods: Things to Keep in Mind
USING: Dermabrasion

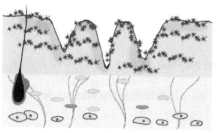

→ Dermabrasion performed on the skin

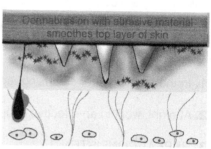

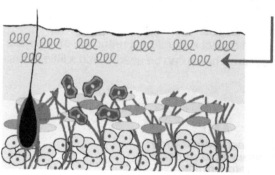

BETTER RESULT:
Follow with SRCPs and dermabrasion
for less redness and
better healing.

SRCPs help activate the stem cells from
enlarged vellus follicles to produce
new skin cells and subcutaneous fat cells.
Total process slowly firms and tightens
skin after dermabrasion procedure.

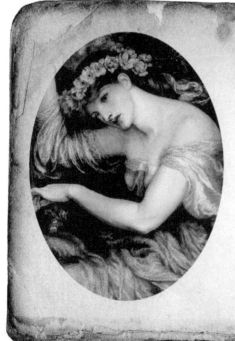

"She will bring, in spite of frost,
Beauties that the earth hath lost...
Where's the cheek that doth not fade,
Too much gaz'd at? Where's the maid
Whose lip mature is ever new?
Where's the eye, however blue
Doth not weary? Where's the face
One would meet in every place?"

—John Keats

USING: Laser Resurfacing

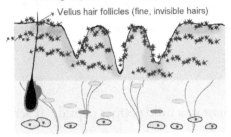

Damaged proteins   • Few fat cells

Vellus hair follicles (fine, invisible hairs)

Laser resurfacing performed

Laser burns off top layer of skin

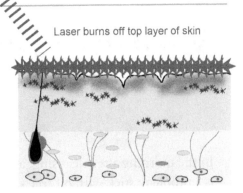

BETTER RESULT:
Follow laser resurfacing with SRCPs
for fewer scars, less redness,
and faster healing time.

SRCPs help activate the stem cells from
enlarged vellus follicles to produce
new skin cells and subcutaneous fat cells.
Total process slowly firms and tightens
skin after laser resurfacing procedure.

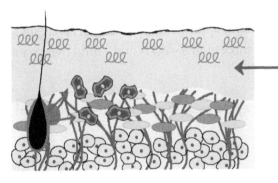

c Loren Pickart PhD

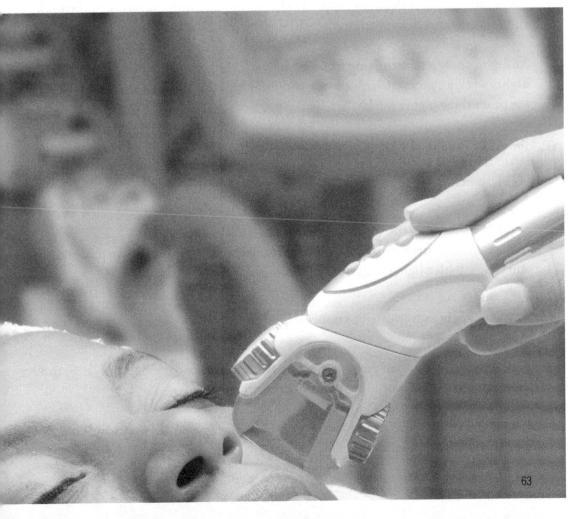

Wrinkle Busting Regimens

The best way to remove wrinkles and damage depends on your skin type. We recommend the following regimens:

Under Age 30

1. In the morning after cleansing, apply a light amount of a mild copper peptide. If acne is a problem, stick with oil-free serum solutions.

2. At night, apply a moisturizing facial cream also containing copper peptides over your face three nights weekly and a mild hydroxy acid leave-on three alternate nights weekly.

3. If dry patches are a problem, use a biological healing oil that does not cause breakouts.

Over Age 30

1. In the morning after cleansing, apply a light amount of a mild copper peptide product, and follow with a light coating of the biological oil of your choice.

2. At night, apply a moisturizing facial cream with copper peptides over your face three nights weekly. Alternate with the use of a mild leave-on hydroxy acid cream or serum the other three nights weekly.

3. After two months, you may progress to a stronger hydroxy acid, such as a 30 percent lactic acid (and a strong copper peptide product). Be sure to use stronger products lightly at first.

Anti-Wrinkle/Rosacea

1. In the morning after cleansing, apply a light amount of a mild copper peptide product, and follow with a light coating of the biological oil of your choice.

2. At night, apply a moisturizing copper peptide facial cream three nights weekly.

3. Sometimes a mild hydroxy acid serum also helps to reduce rosacea. Apply the product lightly at night when not using the copper peptide topical.

4. Remember to only use a mild and gentle cleansing agent that works well on super-sensitive skin with rosacea.

Questions? Email: ghkcopperpeptides@gmail.com

7

TIGHTEN LOOSE & SAGGING SKIN
The Benefits of Biological Skin Tightening

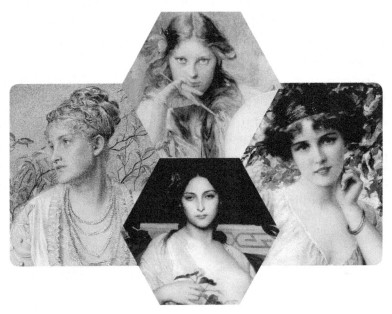

One of the most distinctive qualities of young skin is its ability to stretch and then return to its previous state. Imagine invisible rubber bands pulling the skin back. As we age, those rubber bands weaken until the skin becomes loose. Since the law of gravity is one we all have to obey, our skin eventually begins to sag, forming flaps and folds.

There was a time when the only solution for loose and sagging skin was plastic surgery. The surgeon would cut excessive skin and tighten it up, creating an illusion of wrinkle-free skin. However, anyone who would touch this surgically tightened skin would immediately discover the difference. Even after tightening, such skin would never regain the wonderful plumpness and elasticity of youth.

Recently, new methods of skin tightening have been introduced. For example, skin can be tightened using radiofrequency (RF) and infrared (IR) devices. These types of methods inflict mild damage that triggers a healing response, leading to the production of new collagen. Those methods are usually well-tolerated and produce noticeable improvement. Yet, the skin does not become younger—it only becomes tighter.

"Dr. Pickart, How Can I Tighten My Loose Skin?"

It is no surprise that this is the question I hear most often. This chapter will present you with some natural techniques to tighten the sag that develops with age or as a result of weight loss. As you will soon see, these natural, painless methods can defer your need to go under the knife. Skin-tightening surgery is not only painful, but it costs a bundle. Most importantly, surgical methods have a long recovery period, during which a client must deal with pain, swelling, and redness. Additionally, there is always a risk of side effects, such as inflammation, hyperpigmentation, and scars. It takes at least a year for the rebuilt skin to fully recover. Hence, let's talk about a better approach.

Biological Skin Tightening

What if we could restore those "rubber bands" that worked to pull the skin back when it was younger? If we could do this, not only could we manage to eliminate loose and sagging skin, but we also would achieve overall improvement in its appearance, making it smooth, supple, and elastic.

The first step in achieving this is fully understanding the biological makeup of your skin. There are two kinds of proteins that make the skin resilient, firm, and elastic. They are called collagen and elastin. Collagen molecules look like long spirals that form a supportive net within the skin. They make the skin firm, smooth, and resilient. Elastin molecules look like short coils. They just sit there, doing nothing, but their real power becomes apparent when the skin is pulled or pinched. Yes, it is those elastin coils that act like rubber bands pulling the skin back.

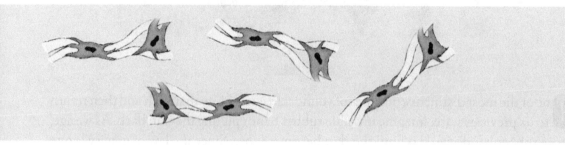

Therefore, both collagen and elastin are required to keep skin firm and elastic. However, it is easier to stimulate collagen synthesis than elastin synthesis. This is why when the skin starts to sag, most methods of rejuvenation fail to restore its elasticity.

If you prefer to use your body's natural systems to tighten skin, you will certainly find this biological approach more appealing. The objective is to help you achieve your skin-tightening goals by working with the skin's natural remodeling system.

We can best demonstrate how the body tightens skin when we observe how wounds heal. Visualize it this way. You fall off a bike and scrape your knee. You put a bandage on the wound. After a very short time, perhaps a few days, the wound closes.

As skin pulls together, new collagen forms to seal the wound. Often during the healing process, the skin-tightening action grows so intense that you can see stress lines on the skin as it pulls the sides of the wound together.

So I'll bet you're wondering, "What pulls the skin together?" Well, it's certainly not spackle, cement, or glue. You knew that? Bear with me. We're just having a little fun here as we learn how to appear sculpted! Wounds are closed by two mechanisms.

First, tissue rebuilds within the injured area; secondly, the skin contracts around the wound. When we use SRCPs, we can enhance the process of healing wounds and thus tighten skin. In my work with SRCPs, one of my first discoveries was that they have a profound effect on tightening wounds. As one example, we treated the skin ulcers of many hospital patients with SRCPs. The results were truly astounding. We often observed strong wound contractions within 48 hours and the development of stress lines in the skin.

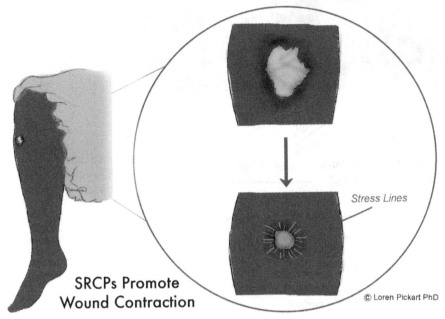

SRCPs Promote Wound Contraction

Stress Lines

© Loren Pickart PhD

These lines result from the intense pulling on the skin by the tightening of collagen strands.

The Natural Way to Tighten Skin

We can visualize young skin as the surface of a buoyant balloon; push it in or pull it out, and it quickly returns to a smooth surface. Like a balloon, biological skin tightening arises as the skin's repair cells and the fibroblasts pull collagen strands together. The fibroblasts biochemically attach collagen strands to each other.

This natural skin tightening process keeps the skin elastic and soft. The fibroblasts use an enzyme called lysyl oxidase to connect the collagen strands, which requires both copper (II) and vitamin C to work. In addition, fibroblasts produce elastin—another essential skin protein. Just like that of collagen, elastin synthesis requires both copper (II) and vitamin C.

Biological Skin Tightening - How and Why It Works:

Youthful, healthy skin (much like the surface of a balloon) will be flexible and enjoy good elasticity. Copper peptides help activate the skin's natural renewal systems to keep the skin that way!

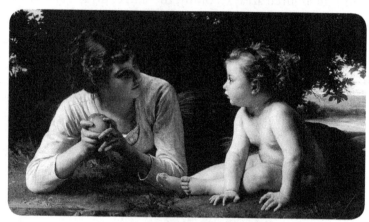

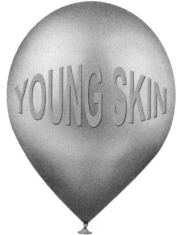

SRCPs *Transfer Copper(II)*

$$\left[\begin{array}{ccc} \text{Loose collagen + ascorbic acid} & \xrightarrow{\text{Lysyl Oxidase + Copper (II)}} & \text{Attached tight} \\ \text{strands} \quad \text{(Vitamin C)} & & \text{collagen + dehydroascorbic} \\ & & \text{strands} \quad \text{acid} \end{array} \right]$$

Your body requires adequate levels of copper (II) and vitamin C in order to tighten your skin. You cannot attain a tightening effect without having a high level of each molecule in your skin. The best way to supply copper (II) is to apply SRCPs to the skin's surface. Topical vitamin C products tend to produce far less collagen than topical SRCPs and so are not recommended. Most vitamin C creams and serums contain forms of vitamin C and pH levels that prevent optimal absorption. We can most easily increase vitamin C levels in our skin by taking 0.5 grams daily as a supplement. For a more extensive discussion on this topic, see **Chapter 19: The Science Behind SRCPs**.

The use of hydroxy acids, such as salicylic acid and lactic acid, also helps tighten the skin. Hydroxy acids remove older cells on the skin's surface by producing a very mild skin damage. This damage assists in the skin renewal process, most likely by increasing the number of fibroblasts.

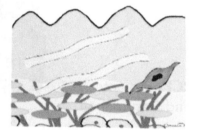

Collagen strands in loose skin:

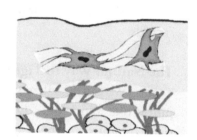

SRCPs can help activate fibroblasts: Attach to collagen strands, and as they contract, collagen strands are pulled closer and are chemically attached...

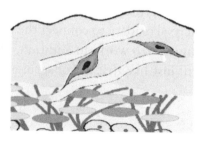

RESULT:
Tightened skin with elastic collagen that retains natural elasticity.

SKIN CARE GUIDE

Recommended Regimen for Tighter Skin on Face and Body

The following regimen has helped many individuals turn back the clock on their skin:

1. Use copper peptide products, vitamin C supplements (0.5 grams daily), and hydroxy acids to tighten the skin. Be patient; this slow process may take several months, and the hydroxy acids can produce a mild irritation. Many apply a 10% hydroxy acid in the morning and a strong copper peptide cream at night. However, some sun lovers opt to reverse the time of day of their regimen since hydroxy acids increase photosensitivity. In this case, they may choose to apply copper peptide creams fortified with titanium dioxide during the day and their 10% hydroxy acid at night. After losing a substantial amount of weight, some have combined these products to effectively avoid surgical removal of excess skin.

2. For maximum effectiveness, other individuals have found it beneficial to apply their copper peptide cream and a hydroxy acid at approximately 4-6 hour intervals. In this case, apply each product twice daily.

3. To speed things up, you might use a stronger hydroxy acid, such as a 10% to 30% lactic acid. Mild microdermabrasion can also help you see faster results.

4. To increase the efficacy of this regimen even more, massage, saunas and steam rooms are recommended. These methods can help stimulate blood flow and dissolve fat pockets that may stand in the way of tightening your loose skin.

5. Take a daily supplement of 1 gram methylsulfonylmethane (MSM), which supplies the nutritional sulfur needed to produce skin proteins.

Achieving a Slight Breast Lift Women can achieve a slight breast lift by following the preceding five-step regimen for tighter skin. A moderate strength copper peptide cream and a 10 to 30% lactic acid product are the best products to use for this purpose. Some women who were planning a surgical breast lift found this mild method gave enough improvement to satisfy them without surgery.

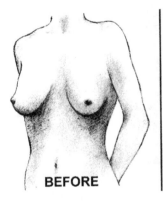
BEFORE

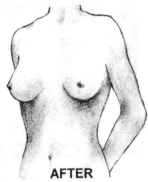
AFTER

Using Controlled Heating Methods to Tighten Skin

Have you ever spilled hot grease on yourself while cooking? Ouch! No one enjoys getting burned. However, you may have noticed that this heat burn caused your skin to contract. In serious burns, the resulting skin contraction can be so severe that it acts as a tourniquet to stop blood flow into the area. When this happens, a doctor may cut open the burned skin to relieve pressure and permit blood flow again.

So what if we could replicate wound healing in a controlled way? Well, that's where lasers, microwaves, and various types of lights enter the picture. These controlled heating methods produce a mild contraction and thereby tighten the skin. So it's out of the hot kitchen and into the weak, not-so-hot fire. However, these methods are far from perfect; the misuse of such methods may actually damage the vellus hair follicles that produce stem cells for rebuilding skin.

Those who use controlled heating methods must take care to treat the skin properly after the procedure. Their effectiveness depends on the skin's ability to regenerate after incurring damage caused by these treatments. To offset the potential harm, application of a mild copper peptide serum followed by a biological healing oil is recommended, beginning one to two weeks after the procedure. By using these products, you will get the results you want. Your skin will rebuild collagen and elastin with less scarring, and you will end up with softer skin.

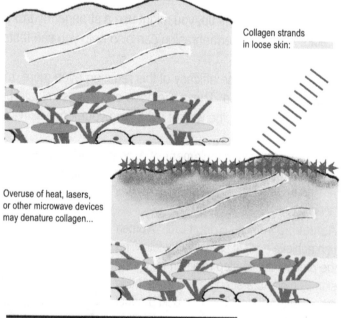

Collagen strands in loose skin:

Overuse of heat, lasers, or other microwave devices may denature collagen...

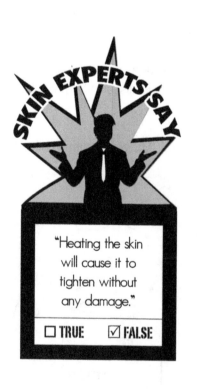

SKIN EXPERTS SAY

"Heating the skin will cause it to tighten without any damage."

☐ TRUE   ☑ FALSE

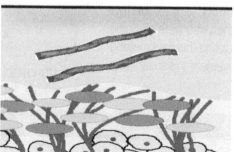

Collagen matrix shrinks, causing a general skin contraction.

RESULT:
Tighter skin with overcondensed collagen

Just as weight training tightens the appearance of loose skin on the body, facial exercise firms the face. Similar to the body, facial skin sags over time. Facial resistance training does for the face what weight training does for the body. Facial exercise can provide a beneficial enhancement to the topical skincare regimen recommended in this book.

When we exercise our facial muscles, we can help strengthen and lift, tone and tighten. Facial exercises create fullness and lift, especially in the cheeks, under the eyes, and around the chin and jaw. It fills in the hollows in the cheeks, flattens the areas under the eyes, and reduces sagging of the jowls, chin, and neck area. The isometric, isotonic resistance training of FlexEffect can be successfully combined with SRCPs to achieve tighter, younger skin.

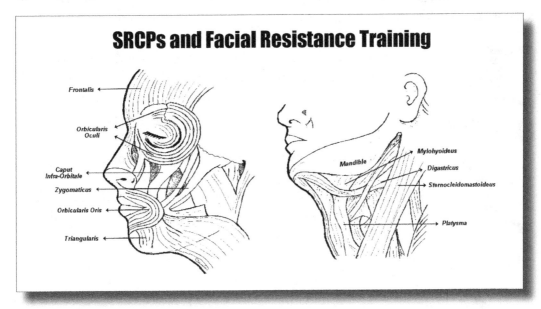

SRCPs and Facial Resistance Training

Information from FlexEffect (Facial Resistance Training: www.flexeffect.com)

Tightening Pores

If clogged and enlarged pores concern you, you may want to know that SRCPs, hydroxy acids, pore cleaning strips, and saunas can help to effectively reduce or tighten pores. Try the following suggestions:

1. In the morning, use a 2% salicylic acid pad (available at drugstores).

2. Apply a light amount of an oil-free hydroxy acid in serum form and leave on the skin without washing off.

3. Apply a light amount of a strong copper peptide oil-free liquid solution (maximum of 4 drops daily when starting and then slightly increasing this amount if needed).

4. Apply pore cleansing strips every two weeks on problem areas as needed.

5. You might also enjoy occasional steam baths or saunas which help with pore size reduction.

Diet and Exercise Helps Tighten Skin

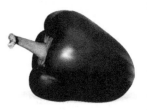

Do not overlook diet and exercise to optimize your skin's natural tightening systems. When you eat a healthy diet, you enhance the body's ability to repair itself. Include plenty of vitamin-C-rich fruit and vegetables, such as oranges and bell peppers, to enhance the benefits of SRCPs.

Get sulfur from tomatoes, kale, broccoli, and brussels sprouts to produce skin protein. Vitamin A in dark greens, carrots, and sweet potatoes are essential for a healthy complexion. When you enjoy almonds and other vitamin E rich foods, you encourage skin to heal and reduce scarring after injuries such as burns.

Add Omega-3-rich fish such as salmon and sardines. Essential fats add luster to your skin. Sardines also contain DMAE, which increases tone in the skin. Minimize high-glycemic, processed foods such as white bread and sugar. Refined foods cross-link proteins, leading to aging skin and wrinkles.

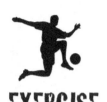

Exercise enhances the skin's natural tightening systems. So build some muscle with weight training to reduce the appearance of saggy skin. If you are overweight, dieting will have a tightening effect on skin.

Consider how people who have been starving for a long time never have areas of loose skin on the body; the body absorbs excess skin when it can't find enough energy producing calories in the diet.

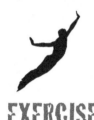

However, when weight is lost too quickly, fat cells will have retained their shape, causing adjacent skin to resemble an empty rubbish bag on the floor. Just as effective skin remodeling takes time, so does weight loss.

Never lose more than one to two pounds a week if you want to minimize loose skin. Follow up weight loss with weight training to rebuild muscle tone and minimize flab.

Aerobic exercise also helps tighten the skin. Regular aerobic exercise tightens the internal muscles and enhances the rebuilding process.

Quick Fixes to Tighten Skin

True skin tightening takes a few months of diligence. Many people who have tried these suggestions rave about their firm, glowing complexions, stating that the journey is well worth it. However, at times, you may yearn for a quick fix to superficially tighten skin while waiting for copper peptides to do their magic. Topical products with a mix of DMAE and algae polysaccharides may be the answer! This type of formulation works as a quick fix elixir that does twice the job of any one product.

Clinical studies show DMAE, first advanced by Dr. Nicholas Perricone, delves below the skin's surface where muscles contract to prevent facial sagging. In contrast, algae polysaccharides work on the skin's surface to immediately tighten the skin.

The algae polysaccharides are carefully fermented to form Pepha-Tight®, which has been proven to not only tighten the skin but also diminish fine lines.

In other words, if you combine DMAE and algae polysaccharides, you will receive the benefits of the synergistic, powered up action of two ingredients.

CONCLUSION There are many reasons to choose biological skin remodeling with topical copper peptides even if you decide to undergo plastic surgery or use RF or IR devices. And there is certainly good reason to use skin remodeling if you do not want to use those intensive methods.

Remodeling allows you to utilize your skin's own natural power to restore elasticity and firmness. It is a fully natural and very safe method that won't accelerate aging. It can even improve the results of plastic surgery or other aggressive methods of rejuvenation, helping you enjoy a young and radiant appearance for many years to come.

Even though skin remodeling is a slow process, you will feel confident knowing that month after month there is an ongoing rejuvenation process taking place inside your skin. As you see your skin becoming smoother and feel its elasticity restored, you will be rewarded with compliments and envious whisper everywhere you go.

So go ahead... fool Mother Nature and cheat Father Time with effective methods of true skin tightening that really work!

Questions? Email: ghkcopperpeptides@gmail.com

8

FROM SCARS AND BLEMISHES TO FLAWLESS SKIN
A BALANCING ACT OF SKIN RENOVATION

We're all of us sentenced to solitary confinement inside our own skins, for life!
—Tennessee Williams

Scars and blemishes from incomplete skin repair deeply affect well-being and self-esteem. No matter how diligently you use concealer or how many layers of makeup you apply, they are hard to hide and even harder to ignore.

So here's the good news: you can eliminate many blemishes and scars by using a combination of hydroxy acids and SRCPs. This painless, low-cost approach utilizes your natural remodeling cycle and thus may take several months to achieve optimal results.

SRCPs provide a delicate balance to the process of removing blemishes. These miraculous molecules help calm and rebuild new skin, allowing skin lesions to be slowly dissolved and replaced by fresh, unblemished skin.

WHAT CAN I USE TO GET RID OF SKIN DAMAGE? Unsightly acne and scars crop up when cellular damage prompts our skin cells to grow in an abnormal manner. Many triggers can disfigure our skin including viruses, bacteria, heat, UV or X-ray radiation, and scar tissue that results from incomplete wound healing. This abnormal skin must be removed so that normal healthy skin can refill the area and create a smooth, unblemished complexion.

First, let's ask ourselves what it is that causes the skin to heal abnormally in the first place? Today, we know that healing requires a certain kind of environment, meaning that a number of molecular factors should be present in the right concentrations to orchestrate and guide the extremely complex healing process, preventing it from going awry.

Caution: These methods are not intended to replace regular skin care by a physician. Lesions that are dark and irregular, those that bleed, or are infected should be promptly checked by a physician.

Selectively remove the blemish as gently as possible while creating an environment that fosters the creation of new healthy skin.

. Blemish develops after skin damage is followed by inadequate healing. Healing process can be further assisted by the following methods...

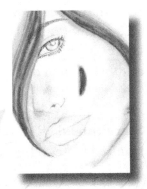

3. Skin Remodeling Copper Peptides help the skin repair itself.

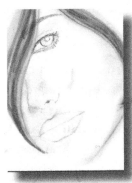

2. Exfoliation with salicylic acid helps to remove damaged skin proteins. Blemish decreases in size and edges may "dry" up and flake off.

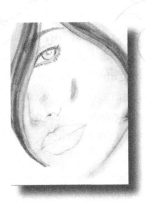

4. Process is repeated over and over again, leaving the skin healthy and unblemished!

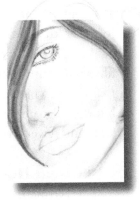

The deficit or excess of such factors can turn healing into pretty messy business, resulting in prolonged inflammation, delayed healing, and hypo- or hyper-pigmentation. So here is the recipe for reversing damage:

What "The Gold Reserve" of Your Skin is and How to Preserve It

Have you ever wondered how skin repairs itself? Why is it possible for it to be reborn, like a legendary Phoenix that burns itself and then rises from the ashes again?

Today, we know the answer. The source of the skin's renovating power, or "gold reserve", is hidden in the lowest part of the epidermis. They are called the stem cells—wonder cells that alone are endowed with an amazing capacity to transform into any cell that your skin needs to rebuild itself. Whenever there is considerable damage to the skin that cannot be filled by existing skin cells, the stem cells start to grow and transform into cells needed for repair.

The problem is that as we grow older, stem cells seem to gradually lose their ability to grow and produce repair cells when needed. That explains why the older we get, the longer it takes for our skin to heal after wounding or skin resurfacing.

The good news is that SRCPs have been scientifically proven to re-charge the regenerative power of aged skin's stem cells by restoring their production of p63, the stem cells' anti-senescence (or anti-aging) protein. The renewed power of skin's stem cells allows the skin to recover after resurfacing procedures more quickly without side effects.

Another way SRCPs help your skin's stem cells is by regulating copper level. Low tissue copper causes skin's stem cells to proliferate, while high tissue copper causes them to differentiate into cells needed for repair.

Decorin—Your Collagen-Building, Anti-Scar Protein!

Scar tissue is formed from coarsely organized loose collagen, while proper skin structure requires well-organized, uniform collagen fibers that are woven into a tight and resilient network. The protein that oversees collagen formation is **decorin**—a small proteoglycan produced by skin fibroblasts. When there is not enough decorin, scars are formed. An addition of decorin to wounds prevents scar formation.

SRCPs have also been scientifically proven to increase decorin production in fibroblasts, thus creating a proper wound healing environment. Not only do they ensure that the skin puts collagen to its proper use, rather than re-creating the scar tissue again, but they also help tighten the skin, making it more resilient and elastic after healing. No scars and fewer wrinkles—now isn't that a dream come true!

First Restore Health, Then Remove Blemishes

No matter which method of scar removal you may choose (whether it is the gentle methods recommended here such as hydroxy acids, retinoic acid, and physical abrasion of scar tissue or more intense skin resurfacing methods), the first step for removing blemishes is to baby your skin back to health.

Before you can remove lesions, you need to heal your skin and strengthen it. Ideally, this is accomplished by using a combination of SRCPs and biological healing oils for two weeks to a month to help nurse your skin and revitalize it. SRCPs used several weeks before scar removal ensure high activity of the skin's stem cells and prompt regeneration. When your skin is in better shape, you can then add the use of hydroxy acid and/or retinoic acid to speed skin-lesion removal. It is preferable to wait before using more aggressive methods and give gentler approaches a fair trial first.

THE BALANCING ACT FOR REDUCING SCARS AND BLEMISHES

Rather than pain outweighing gain, I have found ways to remove blemishes while reducing irritation. It's a balancing act that performs more slowly than some methods. However, it works gently, and you will emerge with a clear radiant complexion. Over years of observation, I discovered a number of routines that help reduce the appearance of many types of blemishes (scars and pitted scars, skin tags, moles, sun damage, stretch marks, warts, hyperpigmentation, discoloration, and so on).

If you use both hydroxy acids and SRCPs, they work together in a balanced way to lessen irritation and eliminate blemishes. It is necessary to alternate applications of moderate-strength hydroxy acids and SRCPs. The hydroxy acids gradually loosen and dissolve the blemished tissue, while the SRCPs help rebuild new skin. This method is slow but effective and does not cause excessive skin irritation.

To remove blemishes, apply an SRCP product in the morning. In the evening, you can rub hydroxy acids into the trouble spots. The most potent hydroxy acids (those higher than 5%) work most quickly, but they can irritate the skin, so use them with caution. Many find that retinoic acid and/or abrasion (such as dermabrasion, pumice stones, or needling/subcision), can also help speed the removal of blemishes.

Perfecting The Balancing Act

The hydroxy acids and SRCPs work best when used daily. Some people with severe scars have experienced radiant results by applying the products up to four times daily (for example, a hydroxy acid at 8 a.m., a SRCP product at noon, a hydroxy acid at 5 p.m., and a SRCP product before bedtime). You should see an improvement in about a month, but some old scars (such as stretch marks and keloid scars) may take six to eight months to slowly fade. Skin usually reverts to its pre-damage color.

Strong hydroxy acids can make your skin more sensitive to sunlight, so use a sun protectant that contains a physical sunblocker such as pure titanium dioxide if you decide to apply hydroxy acids during the day. Or as mentioned earlier, apply hydroxy acids and/or retinoic acids at night and SRCPs in the daytime.

Remember, blemish removal is a balancing act. If you remove too much blemished skin with hydroxy acids, you may end up with a gaping hole marring your beautiful complexion; if you use too few SRCPs, you may not rebuild your skin enough to see results.

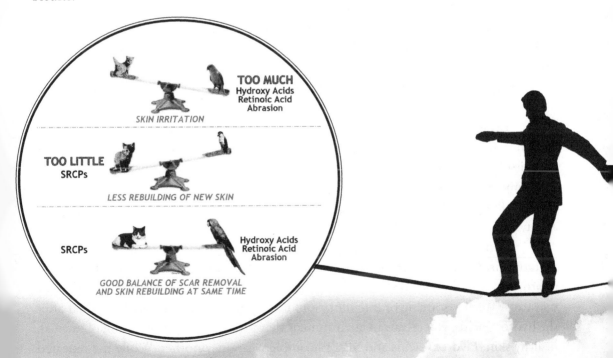

TOO MUCH
Hydroxy Acids
Retinoic Acid
Abrasion

SKIN IRRITATION

TOO LITTLE
SRCPs

LESS REBUILDING OF NEW SKIN

SRCPs

Hydroxy Acids
Retinoic Acid
Abrasion

GOOD BALANCE OF SCAR REMOVAL
AND SKIN REBUILDING AT SAME TIME

Depending on your skin type and condition, you may have to use more or less of the blemish-reduction products. In general, it is best to go slowly. Your skin can only change and improve so fast. When it comes to glowing skin, patience is a virtue.

How Hydroxy Acids and SRCPs Work

In a sense, hydroxy acids do their magic by inflicting damage in order to remove scars and blemishes, which are also forms of skin damage. Hydroxy acids, such as salicylic acid and lactic acid, are widely used as exfoliating agents and for skin peels. They remove dead skin cells and can also loosen and slowly dissolve skin lesions, such as acne scars, skin tags, stretch marks, sun-damage marks, and moles.

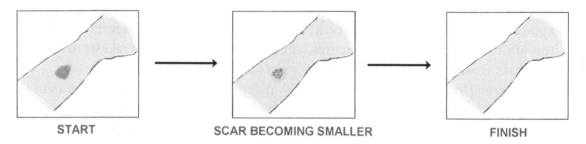

START   SCAR BECOMING SMALLER   FINISH

It may appear ironic that hydroxy acids need to cause damage in order to remove damage. Aaah, life and skin can be an enigma as we balance cosmetic contradictions! So here is the nitty gritty secret behind the action of hydroxy acids. Normal, healthy skin can resist the damage inflicted by hydroxy acids, whereas unhealthy lesions cannot survive this acidic assault. When healthy skin is treated with hydroxy acids, it quickly repairs with the aid of the SRCPs. The only difference is that this time it heals properly without bothering to restore skin lesions and imperfections. This means that your newly restored skin will be healthy, smooth, and blemish-free, provided that this repair process goes through without a hitch. And that's what SRCPs are there for—to ensure correct and flawless regeneration.

The acidic environment created by the hydroxy acids also activates some enzymes and immune cells that help remove damaged skin and lesions. As a result, hydroxy acids will dissolve most skin lesions when used over a period of a month or longer, allowing new unblemished skin to rise to the surface. This approach offers a gentle alternative to normal skin peel techniques that employ a very strong hydroxy acid (or other peeling agent, such as TCA or phenol).

Skin peels work well under perfect circumstances. However, they can severely irritate skin when it is unable to fully regenerate and heal as a result of strong acid treatments. In other words, if too little skin rebuilding takes place, the peeling agent may cause further scarring or inflammation. However, by using an SRCP product after the hydroxy acids, you create an environment that prompts the regeneration of normal, healthy skin. Hydroxy acids and SRCPs complement one another. While the repeated application of hydroxy acids slowly dissolves skin blemishes, SRCPs aid in the rebuilding of healthy, smooth skin. As the skin is rebuilt and scars are removed, the elastic properties of the skin pull it into a smooth surface.

REDUCTION OF ACNE SCARS AND PITTED SCARS

Now, this may sound obvious, but if you want to reduce acne scars, you need to avoid new breakouts.

The following regimen has been found effective by many individuals both for preventing and reducing acne scars and other pitted blemishes. As with all scars and blemishes, the key is to be patient and keep working on the scar.

1. In the morning, wipe your face with a 2 percent salicylic acid pad (available at drugstores).

2. After the salicylic acid pad, apply a copper peptide serum that also contains a small amount of salicylic acid and leave it on. Start with a maximum of four drops daily, and then slowly increase the amount. If you have sensitive skin, start with GHK copper, which is the mildest form.

3. In the evening, apply a light amount of a mix of lactic acid and salicylic acid (in a supportive oil-free liquid) and leave it on.

4. For pitted scars, some people use stronger hydroxy acids and/or retinoic acid at night.

5. About every two weeks, use pore-cleansing strips (available at drugstores) on acne-prone areas. Be careful not to overuse the strips to the point of irritation.

6. Some people use this method one day and anti-acne products on alternate days.

7. Anti-acne products can be somewhat drying to the skin. Biological healing oils, such as emu oil, work well as moisturizing agents and rarely increase breakouts.

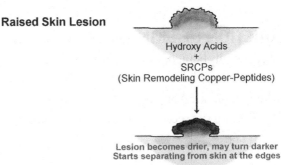

Raised Skin Lesion

Hydroxy Acids
+
SRCPs
(Skin Remodeling Copper-Peptides)

Lesion becomes drier, may turn darker
Starts separating from skin at the edges

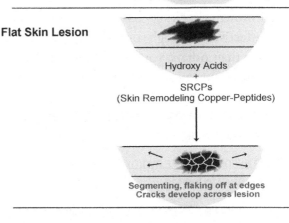

Flat Skin Lesion

Hydroxy Acids
+
SRCPs
(Skin Remodeling Copper-Peptides)

Segmenting, flaking off at edges
Cracks develop across lesion

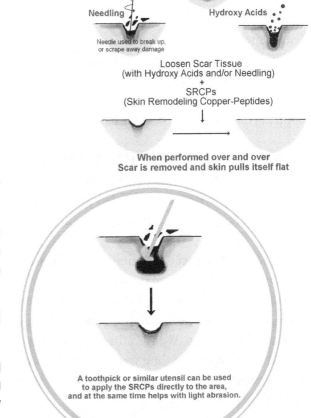

Pitted Acne Scar   Tough Scar Tissue

Needling   Hydroxy Acids

Needle used to break up,
or scrape away damage

Loosen Scar Tissue
(with Hydroxy Acids and/or Needling)
+
SRCPs
(Skin Remodeling Copper-Peptides)

When performed over and over
Scar is removed and skin pulls itself flat

A toothpick or similar utensil can be used
to apply the SRCPs directly to the area,
and at the same time helps with light abrasion.

REDUCTION OF SKIN TAGS Skin tags are small, generally benign skin growths. They often fall off naturally, and hydroxy acids are known to speed up their removal. Applying SRCPs also seems to help by aiding the recovery of normal skin around the skin tag.

The following regimen has been found to be quite effective. Although some skin tags are more resistant than others, you should see significant results in about a month.

1. In the morning, apply a copper peptide serum very lightly on the skin tag.

2. In the evening, apply a hydroxy acid (preferably 10% leave-on acid) to the tag.

3. On alternative evenings, you can apply a stronger copper peptide topical cream as a spot treatment on the area.

Sometimes salicylic acid can irritate the skin tag, and it can become reddened. If this happens, you may want to reduce the frequency of application, but try to find a schedule that allows you to keep applying the cream on a regular basis.

REDUCTION OF STRETCH MARKS Stretch marks arise when your skin needs to stretch rapidly and ends up getting over extended as a result of pregnancy, body building, or weight gain.

Here is another great regimen suggestion for reducing the appearance of these unwanted marks. It will take about a month before you notice an improvement, and the best results may take several months. Be patient. We have had reports from women who said that they were able to remove stretch marks from pregnancy that were up to 30 years old!

1. In the morning, apply a moderate-to-very strong

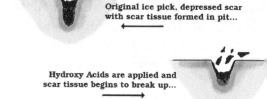

DEPRESSED SCARS
Why Things May Appear to Look Worse Before They Look Better

Original ice pick, depressed scar with scar tissue formed in pit...

Hydroxy Acids are applied and scar tissue begins to break up...

As scar tissue is removed, scar may become deeper for a time...

But this does not last, SRCPs help rebuild healthy skin and slowly the depressed area fills in!

LAYERS OF DAMAGE
What Truly Lies Beneath Your Skin

Damage from acne infection appears on top of skin layer, but reaches deep into skin...

In time, skin may cover and hide damage but scar tissue still lies beneath...

As hydroxy acids + abrasion + SRCP work on the skin, the damage that was below may be revealed...

But this does not last and as scar tissue is removed healthy skin is revealed!

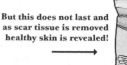
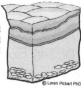

© Loren Pickart PhD

copper peptide cream to the stretch mark.

2. In the evening, apply a hydroxy acid (preferably 10% leave-on acid) to the stretch mark.

3. On alternative evenings, apply another application of the SRCP cream of your choice.

If You Want Faster Results

If you want to see quick results, you may use stronger hydroxy acids with most of the skin-care regimens in this chapter. However, these potent hydroxy acids also increase the chances of irritation or chemical burns. So some opt to use mild leave-on hydroxy acids. For example, a 10% hydroxy acid solution mix (8.5% lactic acid and 1.5% salicylic acid at pH 3.2) or 10% pure lactic acid seems to work very well for daily use. Some estheticians and clinics use 20 percent salicylic acid or 30 to 70 percent alpha hydroxy acids to loosen scar tissue followed by the copper peptide product.

A number of people have had success using the salicylic acid pads (17% to 40%) or salicylic acid solutions (12% to 17%) that are typically used to remove calluses and warts. These work well on many types of skin lesions, but again be cautious to not over use such products. Apply the pads or solutions at one time of the day or on alternative days, and use SRCPs at different times.

Skin Abrasion and Scar Reduction

Methods that mildly abrade skin can also hasten the removal of scars, especially when combined with hydroxy acids and SRCPs. These abrasive techniques and tools include microdermabrasion, microdermabrasion sponges or cloths, and needling (subcision).

Some old scars get especially tough, fibrous, and difficult to decompose. Physically abrasive techniques break down scars and thereby allow the hydroxy acids to start dissolving them.

Microdermabrasion works well for elevated or flat scars. Microdermabrasion sponges

HYDROXY ACIDS
How They Work to Reveal
HIdden Buried Damage

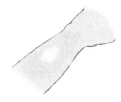

1. Damaged skin with blotchy tone

2. Damage starts to heal and is covered with new skin

3. Years later: Damage seems to fade

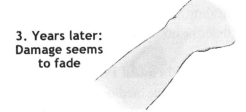

4. Exfoliation with hydroxy acids may uncover scar lines

or cloths work especially well for small skin lesions, since you can focus on abrading a small area. The cloths cost about $10 each. But be careful! They are deceptively potent, and you can easily overuse the product.

Subcision, performed by an esthetician, can break up depressed scars such as pitted acne tissue. In this procedure, a needle (similar to a tattoo needle) disrupts the scar collagen and stimulates its replacement by newly formed collagen. The best results are achieved with several sessions.

Some estheticians tell us that they use a mild copper peptide serum or moderately strong copper peptide cream after the needling and see a much improved and faster clearing of the scar.

However, do not apply the copper peptides until the wound has scabbed over and is no longer open or oozing liquid.

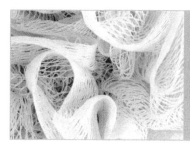

Make the promise to effectively reduce the appearance of your blemishes and marks by adding a method of manual abrasion (using a microdermabrasion cloth, sponge, or loofah) over a consistent period of time to speed up skin renewal and start fading your scars today!

POST-PROCEDURE HEALING
After Peels, Laser Resurfacing, and Dermabrasion

In addition to reducing many types of scars, hydroxy acids and SRCPs can enhance healing after skin peels, laser resurfacing, and dermabrasion. The rest of this chapter will describe how to use hydroxy acids and SRCPs effectively during post-procedure recovery.

After a Chemical Peel

While medium and deep chemical peels may improve damaged skin and promote a rosy glow, they also can produce severe irritation that leads to scars and prolonged redness. Oh no! I can read your mind now. How can a treatment that improves skin also damage it? Well, as we discussed, proper skin care requires a balanced approach. Although medium or deep peels may remove abnormal tissue faster, to ensure that the skin heals properly this time, you need to create the right environment.

After a peel, you will probably want to apply some type of moisturizer and/or anti-inflammatory to reduce irritation. However, petroleum jelly or other simple coverings are not recommended since they do not prevent redness and inflammation. Cortisone, often used as an anti-inflammatory, is also discouraged because it can defeat the healing process since it inhibits skin repair.

Fortunately, SRCPs can rebuild our skin and reduce irritation. So it's good-bye thin skin and hello to a beautiful complexion.

After a chemical peel, some individuals have experienced dramatic results by following these steps:

1. In hot climates, apply a moderately strong copper peptide cream after the peel. Choose a product that contains SRCPs and a high level of squalane and octyl palmitate as skin protectants.

2. In cool climates, apply a mild copper peptide serum followed by emu oil after the peel.

3. The first use of SRCP products should be within two hours of the peel, then on a twice-daily basis. Use the products lightly.

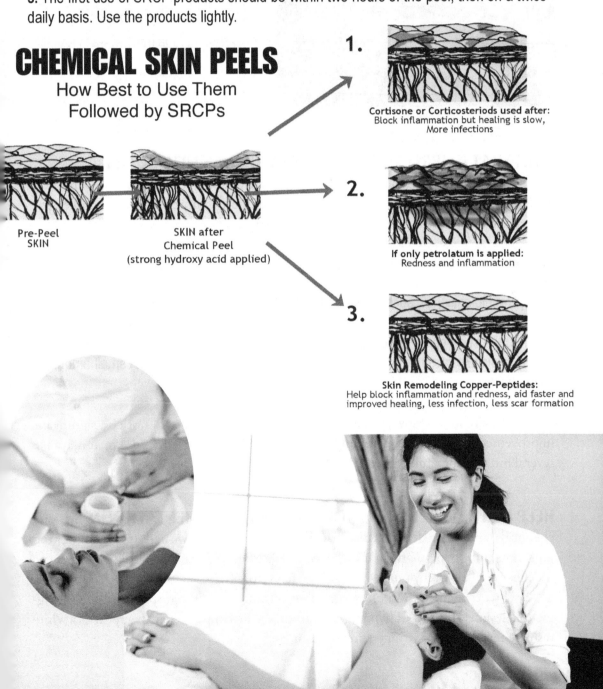

CHEMICAL SKIN PEELS
How Best to Use Them
Followed by SRCPs

Pre-Peel
SKIN

SKIN after
Chemical Peel
(strong hydroxy acid applied)

1.
Cortisone or Corticosteriods used after:
Block inflammation but healing is slow,
More infections

2.
If only petrolatum is applied:
Redness and inflammation

3.
Skin Remodeling Copper-Peptides:
Help block inflammation and redness, aid faster and improved healing, less infection, less scar formation

After Laser Resurfacing and Dermabrasion

Again, some have experienced dramatic results by following these steps:

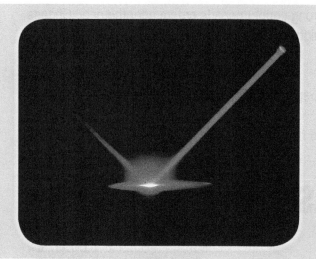

1. Apply a mild copper peptide serum to the skin within two hours of the procedure.

2. Apply a thin coating of the same serum daily to the healing skin. Be careful to use only a light coating.

Too often, people think more is better.

SKIN THAT IS IRRITATED, REDDENED, OR HAS NEW SCARS

As we discussed, chemical peels can irritate the skin and make it sore. This may sometimes lead to visible burns and hyperpigmentation. Unfortunately, this unpleasant phase can last for a year or longer after the procedure.

The following regimen should assist in recovery and hasten healing time.

1. Apply a biological oil, such as emu oil, until all of the soreness is alleviated.

2. When the soreness is gone, apply a mild copper peptide serum followed by emu oil on a daily basis. Be careful to use only a light coating of copper peptides. A small amount is quite effective.

This road to recovery may take time. However, you should notice a significant improvement in a month. If you suffer from severely burned or irritated skin, it may take several months for a full recovery.

HELP FOR <u>HYPERPIGMENTATION</u> AND <u>HYPOPIGMENTATION</u> When sun, chemicals, and other elements discolor and damage the skin, we end up with either too much melanin (hyperpigmentation) or too little (hypopigmentation), which can create the illusion of a blotchy pincushion. Now that's no fun!

Hyperpigmentation often contributes to brown and red spots and highly pigmented lesions. In cases of hypopigmentation, the loss of pigment can appear as a white rash as seen in cases of vitiligo and albinism.

We recommend that you treat hyper/hypopigmented areas in the same manner as you would treat blemishes and scars.

You can remove almost any skin blemish (this includes hyperpigmentation or hypopigmentation) with a combination of hydroxy acids, skin abrasion, and Skin Remodeling Copper Peptides (SRCPs). The hydroxy acids and abrasive methods slowly loosen and dissolve the blemished tissue, while the SRCPs help to rebuild new skin.

Many people have shared their stories with me as they successfully reduced scars and hyperpigmentation. It may take a while, but it has worked for many.

1. If you have oily-to-combination skin, apply a strong copper peptide serum in the morning and a 10% hydroxy acid at night. Start the products lightly, and then slowly increase the amount over time.

2. If you have dry-to-normal skin, use a copper peptide cream with retinol in the morning and a leave-on hydroxy acid at night.

3. If you are not getting enough effect, try a strong copper peptide product and use it consistently.

4. If you still are not getting enough of an effect, then slowly work up to a stronger percentage hydroxy acid product.

5. Microdermabrasion sponges or cloths often work well on reducing scar tissue.

6. Daily supplements of 500 mg Vitamin C, 1 gram MSM, 1 gram of Flaxseed Oil, and 500 mg of Borage Oil also help skin rebuilding.

7. Stress inhibits skin repair and the rate of scar reduction, as it increases blood cortisol. DHEA (75 to 100 mgs daily) may help block the cortisol effect and stimulate skin repair. But only take DHEA for short periods of time, such as one month, if you are experiencing great stress.

8. Regular aerobic exercise increases blood flow into the skin and speeds skin repair and scar reduction. According to recent studies, it also causes the DNA to produce more proteins that are characteristic of young skin, so you get a double benefit—faster healing and younger looking skin.

Skin color will usually revert to its pre-damage color.

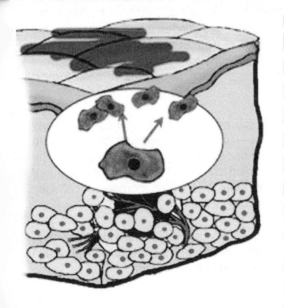
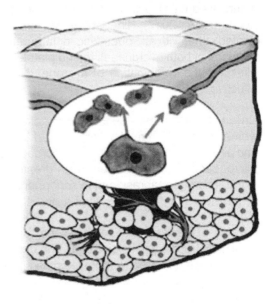

THE ART AND SCIENCE OF MICRONEEDLING

If you look at a scar, you will see that it is very different from surrounding skin. No matter what is the origin of the scar or what type of a scar it is—acne scar, post-injury scar, keloid or depressed scar—it will not have normal skin layers and will always be formed by rough, disorganized bundles of collagen.

All of this makes it very difficult to deliver active ingredients into this area. We have already discussed exfoliating your skin to help penetration of copper peptides. Exfoliation removes the upper layer of dead skin cells, so that active ingredients can be absorbed much more easily. However, if you have thick scars, or if you simply want to ensure that copper peptides are delivered exactly where you want them, you may consider combining copper peptide products with a technique called **microneedling**.

Medical needling has been used for many years by dermatologists to break down scar tissue and help trigger skin regeneration. Even though it is very effective, the procedure of needling the skin must be performed in a clinical setting, requires anesthesia, and may lead to irritation and sometimes hyperpigmentation.

Distinguishing safety features of skin needling include:

Reduced risk of infection

Significantly reduced downtime period for healing

Significantly reduced comparative cost

Microneedling is a gentler and much safer version of medical needling. It is a minimally invasive technique that uses very tiny needles to gently puncture the upper layer of skin and create temporary pores. The microneedling devices—derma rollers—are safe, very inexpensive, and can be used at home.

A recent scientific study confirmed microneedling to be a safe and effective way to deliver copper peptides into skin. Scientists used polymeric microneedles to improve skin absorption of copper peptides through pig skin and artificially grown skin tissue. The rate and depth of penetration of copper peptides increased with the force of application (Li et al, 2015). So, if you have just started using copper peptides with a derma roller, it is always best to be very gentle at first. If you have tougher scars, you may eventually want to apply a bit more force. Always listen to your skin, and when in doubt—start slowly and proceed with caution.

Microneedling, in combination with autologous—a client's own platelet-rich plasma which naturally contains GHK-Cu was shown to be very effective in the treatment of atrophic scars (Ibrahim Z.A., 2017). Ninety patients with atrophic scars were divided into three groups and treated either with microneedling, or intradermal injection of platelet-rich plasma, or alternative sessions of both microneedling and platelet-rich plasma. Although all three approaches were effective, the combination of microneedling and plasma injections proved to be the most effective.

Nassar et al reported success in treatment of stretch marks using microneedling. Forty women with stretch marks were divided to two groups – one was treated with microneedling and another with a combination of microdermabrasion and sonophoresis (Nassar, 2016). The microneedling group showed much greater improvement compared to the second group. If in the "microdermabrasion plus sonophoresis" group, there was a 50% increase of collagen synthesis; in the "microneedling" group, there was a 90% increase!

A review of medical literature shows that microneedling achieves good results with acne scars, wrinkles, atrophic and keloid scars. The procedure improves collagen synthesis, activates skin regeneration and greatly improves delivery of active ingredients.

How does microneedling compare to medical needling? One interesting experiment was conducted using rats. Microneedling alone, or in combination with vitamin C and A, reduced synthesis of "scar collagen" while increasing synthesis of collagen I (or "youth collagen"). The procedure also stimulated secretion of growth factors, increased thickness and vitality of epidermis (up to 658% increase), and restored integrity of dermal tissue. The authors concluded that a microneedling device can achieve, and supersede, the results already shown with medical needling (Zeitter S, 2014).

Skin Needling Plus Copper Peptides

First, always cleanse the area thoroughly with a gentle, neutral pH cleanser. Of course, your hands have to be completely clean as well. If your skin is red, irritated, experiencing an active breakout (or if you have any skin condition), please use copper peptide and biological oils to soothe and heal the skin until the redness and irritation are completely gone. <u>DO NOT USE AROUND THE EYES</u>.

Depending on their skincare goals, many have successfully used skin rollers in various ways. Here is the best technique that works well for the majority:

1. Gently roll on thoroughly cleansed skin, letting the device do the work for you. Avoid pressing too hard or rolling too swiftly. Always start with minimal pressure, then increase when you are sure it is well tolerated.

2. After rolling, apply a light amount of a copper peptide product. Many choose copper peptide serums as they can easily be diluted with water before applying to the area.

3. If needed, soothe skin after rolling with a moisturizing biological oil.

Skin microneedling can be safely performed on all skin colors and types. Those new to skin rolling should always start with a shorter length needle (0.5 mm is perfect for general facial use).

It is very important to give your skin a good rest between needling sessions. Usually once a week, or once every two weeks, achieves excellent results with no side effects. Regular use of copper peptide serums and biological oil moisturizers between sessions will help your skin heal scars and restore smoothness and suppleness.

Note: Use all skin needling rollers as directed by the manufacturer. Do not misuse by performing skin needling more often than the instructions indicate. In the following graphic, it mentions that one could use the device "later" after an application of hydroxy acids. "Later" means the next time you use the device. It does not mean these devices should be used twice a day.

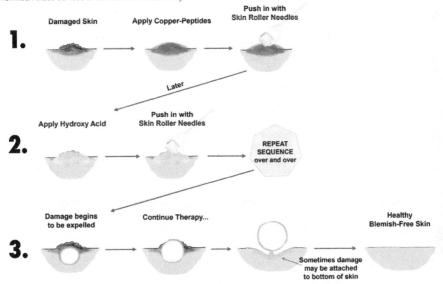

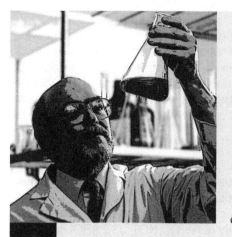

PIGMENTATION PROBLEMS There are at least three mechanisms of skin darkening. The first includes an increase of melanin production in response to skin injury. The second results from local accumulation of dead skin cells (keratosis), which leads to a darkening of the skin color. Finally, abnormal proliferation of melanocytes in response to chronic damage can result in lentigo (or what is commonly referred to as age spots).

Hyperpigmentation that occurs after aggressive cosmetic procedures, such as lasers, deep chemical peels etc., or after acute skin traumas, is usually because of melanin. Stressed keratinocytes (skin cells) produce signal molecules that command pigment cells (melanocytes) to increase melanin production. In the case of very acute or repetitive stress injury, skin cells may become permanently hyper-activated (or "reprogrammed"), and the darker spot will persist.

Keratosis also results in skin discoloration, since areas with thick horny layers look darker. This can be corrected by consistent alpha hydroxy acid application. Dark spots on the skin of elderly people (lentigo) may be the result of decades of sun damage and possibly other damaging factors as well. In case of lentigo, there is an increased number of melanocytes in the darker area. Lentigo may be more difficult to remove than normal hyperpigmentation.

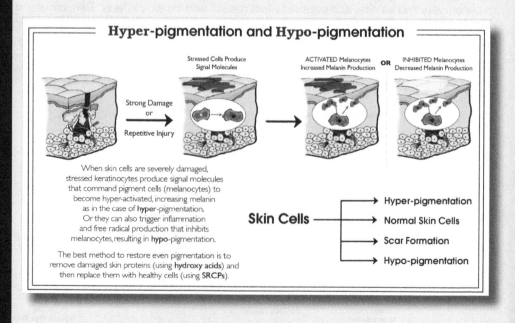

Hyper-pigmentation and Hypo-pigmentation

Stressed Cells Produce Signal Molecules

ACTIVATED Melanocytes Increased Melanin Production **OR** INHIBITED Melanocytes Decreased Melanin Production

Strong Damage or Repetitive Injury

When skin cells are severely damaged, stressed keratinocytes produce signal molecules that command pigment cells (melanocytes) to become hyper-activated, increasing melanin as in the case of **hyper**-pigmentation. Or they can also trigger inflammation and free radical production that inhibits melanocytes, resulting in **hypo**-pigmentation.

The best method to restore even pigmentation is to remove damaged skin proteins (using **hydroxy acids**) and then replace them with healthy cells (using **SRCPs**).

Skin Cells ⟶ Hyper-pigmentation
⟶ Normal Skin Cells
⟶ Scar Formation
⟶ Hypo-pigmentation

WHAT IS "BURIED SKIN DAMAGE"?

At times, removing damaged skin can cause deeply buried scar tissue to become more visible. It is this buried skin damage that is often covered over with normal skin. As such deep damage becomes visible, it is important to focus on the use of SRCPs (to trigger faster production of healthy skin cells) and hydroxy acids (to break down and remove damaged tissue).

Can you see buried skin damage?

Dr. Austin Richards (of Oculus Photonics LLP) is an expert in the field of infrared and ultraviolet imaging. He has years of industrial experience developing invisible-light imaging systems and applications. Dr. Richards developed the UVCorder™ out of the necessity for a digital imaging solution in the near-ultraviolet band. He is the author of the book, *Alien Vision: Exploring the Electromagnetic Spectrum with Imaging Technology*, as well as numerous articles and papers on the subject of invisible-light imaging. For more information, see: www.UVCorder.com.

What can the UVCorder™ reveal?

UVCorder™ is a hand-held digital ultraviolet imaging solution that serves a very practical purpose. In the case of revealing buried skin damage, excess melanin production is much easier to show in the UV light band than in the visible band. Scars and blemishes can be seen in the UV months after they have faded to the naked eye.

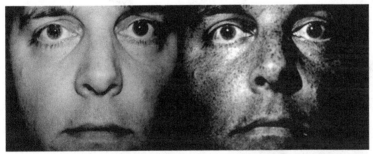

Facial skin with mild sun damage. Left-Visible, Right-UV

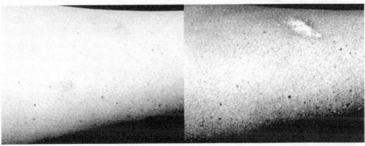

Burn mark on skin. Left-Visible, Right-UV

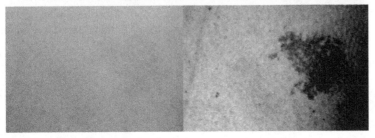

Injection mark on skin. Left-Visible, Right-UV

IN CONCLUSION   Scars and other types of skin blemishes may force people to choose aggressive skin resurfacing methods, such as lasers and deep peels. However, if you treasure your skin and want to preserve its youth and radiance, it is preferable to explore skin remodeling first.

The only natural method to remodel the skin is the removal of buried skin damage and subsequent stimulation of healthy skin cell production. This formula of using copper peptides plus abrasion to repair damage is not a cosmetic cover up or "quick-fix". It takes time, patience, and consistency. But many people have found it effective in helping to remove damage from the inside out—in time, revealing younger, healthier, tighter skin.

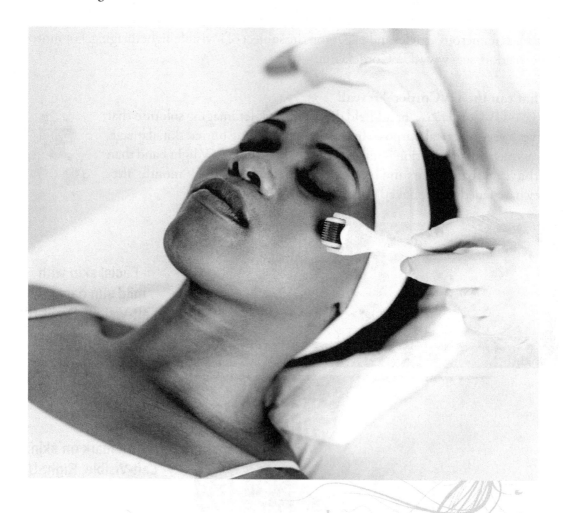

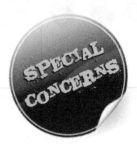

9

WHEN MAKEUP RAVAGES THE SKIN
FOR MODELS, ACTORS, AND MAKEUP LOVERS

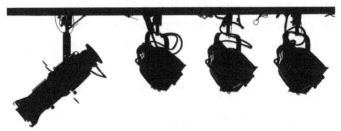

"All right, Mr. DeMille, I'm ready for my close-up." Most of us have that famous quote imprinted in our memories. Gloria Swanson, an aging starlet, walks into a scene of flashing cameras believing she still radiates the glow of her youth. Instead, we see decades of wrinkles earned from wearing too much makeup and acting under hot lights. Yes, unfortunately, many actors, who start out as stunning beauties with flawless skin, end up with skin riddled with moles, spots, or other skin damage. The sad irony is that it is preventable.

Ok, you may think. What does this have to do with me? I do not perform under hot lights, and I definitely do not wear too much makeup! Unfortunately, even if the entertainment industry is not your chosen career, your skin is not immune from damage caused by makeup and makeup removers. The good news is that skin damage is preventable for all of us whether we are stars on a stage or stars of our own successful lives.

"SPOTTED-FACED" BEAUTIES Actors and models lead unique lives. They face the spot light of fans and paparazzi who scrutinize their every move on screen and in magazines. No other profession requires the same dedication to appearance. Sadly, the celebrity lifestyle, which includes the constant application and removal of makeup, the harsh effects of stage lighting and a high level of stress, can take its toll on skin. This especially holds true for actresses and female models. However, makeup and stress plays havoc on all who love cosmetics.

Most damaging of all is the constant application and removal of foundation, eye shadow, blusher, and a whole bucket load of cosmetics. Both makeup (with its colored salts and chemical dyes) and makeup removers (which remove the protective acid mantle) are harsh on the skin.

Actors and models need to quickly change makeup between photos and scenes. And many who don't live under the spotlights still like to change their makeup after work, before going out for an evening of festivities. This requires that they apply, remove and re-apply many coats in quick succession *(See dramatization at the end of this chapter).* Other times, actresses wear heavy foundation for hours at a stretch before they strip away the pasty gook with a makeup remover at the end of the day.

Whatever the circumstances, the frequent application and removal of makeup makes the skin more susceptible to the development of skin damage, warts, moles, sun damage, and skin lesions. Therefore, it is essential for actresses, models, and all who adore makeup to learn how to properly protect and care for their skin.

SKINCARE TIPS FOR ACTORS, MODELS, AND MAKEUP LOVERS

Here are some easy steps to follow that are designed to address the specific concerns you may face...for your beautiful face.

General Guidelines

1. Before putting on makeup, apply a light serum with the milder first generation copper peptides as a base to protect the skin. These types of products help create an invisible shield to gently cushion your complexion against environmental havoc.

2. Hydroxy acids work well to remove dead skin cells and damaged skin proteins, dissolving flaws that impair a beautiful complexion. Use them if you will not be wearing heavy makeup under hot lights. Avoid using hydroxy acids in sunlight since they make skin photosensitive. You may want to use hydroxy acid products in the evening and SRCP products during the day.

3. Morning application of hydroxy acids or first generation copper peptide products with GHK: When using hydroxy acids, exfoliate with a hydroxy acid cream or serum that contains a 10% mix of both salicylic and lactic acid. Apply lightly. When using copper peptide products to counter environmental damage, wash skin with a gentle cleanser especially formulated to be mild and follow with a light application of a serum with GHK copper peptide.

4. Evening use of SRCPs or hydroxy acids: SRCPs repair skin. Spot treat damaged areas with moderate-to-strong copper peptide creams or serums. Serums work best for combination or oily skin, and creams work well for drier skin.

Apply hydroxy acids during the evening if you have used copper peptide products during the day. Some makeup lovers and film stars alternate their evening application between SRCPs and hydroxy acids.

To Protect the Skin After Makeup Sessions

1. Use only biological healing oils (BHOs) to remove make-up. BHOs are much healthier for the skin than harsh chemical removers, which have a drying effect. Oils such as emu oil or squalane work well.

2. To remove makeup, first apply a BHO lightly to the face and then rub gently to remove the makeup. Finally, rinse thoroughly with warm water. Any remaining oil helps replenish the skin's natural oils.

3. After you remove makeup, follow with a mild cleanser. A gentle cleanser formulated for sensitive skin and that has a pH of 7.5 is a good choice. Many soaps and cleansers not only remove surface dirt and oils, but actually damage the skin. Soaps that are alkaline, with a pH of around 10, destroy the skin's acid mantle. These harsh cleansers interfere with the natural protection imparted by the skin's protein/lipid barrier. A gentle yet effective cleanser keeps skin looking its best. Never over cleanse your skin.

4. Next, lightly apply a second generation copper peptide serum to the face to help repair the skin's protective barrier and antioxidant defenses. In clinical studies at the *University of California*, SRCPs were able to stimulate skin-barrier repair within 24 to 48 hours. You may also want to alternate with applications of hydroxy acids, especially if you use SRCPs during the day.

5. When applying a copper peptide serum at night, finish with a light application of a biological healing oil such as emu oil to help the skin retain a healthy glow.

FOR ANYONE WHO LOVES MAKEUP If you act on stage, host TV shows, speak in public or just have a busy social life, you may find wearing makeup unavoidable. And let's face it, you probably enjoy dabbling at the cosmetic counter and may even find your vanity table overflowing with colorful potions. Does this mean you have to put up with skin damage and premature wrinkles? Not at all. If you use our skin care tips, you can keep your passion for makeup while still maintaining your beautiful and flawless complexion. Take care of your skin, and it will take care of you. In fact, if you use quality copper peptide products, you may just find that you look beautiful with or without makeup.

SKIN CARE GUIDE

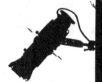

Special Concerns of Models & Actors

Consistent applications and removal of makeup (with its colored salts and chemical dyes) along with makeup removers (which damage both the protective acid mantle and the skin's protein/lipid barrier) are harsh on skin. Long hours of heavy makeup on the skin, scene changes, and touch ups, lights used in the industry and the stress to keep skin looking blemish-free can take its toll.

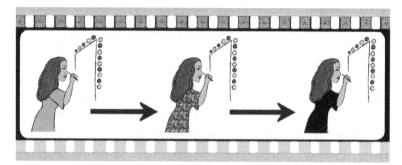

1. Before applying makeup, use a light protective layer of a mild copper peptide serum on the skin.

2. Remove makeup with biological healing oils, instead of harsh makeup removers.

3. Only wash the skin with mild cleansers specifically formulated to be mild.

4. Repair your skin with copper peptides followed by a light application of a biological healing oil.

5. Remove damage marks with daily use of 10% hydroxy acids (lactic and/or salicylic).

6. Repair deeper damage with moderate-to-strong copper peptide spot treatment creams.

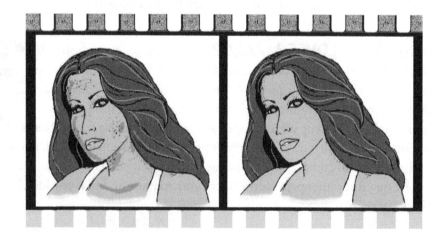

10

GENTLE CARE
FOR DRY AND SENSITIVE SKIN

If you have sensitive skin, there is a chance that you've tried everything—products for sensitive skin, hypo-allergenic cosmetics, botanical oils, and 100% natural, organic products—and yet have found no relief. Creams and serums that looked so soft and luxuriant while in the jar would inevitably turn into stinging, burning, irritating, and drying concoctions the moment they touched your skin. In some cases, burning and tingling sensations in your skin (especially when accompanied by reddening and swelling) are signs of an allergic reaction. If you suspect an allergy, you may want to consult your doctor, who will identify the substances to avoid.

However, if you seem to react to most cosmetic products, but your doctor that believes your skin is healthy, then this chapter is for you! As you will soon discover, with proper care you can strengthen your dermis; eliminate redness; and banish itching, tingling, and burning, achieving smooth, soft, and vibrant skin.

Tell-Tale Signs of a Damaged Skin Barrier

As discussed in Chapter 3, the skin barrier effectively prevents water loss as well as protects the skin from irritating and damaging substances. Unfortunately, it developed millions of years ago, long before we humans invented soap. As it turns out, soap and hot water can disturb your delicate skin barrier by washing away skin protective oils and loosening keratinous scales. You may have a damaged skin barrier if:

- Your skin feels tight and tingly after washing
- Your skin is easily irritated
- You notice patches of red and dry skin
- Your skin feels rough and dry

Complications Caused by Damage to Skin Barrier

Skin barrier damage can be rapidly healed at an early stage of breakdown

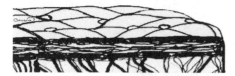

....

IF NOT

Damage to the skin barrier may cause the following:

Irritants may enter, causing eczema, skin allergies, and dermatitis

Viruses, fungi, and bacteria may enter, causing infection

May start skin ulcers (diabetic, bedsores, venous stasis)

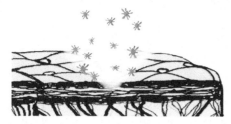

Symptoms of a compromised skin barrier include:

- Irritation
- Skin Allergies
- Dermatitis
- Extreme dryness
- Inflammation

HOW COPPER PEPTIDES CAN HELP If you suffer from extra-sensitive skin, you know that an ounce of prevention is worth far more than the pound of pain you feel from increased skin sensitivity. The key is to prevent such unpleasant consequences with the aid of SRCPs. Healthy skin possesses a strong resistance to irritants and microorganisms, but once damaged, it is prone to infections, inflammation, and allergic reactions. The result is direct damage to the skin itself, an inhibition of the normal repair process, the chronic generation of free radicals in the damaged area, or a combination of the three.

What has been proven particularly effective for those with extra-sensitive skin has been first-generation copper peptides or mild second-generation copper peptides. For example, mild second-generation copper peptides serve as a gentle, safe mineral cream, and many times also contain protective lipids that help the body heal damaged skin. This may offer a safer alternative to cortisone and corticosteroids. GHK-copper, milder than our second-generation products, gently pampers the complexion and provides a sensuous treatment that can help revitalize sensitive skin. The gentle, water-based liquid SRCP products easily spread on the skin. Remember to always use a mild cleansing agent specifically formulated for sensitive skin, and use biological healing oils to replenish natural lipids. This chapter will show you how these methods help improve the health of extra-sensitive skin while repairing damage.

Caution: Topical copper peptide based products are designed to improve skin condition and are not substitutes for regular medical care by a qualified health-care professional. They should not be used on broken skin or large, deep wounds. If skin problems persist or worsen, consult a physician.

*For a detailed discussion on the biology of your skin barrier and acid mantle functions, please see **Chapter 3: Understanding Your Beautiful Skin***

"She walks in beauty, like the night

Of cloudless climes and starry skies;

And all that's best of dark and bright

Meet in her aspect and her eyes;

Thus mellowed to that tender light

Which heaven to gaudy day denies."

—Lord Byron

Copper peptide topicals are designed to adjust the skin's pH level into the acidic range. Copper peptide creams may also contain high levels of such lipids as squalane, cetyl alcohol, glyceryl stearate, and stearic acid, which resemble the fats of the acid mantle. Squalane (or squalene) is the skin's most important protective lipid, but it declines as we age (from levels of up to 15 percent in teenagers' skin to less than 5 percent in adults over age 60), resulting in dryer skin. Effective creams may also contain soothing substances such as allantoin, aloe, vitamin E, and retinol to aid the mantle's protective antioxidant properties.

Extra-sensitive skin is usually skin with a disrupted barrier, and it carries a special danger in that it is prone to infection. Immune cells in the skin naturally produce hydrogen peroxide to fight bacteria. Many users report good results by pre-washing the skin with 3 percent hydrogen peroxide for sterilization and blotting it reasonably dry before applying a copper peptide cream. Some clinicians do not recommend the use of hydrogen peroxide because they say it increases skin damage. In contrast, my review of medical literature has found many reports of improved healing after washes of hydrogen peroxide at low concentrations (1 to 10 percent). However, skin damage is occasionally observed when applying higher concentrations. So any use of hydrogen peroxide on injured skin should be with strengths of 1 to 3 percent and no higher.

Treating Very Dry Skin

As we age, we tend to develop drier, less oily skin prone to cracks and fissures, which causes it to grow irritated, inflamed, and itchy. The condition worsens in areas with relatively few oil glands, such as the arms, legs, and trunk. We develop dry skin more often during the fall and winter due to a combination of low humidity and frequent hot bathing. Some dermatologists believe that dry skin has worsened in recent decades because we take more showers and baths today than in the past. People used to bathe only once or twice a year, allowing their skin a chance to replace its natural oils between cleansings.

Conventional oil/water moisturizers can temporarily relieve parched skin, but they do not address the fundamental problem and can worsen the condition over time by weakening the outer protective proteins. Biological healing oils, such as emu oil or squalane, are the best moisturizers for extremely dry skin.

Rosacea – Beauty and the Beast

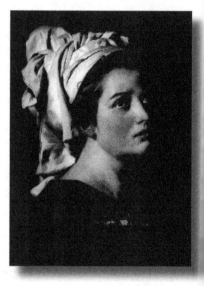

Are you a fair skinned, easily-blushing maiden who seems to descend straight from medieval minstrels' songs? Is your skin extremely sensitive to cosmetics?

Does it respond to cold air, sharp winds, alcohol, and spicy foods with a delicate pink spreading over your nose and cheeks? Have you ever noticed small, reddish bumps on your forehead and nose? Have you ever noticed that your skin can be oily in one area yet dry and flaky in another? If you've answered "yes" to most of these questions, you may have rosacea.

Rosacea is a very common skin disorder that, according to official estimates, affects over 10 million Americans. The actual numbers may be even higher, since many people with mild cases of rosacea never visit the doctor. Rosacea predominantly affects fair-skinned individuals of North European origin (Scandinavian etc.); however, other skin types may be affected as well.

In the beginning, the only symptoms of rosacea may be a poetic tendency to blush easily; an extreme sensitivity to cosmetics; or a rosy glow that appears on nose and cheeks after exposure to cold air, eating spicy foods, or drinking alcohol. At this stage, many people regard those symptoms as one of the characteristics of their skin and see no reason to consult a dermatologist.

Yet, as rosacea progresses, the symptoms become more worrisome—some areas of the skin become dry and covered with silvery scales, while in other areas you may notice enlarged oil glands which resemble acne.

The presence of pink or red bumps that look like pimples may add confusion, and indeed, at this stage, many people think they just have mild case of acne. Until recently, many dermatologists called rosacea "adult acne" or "rosacea acne". However, rosacea is completely unrelated to acne. In fact, many anti-acne cosmetic products and over-the-counter medications may make rosacea even worse.

In some cases, untreated rosacea may lead to fibrous deposits under the skin of the nose and cheeks—causing a red, bulbous nose and puffy cheeks. Don't let your skin condition go that far! Trust me, you can have rosacea tendencies and still be beautiful.

By attending to your skin's needs, you can keep your appearance delicate, rosy and romantic. You have power to preserve your beauty, by taking special care of your very special skin.

Avoid Irritants

If you have rosacea, your golden rule is to avoid irritants. The unpleasant tingling sensation and reddening of the skin that you experience after applying certain cosmetic products is a sign that your skin's defensive mechanisms are activated. Those with normal skin can ignore it. But if you have rosacea, this means that your skin is overreacting. This is not fun, because every time it happens, the condition progresses a tiny step further. Often you may hear at the cosmetic counter that if your skin gets red and start tingling, this means that the product is actually working. Do not believe such statements. For you, the best products are the ones your skin doesn't complain about.

Even though rosacea must be treated by a dermatologist, there is something you can do to relieve discomfort and make your skin appear calm and even. Wash your face with only neutral and very mild cleansers (pH around 7). Avoid harsh alkaline soaps, alcohol based cleansers, and very hot or very cold water. After washing your face, gently pat it with a soft towel—do not rub. Apply a thin coat of a protective moisturizer. Since many cosmetic moisturizers contain irritants, explore natural moisturizers such as squalane and emu oil.

Avoid harsh solvents such as alcohol and acetone. Stay away from artificial dyes and perfumes. Check if a cosmetic product you use contains harsh detergents in it. Components such as sodium lauryl sulfate must be avoided.

What About Sunlight?

If UV-radiation is one of the factors that aggravate rosacea, does that mean that you should avoid sunlight? Not necessarily. In fact, doing so may be a grave mistake. Your skin needs the healing power of the sun, and it needs its vitamin D.

Of course, that doesn't mean you should go to a tanning booth or spend the whole day on the beach baking under the blazing sun. Sensibility is the key. Expose your skin to the healing sun in mid-morning and mid-afternoon hours but not more than 15-30 minutes at a time. Full body exposure is the best, since it allows maximum stimulation of vitamin D synthesis with minimum exposure time. On other occasions, use a physical sunblock with titanium dioxide, and wear a hat with a wide brim to protect your face (See Chapter 17: Your Skin Under the Sun).

THE POWER OF COPPER PEPTIDES Even though copper peptides are not drugs and cannot cure skin diseases, they have been proven to alleviate many factors that contribute to rosacea. In addition, they are very safe and have many other beneficial actions on your skin.

1. SRCPs demonstrate remarkable anti-inflammatory and antioxidant power. They may calm inflammation by lowering the level of inflammatory cytokines such as TNF-alpha and TGF-beta. They also may help replenish copper required for a major skin antioxidant enzyme, superoxide dismutase (SOD).

2. SRCPs increase decorin, an antioxidant, anti-inflammatory, and anti-scarring protein, preventing skin fibrosis.

3. In addition, copper peptides improve the skin barrier (lessening the risk of skin irritation), protect it from adverse effects of UV-radiation, reduce excessive skin oil production, and help the skin deal with microbial infection.

You may also explore natural skin protectors such as squalane, a natural component of skin oil; Emu Oil, a healing oil used by native Australian people; Aloe Vera gel, which has anti-inflammatory and moisturizing effects; and plant antioxidants such as lutein and lycopene. Also, vitamin compounds called tocotrienols, a form of vitamin E, have been shown to accumulate in the skin, protecting it from harmful effects of UV-radiation. In addition, selected essential oils such as lavender and pumpkin have a pleasant smell, while reducing irritation. However, check before you buy, since many cheap essential oils today are adulterated with synthetic compounds and can cause even more irritation.

With proper care, your delicate skin can remain beautiful despite rosacea, and its rosy glow can continue to inspire poetic dreams for many years to come.

If You Have Allergies

Approximately 25 percent of people are allergic to nickel, and many more are sensitive to plants such as poison ivy and poison oak. Many cosmetic ingredients such as fragrances and plant essential oils can cause skin rashes and allergies as well. For example, in Europe cosmetic manufacturers are now required to list on the package the twenty-six common allergens found in plant essential oils if they are present in the formulation. This measure was introduced due to many complaints from customers who developed rashes, skin redness, and other problems after using products with those substances.

Corticosteroids (including cortisone) stop inflammation but produce damaged and thinned skin (often 50 percent thinner) by inhibiting the natural repair process. Overuse of corticosteroids can promote diabetic conditions, thymus involution, immune suppression, the spread of cancers, bone damage, and cataracts.

In one study, a second-generation copper peptide cream both accelerated the recovery of skin after injury and had an anti-inflammatory action on the skin of nickel-allergic subjects who were exposed to nickel salts (See references in Chapter 19). In practical application, many others have also reported rapid relief from insect bites after using similar creams. Because allergies are so diverse, it is always the course of wisdom to test any new product on a small area of skin first.

Skin Care and Contact Dermatitis

Contact dermatitis is an inflammation of the skin caused by direct exposure to an irritating substance. A corrosive chemical agent (an irritant), such as acetone or sodium lauryl phosphate, damages skin cells, causing their membranes to break down, which in turn triggers an inflammatory response from the skin's immune cells.

With repeated exposure, the condition may become chronic. In contrast, healthy skin does not allow entrance to irritants, but as soon as there is some damage to the barrier, there is a high possibility of dermatitis.

This is why contact dermatitis often occurs after we shave or wax our face, arms, or legs; specifically, when we run a razor blade over the skin or pull out hairs with a waxing strip, we remove some of the skin's protective barrier.

These hair-removal methods not only make the skin more prone to dermatitis, but they also allow bacteria and viruses to invade and thus infect our skin. Since viruses can cause warts, we often get these growths in frequently shaved areas, including the legs of women and the beard area in men. The more rapidly we heal our skin barrier, the better we can protect it against viruses and bacteria.

Another common culprit is nail-polish remover, which contains acetone or acetonitrile. This flammable solvent extracts skin fats; damages the skin on the fingers and cuticles; and often produces hangnails, skin flaking, and increased incidence of dermatitis.

If you suffer from contact dermatitis, a mild copper peptide cream or serum applied regularly to the affected area may help healing.

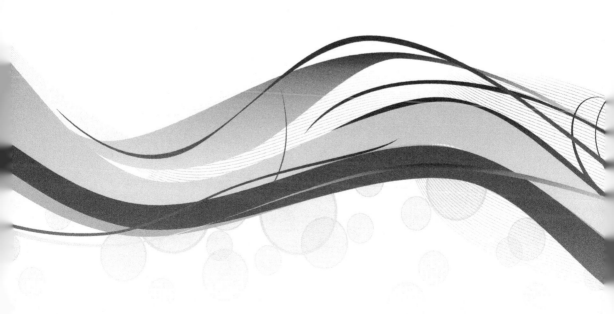

SRCPs Plus Emu Oil—An Effective Skin Enhancement

To enhance the benefits of first- and second-generation copper peptides, it is preferable to follow these SRCPs with a biological healing oil such as emu oil. The fatty acid composition of human skin oil shares a similar profile with emu oil. This similarity may offer one of the factors that enables emu oil to demonstrate such positive actions (Zemtsov et al 1996). Numerous studies have shown the effectiveness of emu oil. A study by Lopez and colleagues found strong anti-inflammatory effects of topically applied emu oil after skin was exposed to a very strong irritant (Lopez et al 1999). Politis and Dmytrowich found that if emu oil was applied two days after injury, it aided the healing process. Researchers at the University of Texas Medical School found emu oil at up to 100 percent concentration in lotions to be non-allergenic, non-comedogenic, bacteriostatic, and to have low irritation potential (Politis & Dmytrowich 1998).

Throughout history, emu oil has been used to help alleviate the discomfort of skin conditions such as arthritis, shingles, eczema, psoriasis, and other inflammatory conditions (References in Chapter 23).

The Art of Being Delicate

I hope that now you can see that sensitive skin is not a curse. When you make sure to strengthen your skin's barrier, avoid inflicting further damage, and take care to understand your skin's uniqueness, you can enjoy being delicate, while remaining strong and resilient.

No matter whether you are dealing with generally sensitive skin, or if you have rosacea tendencies, or if your skin is oily/sensitive, avoiding irritants and toxins, using natural biological healing oils to restore skin barrier, and applying regenerative copper peptides to activate your skin's reparative, antioxidant and anti-inflammatory mechanisms, is your key to comfort. There is no need to put up with burning, stinging and irritation, when it is so easy to start enjoying your healthy, resilient skin, as well as radiant, glowing and youthful appearance.

SKIN CARE GUIDE

Step-by-step Sensitive Skin Help

Sensitive skin requires you to be sensitive to its needs and nurture it as a delicate flower.

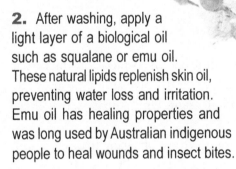

1. Avoid factors that may further disrupt your protective barrier. Wash your skin no more than twice a day, using a mild skin cleanser and warm water. Use a cleanser specially formulated for sensitive skin with pH 5.5-7.5 (from slightly acidic to neutral). Most commercial soaps are alkaline with a pH 9-10 and will cause more irritation.

2. After washing, apply a light layer of a biological oil such as squalane or emu oil. These natural lipids replenish skin oil, preventing water loss and irritation. Emu oil has healing properties and was long used by Australian indigenous people to heal wounds and insect bites.

3. Exfoliate your skin once or twice a week to increase cell turnover. Use only mild exfoliators containing lactic acid. Don't forget to assist your skin healing with emu oil after exfoliation.

4. Use SRCPs to strengthen skin barrier, speed up skin repair, and restore your beautiful and radiant complexion.

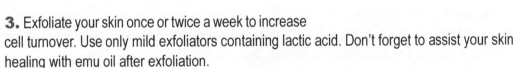

A PERSONALIZED HOW TO GUIDE - DESIGNED FOR MY SKIN

(11)

ACNE & OIL CONTROL
Oily Skin Concerns and Solutions

If your skin is oily, you may be willing to try anything that promises to reduce oily sheen. And this is why nowhere else will you find such a wide assortment of burning, stinging, drying, and overall irritating substances as in sections of cosmetics and drug stores devoted to oily skin care. Let us review a much gentler as well as more effective and natural approach to oily skin care.

Reducing Oiliness

You may be very tempted to battle excessive oiliness with cosmetic products that contain drying solvents such as alcohol or acetone. As you dissolve and wipe away the oil, your skin becomes drier and feels so smooth and pleasant. Unfortunately, this effect does not last for long.

Very soon, the oil is back, and you have to dry and wipe it off again. In desperation, you wash your face with hot water and soap several times a day, and you keep wiping it with alcohol-based cleansers in the hope that this pesky oil will go away for good. Only it never happens. In fact, in the long run it makes your skin even oilier, since by wiping your skin with alcohol and washing it with hot water and soap, you disrupt its barrier, opening the gates for irritants. Skin oil contains protective substances, so in response to irritation, skin often increases oil production.

Oily Skin Can be Sensitive

You may be surprised to know that even though your skin is oily and, yes, may appear thick and tough, in reality it is just as sensitive and delicate as skin that produces much less oil. Unfortunately, oily skin often develops sensitivity and even becomes dehydrated due to the fact people are less inclined to treat it gently. Any cosmetic product that is irritating and toxic to your skin will inevitably worsen its condition.

No matter what you believe about your skin, the truth is that you'll never make your skin prettier (nor healthier) by stinging or burning it. On the contrary, every time your skin gets irritated, it starts producing special kinds of chemicals called neuropeptides. They are first response molecules that cause your skin to itch and burn. It may be annoying, but it provides you with a warning signal that something potentially dangerous has come into contact with your skin. For example, if you spill some acid on your skin, you need to wash it off as soon as possible before it damages your skin too much. Neuropeptides alert you about this unpleasant chemical on your skin, so that you can take action.

However, neuropeptides can also trigger inflammation and increase oil production (since oil is protective), thus making your skin even more oily and blemished.

Unclogging Pores

You probably have tried many products that claimed to refine and unclog pores. Unfortunately, many of them contain substances like camphor or menthol that produce a temporary tightening and skin refreshing effect but really do nothing to your pore size and may be irritating.

To actually reduce pore size, you need to supply your skin with unsaturated fats such as omega 3. Even though it seems strange to you to apply oil based products on oily skin, these oils will help your skin to make more liquid oil that will flow out easily. When your pores are free from excess oil, you can then tighten them with collagen-stimulating agents such as copper peptides. When skin becomes firmer, pore size will visibly decrease.

In addition, clay and mud masks can be used to soften the pore plugs and to absorb oil excess.

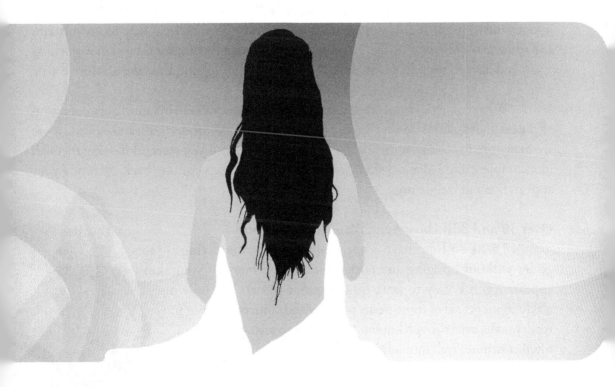

Skin Exfoliation

When you have comedones and clogged pores, you need to apply substances that can unglue the skin cells. You also need to remove dead skin cells from your skin's surface to prevent further clogging. This can be achieved by exfoliating acids such as salicylic and lactic acid. To avoid irritation, use low concentration of acids—around 10 percent.

Lactic acid is a normal component of your skin's acid mantle. This mantle creates a favorable acidic environment for beneficial skin bacteria that keep bad germs away. When you wash your skin with soap, you can make it alkaline, and this may give the advantage to harmful bacteria.

By applying lactic acid, you strengthen your skin's defense system. Also, it is an effective exfoliator that is much less irritating than glycolic acid. Salicylic acid dissolves well in oils, therefore it can penetrate oil glands, helping to dissolve the plugs in your pores. It also has anti-inflammatory action.

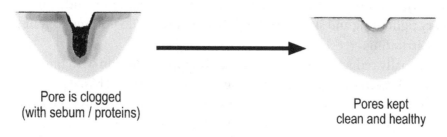

Pore is clogged
(with sebum / proteins)

Pores kept
clean and healthy

WHY ACNE REMEDIES DON'T WORK If you are suffering from acne, you probably have tried enough "magic" remedies that have left you frustrated and in despair.

Every remedy claims to be the "magic bullet" that will leave your skin flawlessly smooth and blemish-free. And although most anti-acne products may help to some extent, and some may even clear up acne for a while, many people soon see their skin worsening again and have to resume what seems to be a never-ending quest for the all elusive acne cure.

What cosmetic companies do not tell you is that acne is an inflammatory condition of the oil gland, and it doesn't appear out of nowhere. As modern research shows, there are many predisposing factors that lead to acne, and until you start addressing them all in a complete and balanced skin care routine, it will keep coming back, affecting your appearance and well-being.

Over 30 and Still Have Acne? You Are Not Alone

"Why do I *still* have acne?", you may start wondering as years go by, without bringing any noticeable improvement in your skin's appearance. It is easy to start thinking that you are the only one who cannot get rid of those pesky pimples and comedones. But in reality, acne, even though known as primarily a teenage problem, often continues well into adulthood.

The Best Method to Keep Pores Open and Clean

The pore is an opening of an oil gland. When oil glands function properly, pores are not visible. Problems begin when there is an increase in sebum production that fills and enlarges the pore so that it becomes visible. Bacteria that feed on sebum can invade and change its quality. Skin irritation increases sebum production even more, resulting in a clog of the opening. The pore plug is formed from dead skin cells that are not properly exfoliated and sebum lipids. When lipids get oxidized, the plug turns black.

In order to keep pores open and clean, several things are needed:.

- **Suppress sebum production**
- **Help dead skin cells exfoliate**
- **Reduce inflammation**
- **Fight bacteria**

HOW TO AVOID: →

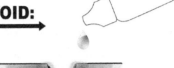 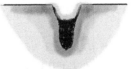

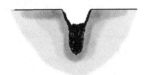

Pore is clogged
(with sebum / proteins)

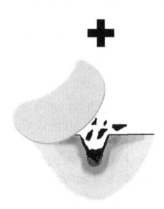

Apply an hydroxy acid serum
Leave on to loosen compacted blockage

+

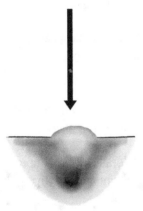

Bacteria
infects the area

Cleanse once daily
with 2% salicylic acid pads

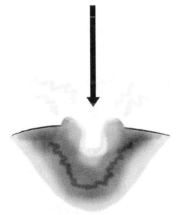

Bacteria infection
results in pimple rupture

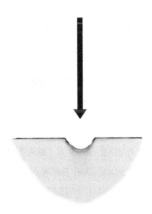

Pores kept
clean and healthy

SKIN CARE GUIDE

Skin Care Routine for Oily, Acne-Prone Skin
Easy-to-follow tips you can do today that will save your oily skin!

1. Cleanse your skin using warm water and gentle facial cleansers. Never use soap. Avoid irritation. Use cleansers with neutral or acid pH, free of harsh detergents and solvents. This step alone can make a huge difference in acne severity. Harsh cleansers disrupt skin barrier and strip away protective acid mantle, opening the way to bacteria and irritants.

2. Exfoliate your skin weekly using salicylic acid and alpha hydroxy acid (lactic acid is best) products. It is important to regularly dissolve plugs made of oil and dead skin cells to clear up whiteheads and blackheads. Salicylic acid is the best since it can work its way deep into the oil glands. Lactic acid (an alpha hydroxy acid) helps remove dead cells from the pore openings, allowing free flow of sebum.

3. Use natural antibacterial remedies such as tea tree oil which can help reduce inflammation and prevent bacterial growth. You can apply pure or diluted tea tree oil directly to inflamed lesions.

4. Natural clay, such as white clay and green clay, absorbs excess oil and inflammatory cytokines from the skin surface. Once a week, use clay masks to purify your skin.

5. Even though excessive sun exposure can damage your skin, moderate sunlight improves immune defense and activates important enzymes. Fifteen-to-thirty minute sunbaths in the mornings can help reduce acne.

6. Use over-the-counter anti-acne remedies such as benzoyl peroxide and salicylic acid. However, remember that, by themselves, they bring only temporary improvement.

7. During the summer, be careful with sunscreens. Many of them increase pore clogging and can worsen acne.

8. Use stress management techniques. Stress increases inflammation and oil secretion, which worsens acne.

Above all, give it time. It takes weeks and even months of carefully designed skin care to slowly bring your skin back to balance and improve your appearance. But it's well worth it, as it will help you maintain a youthful and radiant appearance for years to come.

Oil-free is a Lie!

Oil-free cosmetic lotions and creams often contain synthetic emollients that are highly comedogenic. This means that even though these products do not contain "oils", they have in their formulations a number of oily chemicals that disrupt normal cell shedding in your oil glands, resulting in pore blockage. Even though, "oil-free" products may feel good on skin, they often cause more clogged pores. As a matter of fact, your oily skin often needs oil – a special kind of protective and nurturing oil that can improve sebum quality and make it flow more easily to eliminate pore clogging.

Reducing Inflammation

Copper peptides may help by reducing inflammation and improving the antioxidant defense of your skin. The copper peptide GHK-Cu lowers NFkB, TNF-alpha, and Interleukin 6, the cytokines that trigger inflammation. It also increases superoxide dismutase, the master antioxidant, and prevents inflammation by blocking iron release from ferritin. In addition, you may use many plant substances that have anti-inflammatory and antioxidant effects such as aloe vera gel, beta-carotene, lutein, lycopene, lavender oil, tea tree oil, or white willow bark extract.

Reducing Acne Marks

When you have acne marks, you may reduce them by alternating controlled skin damage with stimulators of regeneration. First, apply exfoliating agents such as lactic or salicylic acid, or use a microdermabrasion cloth. Then use substances that stimulate skin regeneration and reduce scar formation.

Copper peptides have been proven to speed up skin healing and remodeling. They reduce risk of scarring by increasing decorin (anti-scarring protein) and decreasing TGF-beta (a cytokine that increases scarring).

WHAT ABOUT COMEDONES?

Many cosmetic moisturizers boast "oil-free" formulations as a lure for those who are afraid of unsightly comedones. Could biological skin oils increase comedones? You may be surprised, but in a scientific study of comedogenic cosmetic products, the strongest comedone-inducing substances were not natural oils, but fatty acid esters and other chemicals that impart the soft feel to oil-free cosmetic formulations.

1. Cleanse with a gentle, mild cleanser specifically for sensitive skin.

2. Apply an oil reduction serum, perhaps containing cinnamon bark extract.

3. Repeat at night to prevent oily sheen in the morning.

A **comedone** is usually formed when a skin pore (which is actually an oil gland opening) gets plugged by a thick paste comprised of sebum and dead skin cells. This can happen when an increase in sebum production is combined with a buildup of dead cells at the oil gland opening.

There are many reasons for an increase of oil production, including hormones and weather conditions (skin produces more sebum in hot, humid weather). But there is one cause that you can easily avoid, and that is skin irritation. As latest research shows, skin irritation triggers the production of neuropeptides that stimulate oil production. Dead skin cell buildup is caused by insufficient exfoliation and by certain cosmetic ingredients that disrupt skin cell turnover.

At first, the sebum is white, and the comedone is called a **whitehead**. But then the sebum can become oxidized, impregnated with melanin and other pigments that turn it an unpleasant dark color, creating a **blackhead**. Excessive sebum provides a fertile breeding ground for a special kind of oil-eating bacteria—*Propionibacterium acnes*. These tiny pests break down the oil, releasing skin irritating fatty acids that trigger swelling and inflammation. This leads to the development of inflamed comedones or **acne**.

However, acne is a dermatological condition that often requires a combined antibiotics and retinoids treatment. So if you have acne, please consult a medical professional first.

While almost everyone develops clogged pores as well as occasional blackheads and pimples from time to time, to prevent this from happening, you need to (1) avoid skin irritating comedogenic cosmetic products, (2) take care of your skin barrier structure as described in this chapter, (3) and exfoliate your skin regularly using alpha hydroxy acids—salicylic and lactic acids being the best.

SRCPs have been scientifically proven to reduce excessive sebum production in the oil glands, thereby preventing comedone formation.

BEING GENTLE If you want long-term improvement in your skin's appearance, you must learn to be gentle and patient.

If you avoid irritating and drying substances, don't fall for quick-fix solutions; wash your face using mild cleansers with neutral or slightly acidic pH, exfoliate regularly, and use skin remodeling copper peptides to speed up skin regeneration. Then you will enjoy blemish-free and smooth complexion regardless of your skin type.

> **DO YOU REALIZE?** The gentler you are with your skin, the more success you will have controlling breakouts. Baby your skin and even the most breakout-prone skin will respond!

Remember, if you have severe acne and acute inflammation, you may need medical treatment such as prescription antibiotics and retinoids before you can receive any benefits from cosmetics. If you have acne, please consult your dermatologist first.

Questions? Email: ghkcopperpeptides@gmail.com

KEEPING YOUR SKIN YOUNG & BEAUTIFUL
WITH COPPER PEPTIDES

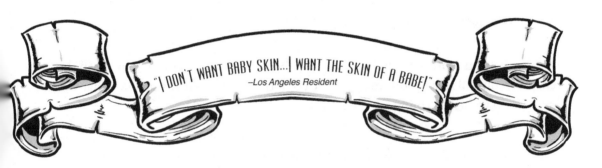

"I DON'T WANT BABY SKIN...I WANT THE SKIN OF A BABE!"
—Los Angeles Resident

In every culture, the most coveted complexion can be observed on a young person between the age of 10 and 20, often admired for resembling that of a baby.

People with young, clear, blemish-free skin possess the power to impact others. Psychological studies covering 170 human cultures have found beautiful skin to be the number one factor in interpersonal attraction.

Beyond the musings of poets, gorgeous skin can be characterized as follows:

✔ • *A clear, vivid look*

✔ • *A firm, elastic tone*

✔ • *Smooth and free of defects*

✔ • *Often has some lingering traces of "baby fat"*

✔ • *Free of skin breaks and cracks*

✔ • *A reddish tint (regardless of skin color) from profuse blood circulation*

Biologically, these characteristics translate into healthy skin as follows:

✓. *A healthy acid mantle and strong protein/lipid skin barrier*

✓. *A rapid turnover of skin cells*

✓. *Collagen and elastin fibers in excellent repair*

✓. *A constantly renewed blood circulation, ensuring an adequate flow of nutrients to the skin*

✓. *Ample levels of water-holding molecules such as proteoglycans and glycosaminoglycans*

✓. *The ability to heal itself rapidly after injury*

✓. *High antioxidant levels (and anti-inflammatory proteins, superoxide dismutase and decorin)*

✓. *Adequate but not excessive natural skin oils*

✓. *A high level of subcutaneous fat cells*

With the proper skin-care regimen, beautiful skin is within your grasp. In this chapter, you will learn about many of the components of healthy skin and what you can do to keep your skin young and beautiful.

QUOTABLE QUOTES: *The skin of a delicate woman is an example of softness and smoothness united.*
—*Uvedale Price*

KEEPING YOUR SKIN IN GOOD REPAIR Although treating your skin gently and protecting it from environmental assaults is very important, it is even more important to keep it in good repair. And this is where SRCPs can do their magic again.

To preserve a protective skin barrier, you need to maintain good skin cell turnover—a constant flow of cells moving outward in the skin to supply new proteins and lipids to replace the older, outer layers. As we age, this revitalizing flow slows down, making skin more vulnerable to assaults and less able to repair damage.

However, as you learned in previous chapters, the aged appearance of our skin can be deceptive, because even in very old skin, there is still a good supply of never-aging, eternally young skin stem cells residing in the lower layers of the epidermis.

According to the recent studies (see Chapter 19), SRCPs can revive the skin stem cells by stimulating the synthesis of p63—an anti-senescence protein. This allows us to use SRCPs to restore proper skin turnover and to ensure speedy restoration of the disrupted skin barrier.

SRCPs also aid in dermal restoration, stimulating the production and repair of the elastic strings of our skin—collagen and elastin fibers. They also ensure that collagen strands properly assemble by stimulating the synthesis of a collagen quality control proteoglycan—decorin.

By keeping your skin in excellent repair, SRCPs not only ensure strong barrier formation but also smooth, resilient, and wrinkle-free skin.

For those of you over age 30, it is known that regular use of SRCPs along with the skin's natural hydroxy acids will speed skin-cell turnover. For skin maintenance, use the following products weekly: Apply mild or moderate strength SRCPs 3 to 4 times a week and an exfoliating agent such as 7 to 10 percent lactic acid or 1 to 2 percent salicylic acid (three times weekly should suffice). Additionally, many people use retinoic acid 2 to 3 times a week.

Manual exfoliation also works well. As we discussed earlier in the book, you can use a skin brush, a pumice stone, or a buffer. Some individuals abrade with a spot scraper to flake-off damage. Microdermabrasion and needling can also prove successful in removing damaged skin.

YOUR ROSY CHEEKS Regardless of the skin color, young skin has an attractive reddish tint indicative of good blood circulation. When the roses and peaches of youth start to fade, which usually happens after the age of 30, many women just start using more makeup.

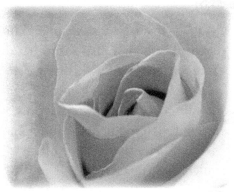

Although makeup is easy to buy and masks the deficiency of circulation splendidly, it is not a solution. Profuse blood circulation of youthful skin is more than just a pretty color. It is an essential factor in determining the skin's well being and its ability to repair itself.

Sad examples of the grim consequences of deficient blood circulation in the skin are bedsores and skin ulcers in elderly residents of nursing homes.

You can think of it like this: Let's imagine a busy home construction site. To make the work go smoothly and without delay, you have to have a constant supply of building materials. As soon as there is an interruption or insufficient delivery of the materials, the work stalls.

The same happens in your skin when the blood supply is not adequate, because skin receives its nutrition and oxygen through the blood.

SRCPs re-establish new blood vessel growth in aged and damaged skin, speeding up skin repair and restoring its youthful glow. They also dilate constricted blood vessels, which increases oxygen perfusion of the skin. As a result, skin repairs itself more quickly and acquires an unmistakably clear and vivid look that indicates perfect health.

We must acknowledge though that, due to the spread of misinformation based on a lack of deep knowledge of skin biology, some have expressed concern that stimulation of blood flow may somehow lead to an increase of skin tumors.

However, it should be pointed out that good blood circulation is found in the skin of babies and healthy, young people. It is an essential attribute of healthy skin. If it were true that excellent blood circulation itself could cause cancer, young people would get cancer much more often than older folks, which is not the case.

Although it is true that tumors are notorious for their extensive circulation, this is very different from normal blood circulation of healthy skin in the same way that skin repair is different from the abnormal cell growth of tumors.

BUILDING UP DERMAL PROTEOGLYCANS Biological oils can restore your skin barrier, but you will also need to increase production of water-holding molecules in the dermis—**proteoglycans** and **glycosaminoglycans**. These substances act as molecular sponges, taking up water and holding it inside your dermis. The most popular glycosaminoglycan in the dermis is hyaluronic acid, which is often found in cosmetic moisturizers.

However, large molecules of hyaluronic acid cannot penetrate the skin. Moreover, when pure hyaluronic acid is injected into the skin, it is quickly dissolved by dermal enzymes.

That is why all wrinkle-filling products based on hyaluronic acid usually contain a chemically modified form that dissolves more slowly. It plumps up the skin, at least temporarily, but does nothing else.

Since SRCPs have been scientifically proven to stimulate the synthesis of water-holding molecules of the dermis, with copper peptide-based products, you can avoid chemically modified skin plumpers and plump your skin with its own proteoglycans instead. For the best result, it should be combined with alpha hydroxy acids or microdermabrasion.

REDUCING PORE SIZE As we age, our skin grows thinner, but our bodies gain girth. How unfair! Most of us want the reverse. Not only that, but thin skin makes pores appear more prominent. Contrary to what magazine advertisements tell you, oil removers do not reduce pore size but rather cause the skin to produce more oil and larger pores to compensate for the removed oil.

In contrast, both retinoic acid and lactic acid reduce oil production and pore size. When you increase the rate of skin renewal, this also reduces pore size, since the firmer and thicker skin helps squeeze the pore downward and inward.

Skin renewal serums and creams that increase collagen, elastin, proteoglycans, and the amount of subcutaneous fat (the very thin layer under the skin) both firm the skin and increase its thickness. Many individuals have found that copper peptide serums work well for this purpose.

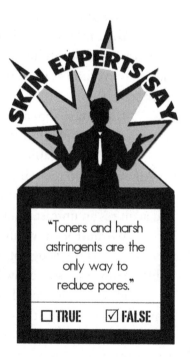

SKIN EXPERTS SAY

"Toners and harsh astringents are the only way to reduce pores."

☐ TRUE   ☑ FALSE

BIOLOGICAL SKIN OILS vs. COSMETIC MOISTURIZERS
THE REAL SKINCARE SHOWDOWN

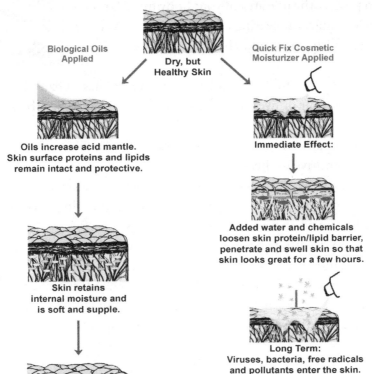

Biological Oils Applied

Dry, but Healthy Skin

Quick Fix Cosmetic Moisturizer Applied

Oils increase acid mantle. Skin surface proteins and lipids remain intact and protective.

Immediate Effect:

Skin retains internal moisture and is soft and supple.

Added water and chemicals loosen skin protein/lipid barrier, penetrate and swell skin so that skin looks great for a few hours.

Long Term: Viruses, bacteria, free radicals and pollutants enter the skin.

Using SRCPs and biological oils reduces water loss and increases water-holding proteoglycans and glycosaminoglycans.

Less protective skin accumulates more moles, warts, lesions, and sun damage.

Methods of Skin Moisturization

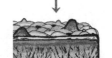

METHOD	HOW IT WORKS	Time to be Effective	PROBLEMS	RECOMMENDED
SRCPs	Mimic natural repair, repair skin damage, and increase the skin's proteoglycans and GAGs	About 2-3 weeks	None	YES
Waxes and Greases	Heavy oils such as petrolatum seal skin surface to water loss	Immediate	May disrupt the skin barrier	NO
Biological Oils	Oils such as emu oil, squalane, octyl palmitate, and cholesterol & lanosterol esters help reduce water loss. Oils similar to human skin oils: emu oil and squalane	Immediate	Not as durable as waxes and greases but stimulates skin repair	YES
Retinyl Palmitate	Increases natural skin oils	2 weeks	Avoid acne-prone areas	YES
Quick Fix Cosmetic Moisturizers	Designed to improve the look of skin at cosmetic counters, mixtures of oils, water, and surface-active chemicals quickly swell the skin by rapid water uptake	5 minutes	Acts like irritant to loosen protective skin barrier, skin more susceptible to infection	NO

PROTECTING YOUR HANDS   There are specific things you can do to protect the one area of your body most exposed to aging elements. Start by wearing vinyl gloves whenever you come in contact with household chemicals and other harsh elements.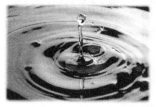

Wear gloves when folding laundry, peeling vegetables, or handling citrus fruits or tomatoes. Purchase four or five pairs and keep them in the kitchen, bathroom, nursery and laundry areas.

Have other pairs for non-wet housework and gardening. Avoid latex gloves since many people are sensitive to them.

Dry out the gloves between cleaning jobs. When outdoors in cool weather, wear unlined leather gloves to protect against dry and chapped skin. Since you can't always wear gloves, take care when washing dishes or clothes.

Just say "no" to dish pan hands! Avoid hand-washing items if you can, but if you must, keep your hands out of the soapy water as much as possible.

Using an automatic dishwasher will protect your hands and also effectively sterilize your dishes. Remove rings whenever washing or working with your hands. When you wash your hands, use lukewarm water and very little soap.

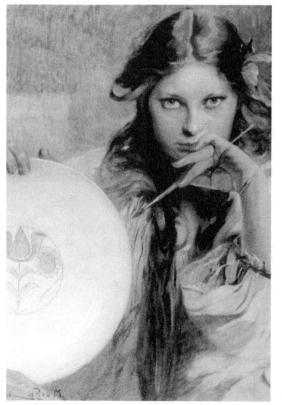

SPECIAL NEEDS OF THE EYELIDS

Your eyelids, the thinnest skin on the body, require special attention.

Before you apply eye makeup, add a light protective layer of a mild copper peptide cream.

As your skin grows thicker and stronger, progressively but slowly move on to stronger products. If any product feels too strong for your sensitive skin, try the super-mild GHK form of copper peptide creams or serums.

Such gentle products provide a protective coating with antioxidant protection. Since makeup can irritate and damage your eye area, use as little eye shadow, eye liner, and mascara as possible.

You may discover that less is more when you emerge with beautiful skin. Remove eye makeup with a biological healing oil, such as emu oil or squalane.

Aerobic Exercise Improves Skin Health

Aerobic exercise can imbue you with a rosy glow. It markedly improves skin quality and overall body health. Aerobics prevent bloating and puffiness, acne, and loss of muscle tone. Exercise brings more oxygen and nutrients to the skin to make it firmer and better nourished. Aerobic exercise can also slow down aging. Mail carriers, who spend their days walking, have the longest lifespan of any occupational group in the United States. Many people who live to a ripe old age walk, hike, or run daily.

Physical ability decreases less with age than commonly believed; the body wears out faster from a lack of use than overuse.

The benefits of aerobic exercise are too numerous to list here. Exercise increases the blood capillary density in the skin and improves the nutrition of skin cells. It increases overall body metabolism and retards many of the effects of aging. In one study, healthy men in their 50's who exercised vigorously displayed a tissue oxygen uptake capacity and cardiovascular function that was 20 to 30 percent higher than sedentary young men (Paffenbarger et al 1978).

Ideally, you should get between three and five hours of vigorous aerobic exercise a week. Researchers have found that when you perform moderate work outs, you get the same health benefits as high intensity aerobics. It doesn't have to be hell to be healthy! The best forms of exercise are fun and reduce your stress level. Do what makes you happy and feel good. Golf, hiking, walking, hunting, fishing, and even gardening are all good options.

Once you establish an exercise routine that works for you, keep it up! Unless you are an elite athlete, if you start skipping workouts, your aerobic capacity will rapidly decrease, dropping by 50 percent in just one week. After five to 12 days, your capillary density will decrease by 10 to 20 percent, and the capacity of your heart to pump blood will also diminish. Two months of inactivity will wipe out about 90 percent of the conditioning gained through exercise (Coastal 1984).

DO YOU REALIZE? The new exercise idea is that very brief periods of intense exercise (for example 30 seconds) followed by a few minutes of very light exercise, then repeated, is all you need to switch your gene output to younger-type proteins.

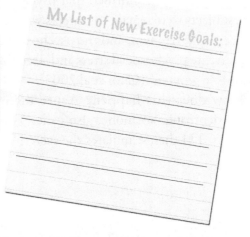

My List of New Exercise Goals:

PSYCHOLOGICAL STRESS DAMAGES SKIN We've all suspected that stress can age us. Just take a look at some of our past presidents after four years in office. Well, now we have proof. Psychological stress ages the skin.

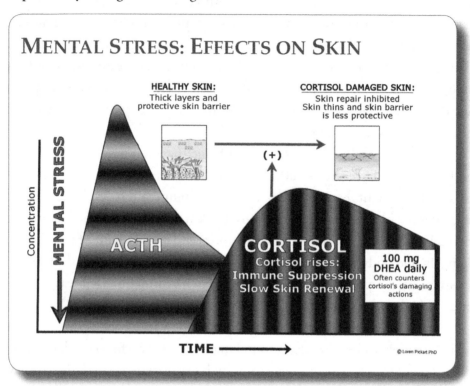

A study measuring the skin barrier recovery of students before and after exams demonstrated how psychological stress adversely affected their skin. The study assessed the skin barrier recovery of medical, dental, and pharmacy students starting at four weeks before final examinations through four weeks after final exams during spring vacation. There was a noteworthy decline in skin barrier protection and healing during the stressful period that they studied for exams. But during spring vacation, their skin health recovered. According to researchers of the study, "the greatest deterioration in barrier function occurred in those subjects who demonstrated the largest increases in perceived psychological stress" (Garg et al 2001).

Another study confirmed that psychological stress has a negative effect on the skin. The subjects were female volunteers who underwent a night of sleep deprivation, a three-day exercise regimen, and the psychosocial stress of an interview. The conclusion was clear: "Acute psychosocial stress and sleep deprivation disrupts skin barrier function homeostasis in women" (Choi et al 2005).

How does this happen? Acute mental stress raises the level of ACTH (adrenocorticotropic hormone, also called corticotropin), the body's stress response hormone. ACTH then stimulates the secretion of cortisol, which in turn inhibits skin repair.

PROTECT YOUR SKIN, RESTORE ITS BEAUTY   As you see, keeping your skin young and beautiful boils down to one simple phrase: "Protect your skin; restore its beauty." It is really that simple! It is true that you can avoid many skin problems just by keeping it out of harm's way—treating it gently, preserving its protective barrier, and avoiding unnecessary assaults from the environment and unhealthy cosmetic products.

However, protection alone is not enough. You need to take special care of your skin's reparative and restorative mechanisms to ensure its speedy recovery from occasional damage and stressful influences.

Remember, babies and young children are not particularly careful with their skin, and yet their skin is perfect because of excellent repair systems. If we only could retain this outstanding reparative power of our skin, we would never grow old.

Today, we know that the main reason for losing this power is age-related depletion of central regulators of the repair process. By protecting the skin from damage while supplying it with those magical molecules, Skin Remodeling Copper Peptides, we can reverse skin aging, making it radiate health and alluring beauty.

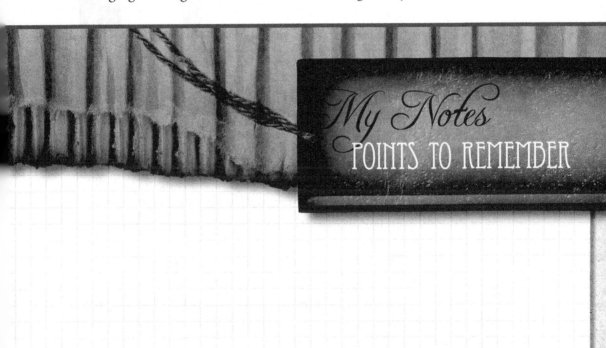

My Notes
POINTS TO REMEMBER

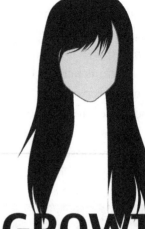

"LONG LET ME INHALE, DEEPLY THE ODOR OF YOUR HAIR, INTO IT PLUNGE THE WHOLE OF MY FACE, AS A THIRSTY MAN INTO THE WATER OF A SPRING, AND WAVE IT IN MY FINGERS LIKE A SCENTED HANDKERCHIEF, TO SHAKE THE MEMORIES INTO THE AIR." –CHARLES BAUDELAIRE

(13)

HEALTHY HAIR GROWTH
STRENGTHEN, THICKEN, LENGTHEN FROM ROOT TO TIP

Your hair, like skin, starts life's journey renewing itself with youthful vigor. When you are young, you flaunt your thick, well-pigmented, fast growing hair. But the passage of time takes a toll, and your hair begins to thin or vanish, grow more slowly, and turn gray. While the search for methods to restore healthy, younger hair is ancient, the reality is that even today, in the era of Rogaine® (minoxidil) and Propecia® (finasteride), the therapies that profess to restore hair health give a marginal result at best.

While far from a miracle therapy, research on SRCPs has uncovered an unexpected benefit: they stimulate hair follicle growth and function. More and more, SRCPs are being used to improve hair growth and condition, with promising results.

Why the Big Apple is a Bad Hair Town

The effect of the hair-care industry on hair health has been disastrous according to many scientists, including Russian physician George Michael. Dr. Michael immigrated to New York City with his family after the 1917 revolution and later set up a medical practice. Despite the city's abundance of beauty salons and other businesses that catered to hair, Michael was immediately struck by the poor quality of women's tresses. He reminisced that in the Russia of his youth, many women in their 60's and beyond displayed healthy, well-pigmented, waist-length locks; in contrast, in New York

City the women had difficulty growing their hair longer than six inches. Dr. Michael concluded that the excess of dyes, cutting, blow-drying, and relaxers was damaging the women's hair. He went on to emerge as the guru of long-hair care, opening a chain of Long Hair Clinics and working with famous long-haired beauties such as Crystal Gayle (For more information on Dr. Michael, visit Jennifer Bahney's www.longhairlovers. com).

WHY MEN GO BALD AND WOMEN GET THIN HAIR No matter how bitterly women complain about hair loss and thinning, they do have to admit that a woman who has gone completely bald is a rare sight, one that is usually associated with certain medical conditions. The long-known fact that so many men go bald, while women do not, prompted scientists to suspect that baldness is caused by male sex hormones, or androgens. Eventually, the male hormone testosterone was blamed as the main culprit in male-pattern hair loss. However, further research revealed a much more complex picture. Even now, there is still no complete clarity on why people lose their hair.

Each hair follicle goes through three distinctive phases of growth and decline. The phase of hair growth is called **anagen**, and it lasts for several years. Then a hair follicle enters the short phase, or **catagen** (about two weeks), during which the follicle shrinks and pushes hair out. The resting phase, during which hair follicles are not producing hair, is called **telogen**, and it lasts for several weeks. Then the whole cycle is repeated.

Testosterone that is found in blood is a weak androgen and has little effect on hair growth. However, in hair follicles testosterone can be converted into a much more potent form—dihydrotestosterone or DHT. Normally, DHT stimulates body and facial hair but has no effect on scalp hair follicles because they lack specific DHT receptors.

Normal Aging and Other Damaging Actions

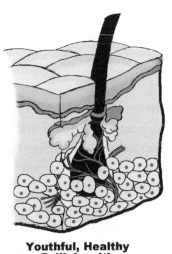

Less Protective Skin Barrier
Longer Telogen Phase
Permanents / Relaxers
Miniaturized Follicles
Auto Immune Attack
Color Cosmetics
Scalp Damage
Excess Heat
Thinner Scalp

SRCPs
Highly Protective Skin Barrier
Rebuild Capillaries to Follicle
Increase Melanin Synthesis
Increase Subcutaneous Fat
Longer Anagen Phase
Inhibit DHT Formation
Increase Follicle Size
Repair Scalp Damage
Inhibit Inflammation
Thicker Scalp

Youthful, Healthy Follicle with Thick, Pigmented Hair

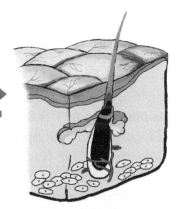

Aged, Damaged Follicle with Thin Gray Hair

The problems begin when certain scalp hair follicles start responding to DHT (develop DHT receptors). In this case, DHT shortens their growth phase (anagen) and eventually causes miniaturization (progressive shrinkage) of the hair follicles. As a result, with each hair cycle, the hair grows thinner and thinner until the follicles start producing thin, barely visible vellus hair instead of thick, beautiful terminal hair.

Men usually have DHT-sensitive hair follicles all grouped together, typically on the forehead and on top of the head. These are the areas where hair loss is often profound and noticeable (male-pattern baldness). In some cases, every single one of the hair follicles on a man's head is DHT-sensitive, eventually resulting in complete baldness.

Women, on the other hand, have diffuse distribution of DHT sensitive follicles. That is why women rarely go completely bald and may just develop thinning hair instead. Since the degree of DHT-dependent hair loss is determined by DHT sensitivity of hair follicles, it is quite possible for a man to have a full head of hair regardless of a high level of DHT.

An enzyme that converts testosterone into DHT is called 5-alpha-reductase (5AR). Normally skin and hair (as well as the liver) contain 5-alpha-reductase Type I, while the prostate contains 5AR Type II. However, it was found that hair follicles in a balding scalp often contain both types of 5AR—Type I and II. That explains why male pattern hair loss can somewhat be reduced by the drug finasteride — a selective inhibitor of 5AR Type II. Unfortunately, finasteride has little effect on female hair loss.

Yet, while the role of DHT in hair loss seems so well established, recent studies have indicated that it is not the whole story (Ellis et al 1998). Today, other factors such as follicle inflammation, poor circulation, and disrupted skin remodeling have started to come forward as true forces behind the age-old hair loss problem.

WHAT IS BEHIND HAIR LOSS? The causes are far more diverse than many people realize. The following is a description of the factors that can inhibit hair growth.

Hair Loss and TGF-beta. Miniaturization of the hair follicles is the most distinctive finding in individuals experiencing balding or thinning hair, so it is natural to assume that DHT is the cause of it. However, some researchers now believe that DHT causes miniaturization of hair follicles *indirectly*, and that its main action is to raise the level of TGF-beta (a scar-promoting and pro-inflammatory cytokine). In turn, TGF-beta causes inflammation and accumulation of excessive collagen around hair follicles, restricting their growth and impeding circulation. It has been demonstrated that miniaturization of hair follicles is usually associated with inflammation, increased level of TGF-beta, and accumulation of fibrose tissue around the follicle (Uno 1988).

Inadequate follicle microcirculation. The blood flow of older follicles slows down as we age, which diminishes synthesis, the formation of necessary compounds. As a result, the follicles shrink in size and function. The synthesis of new hair necessitates a very high nutrient flow to the follicle bulb. Morphological studies that measure structures of aged follicles often observe a markedly diminished capillary blood supply in aged, miniaturized follicles. This alone may be the cause of follicle miniaturization and inadequate hair synthesis (Stenn et al 1991).

Decreased subcutaneous fat layer. The layer of fat at the base of the skin, known as subcutaneous adipose tissue or baby fat, diminishes with age. Researchers have noted that fat accumulates around healthy follicles that vigorously grow hair. In contrast, they observed a lack of fat around dormant follicles. They postulate that these fat cells serve a supportive function for the hair follicle. Conditions that inhibit hair growth, such as chemotherapy and starvation, also decrease the subcutaneous fat layer (Stenn et al 1991).

Supplements of MSM may greatly help me to grow out my hair!

Lack of sulfur donors. Hair is composed of 35 percent sulfur-containing amino acids. Only bird feathers boast a similar level of amino acids. Nutritional sulfur supplements, such as methylsulfonylmethane (commonly known as MSM), have long been shown to beautify the manes of racehorses, and many individuals rave about how MSM adds health and luster to their hair.

Damage from relaxers, excessive heat, coloring agents, and dyes. As we discussed, an array of razzle-dazzle hair products that are designed to beautify can actually inflict more harm than good as they damage the scalp and frazzle the follicles. Relaxers, permanents, color cosmetics with their organic dyes and metallic salts, and excessive heat from blow dryers and hot oil treatments can literally boil the follicles and also damage the hair shaft's hard outer layers of keratin. When we combine these treatments, it's like adding oil to a fire, as these procedures ravish hair follicles and reduce hair growth. This follicle onslaught is most noticeable when some women lose their eyebrows and eyelashes by age 40. Such self-inflicted damage can also result in hair loss via excessive breakage, when hair shafts become so badly damaged that they break, leaving only short stumps like those in a heavily logged forest. This form of hair loss can often be reduced by the regular use of a good, well-formulated conditioner. But avoiding the damage in the first place would be a much better strategy.

Excessive hair cutting. If long, lush, healthy locks are what you crave, I have good news for you. According to Dr. George Michael, long hair is healthier than short hair. He contends that the longer you grow your hair, the stronger your roots. It is possible that the hair follicles thrive from the tension produced by the weight of a heavy hair shaft in the same manner that muscles and bones respond to exercise. So cut your hair less, and get more out of your hair.

ESTROGENS AND HEALTHY HAIR Estrogens are female hormones that inhibit the growth of facial hair (with the exception of eyelashes) and body hair (with the exception of underarm and pubic hair) while stimulating scalp hair. Estrogens counteract the effect of androgens. That is why a hormonal shift can have a profound effect on a woman's hair:

Extreme exercise. Severe exercise tends to reduce estrogen and raise testosterone. This hormonal shift can stop the menstrual cycle. It may also lead to brittle bones and hair thinning or loss. While there are many positive aspects of exercise, there can be too much of a good thing.

Sudden hormone shifts. Hair loss can intensify after a woman gives birth or discontinues oral contraceptives. In these cases, a brief therapy with hair stimulators is recommended; they can usually restore hair to its previous condition. Such hair stimulators include SRCPs and other supplements such as MSM and Flaxseed Oil.

Effect of menopause. Pre-menopause and menopause are associated with a progressive decline of the estrogen level, which can result in hair loss. In this case, herbal supplements containing phytoestrogens such as red clover, soy, flaxseed, pomegranate, and others can be recommended.

Using SRCPs to Stimulate Hair Growth—A Hair-Raising Discovery

      One of the most exciting discoveries from stem cell researchers, truly hair raising, reveals that hair follicles provide the source of stem cells for skin. This vital finding links hair follicles with skin repair. However, long before this discovery, I observed that after applying GHK-Cu to a wound, hair follicles enlarged dramatically at the edge of the wound.

Since then, SRCPs have been proven to:
- Increase hair growth in humans
- Increase hair follicle size in humans
- Improve the "take" of transplanted hair plugs
- Reduce hair loss caused by chemotherapeutic drugs
- Increase the recovery of hair loss due to chemotherapeutic drugs

An in-depth discussion of the above actions can be found in Chapter 19, "The Science Behind SRCPs".

IMPROVING HAIR VITALITY WITH SRCPS While recent studies hold promise, SRCPs are not the panacea for hair loss. A more important future use of SRCPs may be as a regular scalp treatment or hair tonic, used once or twice weekly, for the enhancement of hair and scalp health. SRCPs have numerous actions that may improve the hair and scalp. These include:

Reducing DHT formation in hair follicles. An enzyme which converts testosterone to DHT (5-AR) damages hair growth. It exists in two forms: type-1, which functions in hair follicles, and type-2, which acts in prostate tissue.

Follicle-damaging DHT is produced in the hair follicles. Propecia (finasteride), a prescription treatment for hair loss in men who have male pattern baldness, inhibits 5-AR throughout the body and improves hair growth. But it works best on the type-2 form and is better suited for controlling prostate enlargement. It also must be administered by pills that spread the drug throughout the body.

A superior way to inhibit the type-1 5-AR that damages hair growth may be to increase copper ions in the skin. Sugimoto et al found that copper (II) ions could give up to a 90 percent inhibition of type 1 5-AR. At 1.2 micrograms copper ion per milliliter, type-1 5-AR activity reduced by 50 percent, but copper (II) ions were 10-fold less active on inhibiting the type-2 prostate form. Thus, copper ions are more specific inhibitors of 5-AR than Propecia.

Human transdermal studies have found that concentrations of up to 0.50 micrograms per milliliter of copper ion can be introduced into the skin with SRCPs without irritation. For comparison, the blood plasma copper level is approximately 1 microgram per milliliter (Sugimoto et al 1995).

Blocking TGF-beta Formation. SRCPs block production of TGF-beta, a cytokine closely involved in the processes that leads to miniaturization of hair follicles. Copper peptides inhibit TGF-beta directly by stimulating the production of decorin —a molecule that also inhibits TGF-beta production (see Chapter 19).

Improving microcirculation to hair follicles. Hair follicles have extreme rates of metabolic activity. However, morphological studies of aged follicles often find an inadequate capillary circulation. As a result, some researchers have suggested that the reduced nutrient flow may cause hair shafts to thin as we age. SRCPs have angiogenic activity (growth of new blood vessels from pre-existing vessels) that may correct this problem. See Chapter 19, which goes into more depth about the science behind SRCPs.

Protective anti-inflammatory actions. The final event in the sequence of degenerative changes produces non-functional hair follicles which have involuted (rolled inward). These changes cause tissue damage, auto-immune inflammation, and free-radical reactions around the follicle.

SRCPs reduce inflammation and free radical formation in hair follicles since they block the inflammatory actions of both interleukin 1 and Transforming Growth Factor beta 1. Also during tissue injury, the release of ferrous iron from ferritin increases the formation of tissue-damaging free radicals, but SRCPs block the release of iron from ferritin. Finally, only about 50 percent of copper zinc superoxide dismutase is activated due to a lack of copper in the protein. SRCPs can supply additional copper to zinc superoxide dismutase and increase its antioxidant effectiveness as well.

Autoimmune damage causing hair loss exists in conditions such as alopecia areata, diabetes, vitiligo, certain types of thyroid disease, and pernicious anemia.

Physicians normally treat these conditions with a short course of any cortisone-type drug, which often restores hair growth. However, when we inject cortisone into bald spots, the hair regrowth is temporary. Here's the problem: corticosteroids inhibit skin repair, thereby producing thinner, less functional skin left unable to support hair follicle functions. In studies on nickel allergic patients, Zhai et al wrote that SRCPs were effective in reducing redness and inflammation after allergic reactions while also stimulating skin repair. See Chapter 19 for details.

To take care of the health of my hair, I first need to take care of my scalp!

Enhancing the skin's subcutaneous fat layer and thickening of the scalp. Newborns and small children have ample padding of subcutaneous fat underneath scalp skin, which protects their little heads from injuries. As we age, some of us grow stubborn and thick-headed, while our scalps get thinner. None of us mind a thin waistline—but a thin scalp? The scalp becomes thinner in part because the subcutaneous fat layer that surrounds hair follicles diminishes with age. Pathologists have noted that large subcutaneous fat cells are associated with large, healthy hair follicles and have postulated that the fat cells provide nutritional support to the follicles. Conditions that cause hair loss, such as cancer chemotherapy, are associated with a sharp decrease in the volume of subcutaneous fat cells. SRCPs increase both hair follicle size and the amount of subcutaneous fat.

SRCPs also help increase skin thickness by boosting the dermal levels of collagen, elastin, and the water-holding proteoglycans (carbohydrate molecules linked to protein) and glycosaminoglycans (unbranched polysaccharide molecules composed of many carbohydrates). See Chapter 19 for further information.

Reviving hair follicle stem cells. SRCPs have been shown to restore the vitality and reparative ability of skin stem cells (see Chapter 19 for more details). Since hair, just like skin, requires an adequate supply of stem cells in order to grow, stem cell health is an important attribute of long and lustrous hair.

Repairing damaged scalp. Women often lose hair as a result of numerous assaults inflicted by relaxers, permanents, coloring chemicals, and excessive heat from blow dryers and hot oil treatments. SRCPs work wonders to speed up the repair of scalp damage after various hair procedures.

Reducing graying of hair. Hair grays with age, but the speed at which this occurs may depend on the availability of copper in the scalp. Melanin and other hair pigments are produced from the amino acid tyrosine by the action of tyrosinase, a copper-containing enzyme. Additional scalp copper might slow the graying process. In fact, over the years, many individuals have reported the re-pigmentation of gray hair after using SRCP products.

USING COPPER PEPTIDES TO IMPROVE HAIR HEALTH

My research in the 1980's led to my earlier inventions with products such as Tricomin™, which was demonstrated to increase hair growth in humans, and GraftCyte™, which was proven to increase hair transplant success in humans. For more specifics, see Chapter 19. The latest inventions of copper peptide topical scalp products have taken hair repair to the next level. These began as an SRCP skin repair cream that was tested in the Dermatology Department at the *University of California San Francisco*. A 41-year-old woman with severe hair loss tried the skin repair cream on her head because nothing else had worked to restore her lost hair. Over the next two-and-a-half months, she regained all of her lost hair. Word spread, and other people began using the skin repair cream to counter hair loss. In time, copper peptides emerged as a distinct product line designed to repair hair. Their biological effect is similar to the results achieved by my earlier line of hair products; however, the new generation of products appear even more effective, as demonstrated in my basic tests on hair function.

Second-generation copper peptide scalp products generally are available in two forms: creams (which work well on hairlines or denser areas) and sprays (a fine mist that can be sprayed directly on the scalp). Copper peptides can also be found in formulations of mild shampoos and conditioners.

Many people have used such products to calm scalp tissue irritated by other hair growth stimulators, such as minoxidil and retinoic acid. When you rub on a copper peptide product to calm your scalp, start with a light application. If your scalp is irritated, you may experience a brief stinging, but as your scalp repairs itself, it will become more protective and less sensitive to irritation by minoxidil, retinoic acid, and other products.

My Hair Regrowth Recommendations

The following regrowth products and procedures are preferable, based on reports from people who have used copper peptide products, to help restore lost or thinning hair. Women often lose hair as a result of stress or hormonal shifts caused by menopausal changes or discontinuation of birth control pills. Another frequent cause of hair loss is extreme dieting that can result in hormonal shifts (sometimes to the point of even disrupting the menstrual cycle) and essential nutrient deficiency. Fortunately for women, their hair loss is easier to reverse than for men.

1. Apply an SRCP product in the version best suited for the area of concern (either a cream or spray). The recommended frequency is four to five times a week, applied as a light coating before bedtime. Individuals usually report that copper peptides help markedly reduce hair loss in about three weeks, improve scalp health, and reduce irritation, resulting in a thicker head of hair in about four months.

2. Apply emu oil on the scalp. The combination of SRCPs and emu oil often produces drastic reductions in hair loss and increases hair growth. Recently, Dr. Michael Holick of *Boston University Medical Center* reported a clinical study that found emu oil to accelerate skin regeneration and also stimulate hair growth. He wrote, "The hair follicles were more robust, the skin thickness was remarkably increased...Also, we discovered in the same test that over 80 percent of hair follicles that had been 'asleep' were awakened and began growing hair."

3. For added stimulation, apply minoxidil (2 to 5 percent). Start by using 2 percent minoxidil and progressively increase to 5 percent. At times minoxidil can irritate the scalp. If this occurs, stop using the product and only use copper peptides until your scalp health is restored. Then, resume the use of 2 percent minoxidil and eventually 5 percent if your scalp remains healthy.

Hideo Uno, who wrote the textbook on Rogaine®, found that both SRCPs and minoxidil work synergistically to improve hair health. While minoxidil primarily stimulates new vellus hair growth, SRCPs prove more effective in thickening the hair shafts.

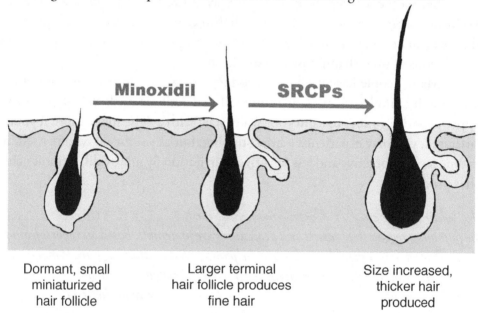

| Dormant, small miniaturized hair follicle | Larger terminal hair follicle produces fine hair | Size increased, thicker hair produced |

4. Retinoic acid (0.01 to 0.05 percent) also stimulates hair follicles. Retinoic acid helps produce thicker hair shafts when combined with minoxidil, but this combination may irritate the scalp. When used lightly, copper peptides can greatly reduce the irritation.

5. If your hair thins or falls out as the result of low estrogen caused by menopause or other hormonal shifts, you may benefit from estrogen supplements. However, be mindful that recent studies have shown that there is a link between hormone replacement therapy and certain cancers, so make sure to talk to your doctor first (Sugimoto et al 1995). Phytoestrogens, such as soy isoflavones or red clover, may soften the sharpness of estrogen decline and reduce hair loss. Since subcutaneous fat becomes an important site for estrogen synthesis in pre-menopause and menopause, steer clear from extreme dieting, and consider keeping a few extra pounds instead of trying to slim to the bones.

6. For those who prefer an all-natural approach, there are several non-drug DHT blockers. These include saw palmetto oil, pygeum and nettle root extract, the soybean isoflavones genistein and daidzein, ginkgo biloba, and gamma linoleic acid.

Saw palmetto oil has been used for more than 400 years as an herbal treatment for enuresis, nocturia, atrophy of the testes, impotence, inflammation of the prostate, and as a mild aphrodisiac for men. Women used the berries to treat infertility, painful periods, and problems with lactation. Extracts of two plants, pygeum bark (Pygeum africanum) and nettle root (Urtica dioica) are widely used to treat prostate hyperplasia.

Isoflavonoids, such as genistein and daidzein, are weak estrogens and may lessen the risk of osteoporosis and heart disease. Several studies have found that isoflavones can protect against the development of cancer. A report from China indicates that daidzein exhibits hair-growth and hair-color-promoting activity.

Ginkgo biloba is a popular herb used worldwide to improve cerebral blood flow and general blood circulation.

QUOTABLE QUOTES: *And Delilah made Samson sleep upon her knees; and she called for a man, and she caused him to shave off seven locks from Samson's head; and she began to afflict him, and Samson's strength went from him.* —Capture of Samson, Judges 16

Getting Rid of Any Green
No one wants to hear that "the dye is cast" if it means turning blond hair green. Blond hair may pick up a green tint when exposed to copper peptides, just as when it is dipped in chlorinated water from a swimming pool. In order to reap the benefits of such products without tinting hair, be careful to keep the products on the scalp and off the hair. If you notice a green hue, blend a solution of one part lemon juice and four parts water to remove the green color. Or look for tin peptide based scalp products that present no color problems and often work to reduce hair loss.

COPPER PEPTIDE SHAMPOOS & CONDITIONERS Designed as relatively low pH products, shampoos and conditioners fortified with copper peptides work well to clean hair with a minimum amount of damage and then tighten up and re-seal the hair shafts. The addition of SRCPs enhances the vitality of the hair follicles and scalp.

Hair contains a high sulfur content from the amino acid cysteine and can easily form cross-links to other cysteines in the hair molecule. These bonds keep the hair tough and strong and thus able to resist abrasion. The cross-links hold the hair fibers together. As long as this organization is not disrupted, the fiber remains robust and appears "healthy".

Shampoos with a high alkaline pH may work better to clean the hair and scalp, but they also strip away too many natural scalp oils and extract the glues that help hold the hair shafts together. An effective shampoo that is also healthy for the scalp should not contain flash-foamers (foaming chemicals that add lather). These do nothing for the hair and damage the hair shafts and scalp.

Conditioners are formulated to re-acidify the hair after shampooing. When you restore this natural acid environment to the hair and scalp, you keep your hair proteins hard and thereby prevent the growth of foreign bacteria. An effective conditioner should also contain the highest-quality amino acids and pantothenic acid (vitamin B-5) to re-seal the hair cuticle. It should also be designed to help de-tangle the hair and add a lustrous shine. The addition of SRCPs to a conditioner helps enhance the health and vitality of the hair, scalp, and hair follicles.

Many quality shampoos and conditioners will be in a concentrated formula, so you may want to mix the products with a small amount of water to make them easier to use.

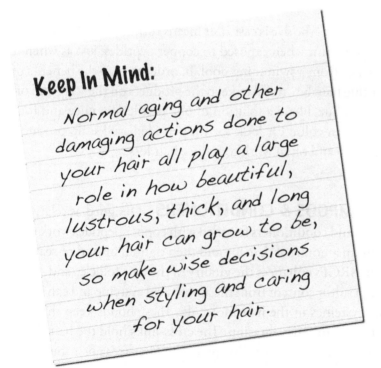

Overwashing my hair can cause more damage than it may help!

Keep In Mind:
Normal aging and other damaging actions done to your hair all play a large role in how beautiful, lustrous, thick, and long your hair can grow to be, so make wise decisions when styling and caring for your hair.

Questions? Email: ghkcopperpeptides@gmail.com

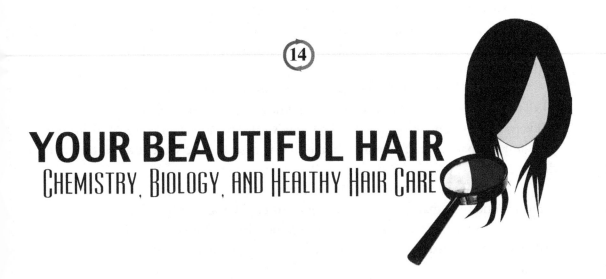

YOUR BEAUTIFUL HAIR
Chemistry, Biology, and Healthy Hair Care

Throughout history, women have woven a tapestry of desire with their alluring tresses. Legend has it that mermaids and sirens lured sailors to their deaths while combing their long, lustrous curls. Indigenous people of Australia saved their wives' hair clippings as a prized possession. Even today, some orthodox Jewish women only allow their husbands to see this most enticing treasure, their crowning glory. Nowadays, a dazzling variety of hair styles and colors allow us to express our individuality, lifestyle, beliefs, social status, and much more.

Yet, despite the cultural tapestry of diverse hair styles, the universal barometer for a beautiful head of hair is youth. Just as a child's skin radiates with newborn freshness, young hair reigns supreme as the ideal crown to frame your dewy complexion. Sadly, our hair moves away from that ideal as we watch it grow thin, lose pigment, and become more and more damaged over time. Unfortunately, gray, thin, or receding hair will make you look older even if your skin is in top condition. However, proper hair care can reduce, and in some cases, even reverse the effects of the passing years.

WHAT IS HAIR? I can't count the number of times I've heard people say they wish for long, beautiful hair. The question is, how many beautiful hairs does it take to make up one lovely head of hair?

Well, a single hair has a thickness of 0.02 to 0.04 millimeters, so it takes 20 to 50 hair fibers stacked next to one other to span about one millimeter. We have about five million hairs on our bodies, with about 450,000 of them found above the neck. Now that's a whole lot of hairs, isn't it?

Most people have about 150,000 hairs on their head and normally shed 25 to 100 a day while growing an equivalent number of new hairs. Another 30,000 hairs reside in men's mustaches and beards. Blondes usually have more scalp hair than those with dark or red hair.

Mature hairs are filaments composed primarily of proteins (88%) that form a hard, tough, fibrous specific type of protein known as **keratin**. You may be surprised, but keratin is the same protein that is found in your skin. Your hair emerges from your skin and is a part of it. You would agree that it deserves the same level of care and dedication.

Proteins are composed of a long chain of amino acids that link together. The keratin found in human hair is also a major protein in fingernails.

Hair contains a tough outer coating, the cuticle, that consists of overlapping, scale-like bits of hard keratin. Inside the hair shaft, or cortex, resides a core of softer protein filaments.

Hair proteins have a high sulfur content from the amino acid cysteine, which forms cross-links in the hair proteins that are responsible for the hair's toughness and abrasion resistance. You would never guess when looking at all the hairs that collect in your brush, but human hair is as strong as a wire of iron. Nevertheless, it rips after being damaged or stretched 70% beyond its original length.

QUOTABLE QUOTES: *If a woman has long hair, it is a glory unto her.*
—St. Paul, 1 Corinthians

HAIR'S MANY HUES The sumptuous shades of human hair are too vast to count. This colorful rainbow ranges from black, brown, red and blond with countless subtle variations between like burgundy, strawberry blond, and copper brown. This rich feast treats our eyes with a smorgasbord of endless hues.

As in a rainbow where light bounces all around us, light bounces off the hair proteins, and this partially influences hair color. However, it is the type and amount of pigment within the hair shaft center that primarily determines the tint. Eumelanin is the pigment found in black and brown hair and, to a lesser degree, in blonde hair. Pheomelanin produces red hair, while a mix of eumelanin and pheomelanin produces the blonde-red combination known as strawberry blonde. The greater the amount of pigment, the darker the hair color. As the amount of pigment decreases, the hair color turns from black to brown and then reddish or blond. When pigment drastically diminishes, the hair appears gray, and when absent, the hair looks white.

As we age, our hair color generally changes. Many "towheaded" children who have blonde-whitish hair as youngsters turn into brunette adults and eventually gray or white-haired elders. Swedes, famous for their blond hair, often grow into brunette adults. Ingmar Bergman, a famous Swedish director, paints his young, innocent, blond characters to grow up as dark, somber, and reflective. So could the transition from blond to brunette have provided him with a useful metaphor?

Under some circumstances, the hair can lose its color prematurely. Severe stress can turn hair white overnight. Legend has it that Marie Antoinette went "white" the night before her execution. In the trench warfare of World War I, there were cases of young men whose hair turned gray within two months after prolonged episodes of severe fighting and artillery bombardments. Malnutrition can also cause hair to prematurely turn gray or white. A lack of sufficient dietary copper can cause the hair to lose its color. Excessive dietary zinc from supplements may drive out the copper needed to synthesize hair pigments and turn hair gray.

HAIR LENGTH AND GROWTH Hair grows faster in the spring and summer. Advertisers often manipulate this fact to "prove" that certain hair-growth remedies work wonders. In actuality, one's age, health, diet, and genetics determine the rate at which the hair grows. The length of time your hair follicles stay in the anagen (active growth) phase determines the maximum length your hair will grow. On average, waist-length hair takes about five years to grow out from a short haircut (with periodic trims included). The following list illustrates the average lengths and growth rates of the hair on the head and body.

HAIRS:	Average Length (cm)	Growth Rate Per Day (mm)
On the head	70	0.35
Eyebrows	1.0	0.15
Mustache (beard or whiskers)	28	0.4
Armpit hairs	5	0.3
Pubic hairs	4	0.2

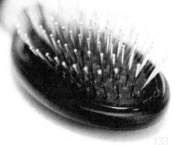

FACTORS THAT DAMAGE HAIR Many factors damage hair fibers, including environmental elements (such as prolonged exposure to sunlight or wind) and chemical and mechanical injuries (such as tight hairstyles, hot rollers, hot oil treatments, and harsh use of hair dryers). The chemicals we use to alter our hair come with a price. Bleaches, dyes, relaxers, and perming agents all cause varying degrees of damage. Some cosmetic products partially repair damaged hair, but a good quality of hair will return only after new hair grows in.

The Damaging Things We Do to Our Hair

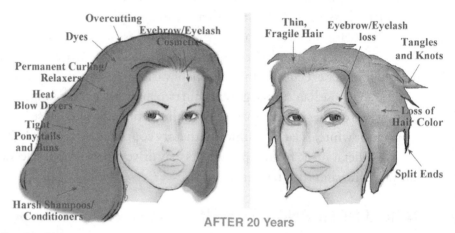

Overcutting
Dyes
Eyebrow/Eyelash Cosmetics
Permanent Curling/ Relaxers
Heat
Blow Dryers
Tight Pony-tails and Buns
Harsh Shampoos/ Conditioners

Thin, Fragile Hair
Eyebrow/Eyelash loss
Tangles and Knots
Loss of Hair Color
Split Ends

AFTER 20 Years

Choosing the Right Shampoo

When you wash your hair excessively, you shampoo out more than grime. You also wash out natural oils which protect your scalp. As a result, too much shampooing damages hair shafts. It is important to choose shampoo carefully. The best shampoos are around pH 6.0, at the high end of the slightly acidic pH of the scalp (4.5 to 6.0). Maintaining the natural acid environment of the hair and scalp keeps the hair proteins hard and prevents the growth of foreign bacteria. Thus, by using the best shampoos and not over-washing, you preserve the hair and skin oils that benefit your scalp.

Shampoos with a higher pH have a negative impact on the hair for several reasons. While more alkaline shampoos work better to clean the hair and scalp, they also strip away many of the hair's natural oils and the glues that help hold the hair shafts together. A high pH shampoo may make hair look great for a few weeks, but eventually it will lead to dry, brittle hair and increased breakage.

Don't be fooled by baby shampoos that claim to be gentle to your hair and eyes. Many baby shampoos have a high pH that can strip hair and are thus not at all gentle. Also be cautious with clarifying shampoos. Formulated to remove buildup of gels, mousses, pomades, and other products that weigh down your hair, they can also remove color and perms. Some hair experts recommend using a combination of plain baking soda and your normal shampoo to remove build-up. Other ingredients to avoid include flash foamers (chemicals that enhance the foaming of shampoo) and added fragrances, neither of which have a positive effect.

Choosing the right shampoo is especially important for those with an oily scalp. Greasy hair is more difficult to manage than normal or dry hair and is often tough to comb. Oily hair is covered with sebum from the sebaceous glands of the hair follicle.

While frequent washing with a stronger, more-soapy shampoo may help remove oil, it can also damage the hair. Some individuals have used retinoic acid to reduce oil production. Retinoic acid should be used sparingly, as overuse can irritate the scalp.

Avoid selecting a shampoo based on its high price tag. Costly shampoos are not a head above the rest! A shampoo's price is generally related to the cost of its advertising.

If the label on a shampoo bottle tells you to wash your hair twice, ignore it; the manufacturer is simply encouraging you to use more of the product. Always use a minimum amount of shampoo.

Some shampoo manufacturers recommend that you comb through wet hair to distribute the shampoo evenly. But wet hair is more easily broken, and you will only end up with damaged hair.

When you are done washing your hair, the shampoo should be *completely* rinsed out to help bring the pH back down to its natural level. If your hair is very dry, only shampoo every three days. Our ancestors went months between hair washings, one of the reasons their hair was so healthy.

Choosing the Right Conditioner

The outer layer of hair, called the cuticle, is somewhat like fish scales made of hard keratin. The cuticle is held together by disulfide bonds and small amino acids.

INSIDE:
Cortex is the soft center of hair shaft.

Cuticle is the outer hard, overlapping scales of protein.

In healthy, shiny hair, the outer layer of scales lies flat which allows for combs and brushes to smoothly glide through it. Hair with a damaged cuticle appears dry, drab, split, brittle, or frizzy.

Quality conditioners add amino acids, peptides, and pantothenic acid (vitamin B-5) into the cuticle to help glue the scales tightly to the hair shaft. If the cuticle stays open, it can start a tear in the hair shaft that leads to breakage of the shaft. This is why it is important to use a conditioner separately.

Conditioners that strengthen the hair have a low pH of about 4.0 to 4.7. The hair proteins remain hard and strong at a low pH. Some conditioners contain a small amount of fat to give the hair a better shine.

The best products are sold in successful hair salons. These salons need happy, repeat customers and usually do not advertise their products.

The longer you leave the conditioner on your hair, the better it works. Some manufacturers recommend leaving conditioner on the hair for only a few seconds, but longer is generally better (one to two minutes).

Is It Important to Use Both a Shampoo and Conditioner?

WHY YOU SHOULD NEVER USE A 2-IN-1 SHAMPOO/CONDITIONER

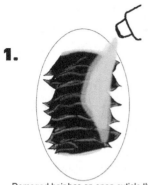

1.

Damaged hair has an open cuticle that causes ripping, tearing, and breakage. Use a mild shampoo and <u>rinse well</u>.

2.

Follow with an acid conditioner to harden and flatten cuticle and apply protective nutrients.

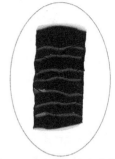

3.

Over a period of time, hair shaft lies flat providing sealed hair shaft with protective proteins that prevent growth of bacteria, split ends, help detangle, and add a lustrous shine to the hair. *SRCPs also help calm scalp irritation.*

TIPS FOR LONG, HEALTHY HAIR In the previous chapter I told you about George Michael (now retired), who became famous for helping women grow their hair to extraordinary lengths. As I mentioned, Dr. Michael believes that longer hair is healthier hair, or as he puts it, "The longer the hair, the stronger the root." Many women are taught that by age 30, their hair should be no longer than shoulder length. Dr. Michael feels the contrary is true. He believes long hair majestically frames a mature woman's features—that it downplays wrinkles and makes her look younger.

When counseling women on how to grow long hair, Dr. Michael taught them that it is important to have hair of one length, without bangs or layers. According to his findings, the body tries to equalize uneven hair by excessively shedding strands.

LONGER HAIR REDUCES SHEDDING - STUDIES BY DR. GEORGE MICHAEL

Hair Length - Inches	Number Hairs Lost Per Day
4	87
12	26
Waist Length	16
Floor Length	2

When working with long-haired clients, Dr. Michael utilized many methods to protect the hair. He set hair dryers at only about 10 degrees F higher than body temperature (most blow dryers reach temperatures of up to 260 degrees and damage hair follicles). When curling the hair, he used large rollers of soft mesh or plastic rather than rollers that grab the hair and can tear it. He took special care to protect the ends of the hair when rolling or setting. Shampoos were kept to a minimum. He recommended vitamin and mineral supplements. Dr. Michael also advised women to cover their hair at all times when exposed to direct sunlight. (See www.longhairlovers.com).

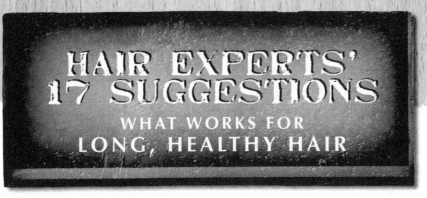

1. Cut dry hair for best results.

2. Detangle dry hair before washing. Detangle the ends first and work your way up. Do not try to remove kinks from top to bottom since this may pull out hair. Before entering the shower, give your hair a few strokes with a comb or brush. This aligns the strands and helps to prevent tangles.

3. When shampooing, use water at room temperature. The lower the temperature, the better it is for your hair. Warm water opens the hair scales, making the hair shaft more vulnerable to damage.

4. When preparing to wash your hair, bring the hair in front of your face before wetting it and leave it there. Let your hair hang down in front during shampooing. Try not to move your hair while you wash it. This keeps the hair strands in position, so they won't move upwards and wrap themselves around other strands, resulting in tangles.

5. Don't try to overwash your hair. The purpose of shampoo is to remove dirt from the top layers. Just let the shampoo penetrate the lower layers briefly as it flows over your hair.

6. Make sure to wash out all of the shampoo. When you think the shampoo is gone, allow another half-minute of constant water flow to ensure the removal of residue. For a final rinse, immerse in cool or cold water.

7. Use an acidifying conditioner with peptides to re-glue the protein scales of the cuticle. Put extra conditioner on your hair ends to prevent split ends. Give the conditioner at least a minute to glue into the hair. For a final rinse, use cool or cold water.

8. Air-dry your hair whenever possible.

9. When you must blow-dry your hair, first wrap it in a special, highly absorbent towel to remove water. Blow-dry the hair for a few minutes, and then let it air dry. A cool setting on the hair dryer helps "set" the hair.

10. Never use a heavy-duty reconstructor on your hair. It does more harm than good.

11. Avoid excessive sunlight and tanning beds, which harm the hair.

12. Apply a non-alcohol hair spray, since alcohol dries the hair.

13. Use wide-toothed combs and picks.

14. Only use coated or snag-free elastics and hair fasteners.

15. Think of your hair as a silk garment and treat it accordingly. Both silk and hair are protein fibers. You wouldn't wash a silk garment with a cheap detergent in a washing machine at a high temperature with a high agitation cycle and then dry it in a dryer at a high temperature.

16. Many hairdressers only cut hair. For long, healthy hair, tell them to keep trimming to an absolute minimum.

17. If someone criticizes your hair, IGNORE THEM. Hair arouses many emotions and jealousies, so arrange your hair in a fashion that pleases yourself.

CHANGING THE LOOK OF YOUR HAIR You can dramatically alter your hair's appearance by changing its shape through permanent waving or straightening. However, both of these procedures cause damage to the scalp and hair. This damage might include breakage, thinning, lack of growth, scalp irritation, scalp damage, and hair loss. If the damage becomes excessive, serious hair loss may occur. Before undergoing any hair treatment, especially one that introduces powerful chemicals to your hair, you owe it to yourself to be well informed about the following procedures.

Permanents

Permanents add depth and richness to limp or frizzy hair. However, they can also be quite harsh. Permanents break the disulfide bonds in the proteins that hold hair together during the process of wrapping hair around a roller to form it into a new texture. As a result, the disulfide bonds are chemically reset and the new, curly texture locks into place. However, when the perming solution is left on too long, is too strong, or applied to chemically-damaged hair, the hair and follicles can get severely damaged. If this happens to you, rub a copper peptide lotion onto your scalp for three to four nights following the procedure to restore scalp health.

PERMANENTS
STRAIGHTENING
RELAXERS
FLAT IRONS
CURLING IRONS
HAIR DYES

Hair Straightening

Many women love the look of straight locks of shiny hair. Thus, straightening is an increasingly popular option. During the procedure, an alkaline-reducing agent breaks down disulfide bonds that keep hair curly. Hair relaxers, typically creams or cream lotions, contain about 2 to 4% of strong bases such as sodium hydroxide, potassium hydroxide, and lithium hydroxide or 5% calcium hydroxide plus a solution of up to about 30% guanidine carbonate. The pH is around 12. Some relaxers contain about 4 percent ammonium thioglycolate as the active ingredient.

Before the straightening procedure, you apply a petroleum-based cream to help protect the scalp. Then rub on the chemical relaxer, and gently comb the hair straight. After a period of time, remove the relaxer with warm water and a neutralizing formula. Finally, apply a conditioner to restore some of the natural oils and proteins removed by the chemical.

As with perms, the harsh chemicals in straighteners can cause severe damage to the hair. It is preferable to follow the procedure with applications of a copper peptide product to restore scalp health.

Only employ a hair-care specialist with a record of success in chemical straightening. It is also strongly recommended that you obtain professional conditioning treatments before and after the process.

Alternatively, you can apply intense heat to reset bonds which straightens curls. Some use a flat styling iron. Others boldly flatten their hair with a clothing iron over an ironing board covered with a smooth towel. And for many years, people have used "hot combs" to press out the hair by running a metal comb (heated either electrically or manually) gently through the hair. However, it is important to note that extreme heat can severely damage the hair. So caution is needed with whichever method of straightening a person may individually decide to use.

Chemical Hair Relaxers

Sit down, relax, and listen to the hair-raising story of hair relaxers. It began early in the twentieth century.

His name was Garrett Augustus Morgan, and he was born the seventh of eleven children of former slaves. He is best known for his invention of the automatic traffic signal and gas mask. Around 1910, while attempting to invent a new lubricating liquid for the sewing machine, Morgan wiped his hands on a wool cloth and found that the wooly texture of the cloth "smoothed out." He experimented on his curly-haired Airedale dog and successfully duplicated the effect. Morgan called his discovery a "hair-refining cream" and patented the first chemical hair relaxer.

Today, Morgan's discovery, lye (sodium hydroxide), is still a common ingredient in chemical relaxers because it provides the strongest and most dramatic effect. However strong drain cleaners also contain this harsh chemical. Try visualizing drain cleaner on your scalp. Not a pretty picture!

Guanidine hydroxide, another chemical commonly found in hair relaxers, is often promoted as the "no-lye" relaxer. However, do not let the name fool you. It still contains strong chemicals. Although this type of relaxer can inflict less damage than its counterpart, your hair and scalp should still be in top condition before you attempt the procedure.

How Chemical Relaxers Work

How can chemicals relax or straighten hair? Both lye and no-lye relaxers contain harsh chemicals that work in the same manner: they both alter the basic structure of the hair shaft. The chemical penetrates the cortex or cortical layer and loosens the natural curl pattern. However, this inner layer of the shaft not only gives curly hair its shape; it also provides strength and elasticity. Once you perform the straightening process, the result is irreversible. Although you end up with straighter hair, you are now left with much weaker strands susceptible to breakage.

CORTICAL LAYER
MEDULLA
MELANIN
CUTICLE

It is easy to over-process hair by using excessive relaxers or by applying more chemicals to hair already processed or relaxed. This over-processing is the most typical misuse of hair-relaxing chemicals. Once you apply the initial relaxer to virgin hair, perform touch-ups to new growth no more than every six to eight weeks.

HAIR REMOVAL 101

Hair Removal Techniques for Women and Men

Surveys indicate that 80 percent of women and more than 50 percent of men have unwanted hair in various areas of their bodies.

Much of this excessive hair is genetic, but sometimes it results from other causes, such as testosterone treatment. Whether or not you want to remove body hair is entirely your choice. However, if you feel that you want to get rid of unwanted hair, you have several of the following options:

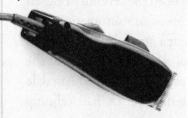

- **Depilation**—The removal of the visible portion of the hair: Shaving, chemical, or mechanical depilation. Hair grows back fast and must be removed regularly.

- **Epilation**—The destruction or removal of the entire hair <u>with</u> its roots: Tweezing, waxing, electrolysis, laser hair removal. Hair grows back slowly, and it is usually thinner and lighter. Some methods allow permanent hair removal.

Keeping It Simple — Shaving 101

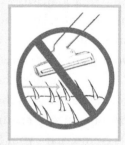

The most popular form of hair removal by far is shaving. However, since shaving must be repeated often to maintain a smooth appearance, the proper technique is vital. Before you start, wash the skin to exfoliate it and lift the hair away from the follicle; this softens the hair and prepares it for the shave. Be sure to shave in the same direction each time (down rather than up); this helps train the hair to grow out straight, making hair removal easier.

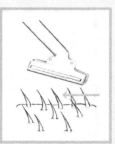

You may notice small bumps appear not long after you shave. These razor rashes may become further irritated, resulting in redness, itchiness, discoloration, or infection. The medical term for bumps is pseudofolliculitis barbae, commonly referred to as ingrown hairs or razor bumps. Many people have found they can decrease ingrown hairs by using an electric razor, although the shave may not be as close as that of a blade. Exfoliate and cleanse your face before shaving to obtain the best defense against ingrown hairs and razor bumps. Hydroxy acid serums, such as 10% alpha and/or beta hydroxy acids, are the best agents to exfoliate your skin. When you gently cleanse your skin and keep it smooth and supple, you moisturize follicles. As a result, the follicles grow in the right direction to prevent razor bumps.

Chemical Depilatories

This type of depilatory contains calcium thioglycolate, a harsh chemical that literally dissolves the hair shaft. The partially dissolved hair then can be removed with a sponge and warm water. Since the root remains intact, hair grows back promptly. Chemical depilatories are found in the form of creams, lotions, or sprays. Many modern formulations also contain additives to soothe irritation or slow down hair growth. However, if your hair is thick, and the skin is sensitive or damaged, painful irritation may develop before the hair finishes dissolving. The result will be red, inflamed skin covered with the remains of the unwanted hair. That is why it is always important to test this method on a small area first. Harsh chemicals that are strong enough to dissolve your hair will not be so gentle on skin either. Those with sensitive, thin skin should be especially careful with this method of hair removal. Since skin irritation leads to increased pigment production, it is important to protect your skin from UV rays immediately after depilation, lest it develop pigmented spots. Also, make sure to apply healing products that calm down irritation and facilitate recovery post hair removal.

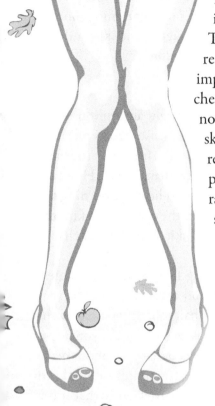

Tweezing

Hair on small areas such as eyebrows can be plucked out with tweezers. This method works well for shaping eyebrows or removing hairs remaining after other methods of hair removal such as waxing. Tweezing does damage hair roots, and eventually the hair grows back thinner and lighter. However, this method causes frequent damage to hair follicles and may lead to inflammation and the development of red bumps. If freshly plucked skin is exposed to sunlight, unwanted pigmentation may also develop.

Waxing

For eons, hair waxing has been used by Asian women for hygienic, cultural, and esthetic reasons. Modern chemistry, in many cases, brought modifications to this method; however, the basic principle remains the same—extraction of the hair from its root with the aid of a sticky substance. The best waxes are those that do not stick as much to the skin as they do to the hair, thus ensuring a relatively painless and complete hair removal. Sadly, the majority of hair waxing products grip the skin as well, pulling it and stripping away thin layers of the stratum corneum. This results in irritation, damage of skin elastic fibers, and disruption of the skin barrier. Those treated with systemic retinoids, such as Accutane, should not use waxing methods because their skin will be fragile and more easily damaged. Additionally, waxing should not be used on anyone with damaged skin, warts, or moles.

Electrolysis

This is a slow and often painful procedure, but it is the only FDA-approved method of permanent hair removal. An electric current is delivered to the hair follicle via a very thin needle that has to be precisely situated in the follicle. If the esthetician misses the follicle, the hair will grow back and the procedure has to be repeated. Since actively growing hair is the most sensitive to the procedure, it takes many sessions (15-30) to target all the hair. Although with patience and time (not mentioning money) hair can be permanently removed using this method, the damage to the skin and hair follicle can result in keloid formation, warts, and skin discoloration.

Laser Hair Removal

The laser hair removal technique utilizes the process of light absorption by the dark hair pigment—melanin. When high energy laser radiation is absorbed by melanin, the hair heats up, burning the hair follicle just as a metal rod in the fire burns the hand that holds it. The result is severe damage to the follicle, which stops hair growth. However, the skin also contains melanin that can absorb laser energy and heat up, burning the surrounding areas. Therefore, the more pigment in the hair, the less in the skin, the better. So those with the contrast of black hair and very light skin have the best chance for successful hair removal with minimal skin damage.

Lasers have revolutionized hair removal, allowing fast, relatively painless elimination of hair from large areas. But this is still a method that you should be very cautious about. The intense heat delivered straight into the hair follicle incinerates not only the unwanted hair but often your skin's gold reserve as well—namely, your stem cells located in the bulge area of hair follicles. You know the saying that you cannot make an omelet without breaking a couple of eggs? Well, in this case, you simply cannot burn down the hair follicle without damaging your stem cells as well. Make sure that it is a price you are willing to pay for smooth, hairless skin.

Although lasers are considered "safe" under the direction of a skilled expert ("safe" in that there may not be any visible or immediate complications), they can turn into a weapon of skin destruction if used improperly. Dermatologists often see disfigurement, burns, scars, and skin discoloration in those who didn't spend enough time researching the credentials of their laser hair removal specialist. Remember, though, that even if no visible complications are present, the skin rarely emerges from such a procedure intact and therefore needs your special attention to recover.

☑ HOW TO REDUCE ANY SKIN DAMAGE AFTER HAIR REMOVAL:

1. USE A COPPER PEPTIDE CREAM TO REPAIR IRRITATION
2. FOLLOW WITH A BIOLOGICAL HEALING OIL TO SOOTHE AND MOISTURIZE

Importance of Skin Healing After Hair Removal

All hair-removal methods (tweezing, shaving, waxing, electrolysis, lasers, pharmaceutical creams, and so on) cause skin damage that allows viruses and bacteria to penetrate into the skin. For example, warts seem to develop from injured or broken skin. In adults, warts tend to grow where hair-removal procedures have damaged the skin, such as the beard area of men and the legs of women. To restore the skin after shaving, many have found success in using copper peptide creams fortified with antioxidants and skin-nourishing lipid replenishers. Such creams help close the skin's surface to viruses and bacteria to help heal the skin.

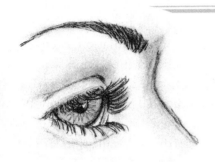

Longer Eyelashes, Thicker Eyebrows The loss of eyebrows and eyelashes often results from long-term use of cosmetics. However, some have reported a reversal of this effect through the light use of an SRCP product followed by a biological healing oil, such as emu oil.

This regimen often helps restore the lost hairs in about two months. For eyebrows: each day, apply a copper peptide cream followed by emu oil. For eyelashes: Do the exact same. Apply a light coating of a copper peptide cream and perhaps follow with a light application of a biological healing oil applied to the skin below or above the eyelashes near the eyelash bed (where the eyelashes would protrude from).

MEN'S CORNER—CARING FOR YOUR BEARD Have you ever felt a twinge of envy when you think about how women don't have to shave their faces every day? They don't have to deal with razor cuts, ingrown hairs, and annoying irritation. They never have to ponder the ultimate question: To shave or not to shave?

If this is how you've been feeling, then read on. You are about to learn why the mere fact that you can grow a beard actually keeps your skin looking younger! You will also learn how your beard can protect your skin from the effects of UV-radiation and other damaging environmental factors. You'll learn that your beard may help you attract women, regardless of whether they think they like bearded men or not. Most importantly, you will learn how to look good with or without a beard.

Your Beard and Skin Health

Nowadays, a beard is no longer considered an essential attribute of masculinity, and most men prefer to shave their faces every day. Yet, shaved or not, the beard continues to play a very important role in male skin physiology.

In female facial skin, small hair follicles produce fine, thin, short vellus hair. In male skin, hair follicles produce thick, terminal hair. Usually, beard hair is coarser and thicker than scalp hair, and it has even larger follicles. Scientists have discovered that those exceptionally large hair follicles and coarse hair shafts found in male skin serve as an additional support, making the skin firmer. When female skin starts losing collagen, elastin, and glycosaminoglycans, it develops wrinkles very quickly. On the contrary, male skin may lose just as much collagen, while remaining relatively smooth.

This interesting fact became apparent when more and more men opted to have their facial hair removed by lasers. According to studies, after laser hair removal, male skin becomes thinner and starts to wrinkle faster than before. This is due to the fact that lasers destroy not only hair shafts but also hair follicles.

Furthermore, if you wear a beard, your skin has additional protection from UV-radiation. Even if you shave, your skin still has better protection when compared with female skin, especially if you have darker-colored hair. This additional protection comes from many large, melanin-loaded hair follicles and thick hair shafts traversing the dermis, offering a good defense from UV-radiation. This also helps preserve male skin and delay aging.

Not many men use anti-aging cosmetic products. But did you know that shaving itself is a very effective rejuvenating process? Every time you shave, you are removing a thin layer of upper skin, which triggers skin renewal.

Unfortunately, the benefits of a beard are counterbalanced by certain challenges of male skin care.

MEN: Successfully Dealing with the Challenges of Shaving

If you shave, you may experience cuts, lacerations, skin irritation, razor bumps, or ingrown hairs. If you grow a beard, you may need to trim it regularly and think how you can best keep it clean and looking great.

Facial hair can easily become a platform for bacterial growth. This is important to recognize, because under the influence of testosterone, male skin produces more skin oil and sweat than female skin.

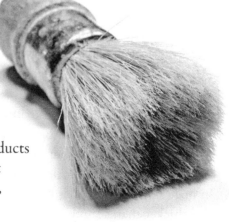

When bacteria feed on a mix of this oil and sweat, they produce chemicals that can give your skin an unpleasant smell.

It is no wonder that the most popular products in the male skin care market are products that improve shaving, prevent shaving complications, soothe irritation, deodorize, and cleanse the skin.

TIPS FOR ^Perfect SHAVING AND A HEALTHY BEARD

CLEANSING

Use a mild cleanser with a neutral or slightly acidic pH. Do not use soaps, since they are too alkaline and may increase skin irritation. If you have a beard, you may use shampoo and conditioner on your beard. Conditioner will help make your beard softer and add an especially well-groomed look.

GROWTH STIMULATION

If your beard doesn't grow as well as you wish it to, you may consider using hair products that improve the appearance and thickness of hair, such as ones that contain copper peptides. Even though the growth of your beard is determined genetically (and of course has nothing to do with masculinity), using hair stimulating products may help achieve the look of a more uniform and full growth.

ITCHING SOLUTIONS THAT REALLY WORK

When attempting to grow a beard, many people experience itching. Also, frequent shaving (especially if you have light-colored, thin skin) may cause redness and irritation. Unfortunately, many after-shaving creams and products only serve to further increase irritation, because they are loaded with skin damaging chemicals.

This is why, when dealing with itchy skin, keep it simple. What you want is to seal and soothe your skin, not open up a chemical warfare on it. Use biological oils and products with squalane and aloe vera to soothe the skin and reduce itching.

PREVENTING RAZOR BUMPS

Razor bumps (or pseudofolliculitis barbae) are small red bumps on the skin that appear soon after shaving. They are caused by hairs that curl back and grow into the skin. This problem is especially common among men with thick, curly hair. To prevent razor bumps, take hot showers before shaving or wash your face with a warm towel—this will help soften the skin. Shave in the direction your hair growth. After shaving, rinse your face with cold water or press a cold cloth to your face.

The thicker the upper layer of dead skin cells (stratum corneum), the greater the chance of developing razor bumps. This is why you may want to try products that contain exfoliating hydroxy acids.

CONCLUSION Your beautiful hair is more than just a skin appendage. It reflects your culture, ethnicity, beliefs, personality, and social status. For many women and men, hair is their pride and glory. Women may treasure their long, thick tresses, and men may grow quite fond of their neatly trimmed beard and mustache. You too may have gone to some lengths trying to change your hair style and color. Unfortunately, many modern methods of hair styling are damaging to hair. When making a decision to color, curl, or straighten your hair, keep in mind that beautiful hair is healthy hair.

Take time to investigate products and/or procedures before you use them, and make sure you know their effects on your hair over the long term. Remember to use SRCP products and biological oils to strengthen your hair's roots, prevent damage to hair structure, and restore its healthy appearance. Discover how perfectly your thick, lush, gleaming hair can frame your smooth, glowing skin and how easy it is to look years younger when you give your hair the care it deserves.

Questions? Email: ghkcopperpeptides@gmail.com

GROW LONG, STRONG, BEAUTIFUL NAILS

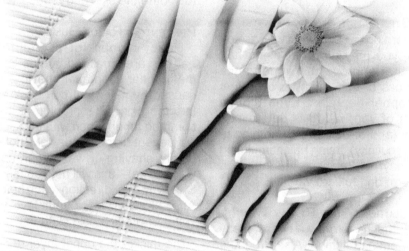

Your nails are like jewels that crown your fingers. Lengthy, exquisite nails have been the envy of women throughout the ages. While nail fashions may change from one century to the next and even from week to week, the desire for long, strong nails has spanned many epochs.

In ancient China, women of high status grew their nails long and painted them with gold lacquer, indicating they never had to toil. Yet in other eras, nails were used as weapons. You have no doubt heard the saying, "I'm going to claw your eyes out!" Nails are vestigial remnants of defensive weapons of our distant ancestors. Our nails evolved as aids for picking up small objects, scratching, and for taking revenge on two-timing beaus!

Today, women make a fashion statement with these functional, yet oh so expressive appendages. One season, women may wear square-cut nails. A few months later, they re-shape these beauties into stylish ovals. From white-tipped French manicures, nail art, shocking crimson, and glitter to naked nails in the buff, your fingernails make a personal statement about how you care for yourself, your sense of style, and who you are. In this chapter, you will learn how to protect, renew, and beautify one of the most expressive parts of a woman's body.

SRCPS, HORSE HOOVES, AND FINGERNAILS Skin Remodeling Copper Peptides (SRCPs) increase the proliferation of the keratin-producing cell, the keratinocyte. Keratin is the protein that makes up our outer protective skin layer and our nails. In animals, it is what composes their horns, claws, and hooves.

Throughout the course of prolonged rainstorms in Washington State, horses often develop severe irritations and infections in their lower extremities—especially where the hair-covered lower leg joins the hoof. During experiments to heal inflamed skin above the hooves, copper peptide creams were generously applied to their legs, but due to the movements of these feisty horses, much product ended up on the hooves. It was no surprise to observe how rapidly the copper healed their skin. However, we were both delighted and amazed to see that the damaged hooves also improved. Later, we experimented with more controlled applications of copper peptide creams into cracks in badly damaged hooves. We found that the copper peptide cream usually produced a remarkable healing in the hooves and closure of the cracks.

Since the hooves of horses and nails of humans are biochemically similar, we experimented with applications of copper peptide creams to damaged human fingernails and toenails. We observed that, as in the horses, human nails grew healthier and stronger than we could have ever imagined. Such types of copper peptides, when applied to the nail matrix and nail bed area, enhance the process of nail growth, resulting in stronger, thicker, and smoother nails.

In an informal study on nail growth in humans, the fingernail growth rates of the index fingers were used as a measurement. In some experiments, copper peptides were applied to the index fingernail and cuticle on the right hand, while the left hand nail was untreated and used as a control.

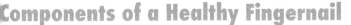

Components of a Healthy Fingernail

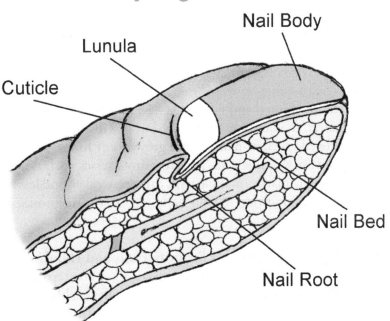

Nail Body

Lunula

Cuticle

Nail Bed

Nail Root

In the second set of experiments, copper peptides were applied to the index fingernail and cuticle on the left hand while the right hand nail was treated with a placebo cream. After four weeks, nail length was measured from the end of the nail bed to the tip of the nail at the center. The effect of nail growth stimulation was similar if either the right or left hand treated group was used.

TIN PEPTIDES vs. COPPER PEPTIDES But a problem arose since copper peptides often stain nails with a greenish tint. I later found that tin peptides, a complex of ionic tin (2+) and peptides, do not tarnish nails and are more effective than copper peptides on nail growth.

Tin peptides also work better than SRCPs in our test systems for hair growth. While tin peptides lack the wound healing actions of SRCPs, they work better at producing keratin, the major protein in nails and hair.

Tin peptides beautify more than your nails. They also rejuvenate hands and hair. Tin peptides make hands appear years younger and repair damage caused by gardening, washing clothes, and other forms of physical labor.

The outer layers of the skin are made of a protein called keratin. High levels of synthetic detergents found in many soaps (or other factors such as dry skin conditions) can strip away the skin mantle and loosen protective keratin proteins. We have found that tin peptides increase the production of keratinocytes that form the outer skin covering, resulting in a softer, smoother surface.

Nail Growth and Health

While the fingernail resembles hair and shares similar attributes, it does not share the hair's cycle of growth and non-growth. Healthy nails grow continuously throughout your life. They grow approximately one-half to one millimeter weekly. It takes five to seven months for the nail to grow completely and replace itself from the time it forms at the root until it reaches beyond the fingertip.

Like hair, nails grow more during the summer. The middle finger nail grows fastest, with the growth rate progressively decreasing on the fourth, second, fifth fingers, and finally the thumb. Toenails grow at a snail's pace, about a third to half the growth rate of fingernails.

When a nail gets injured and falls off, a new nail grows in at the normal rate. With a damaged matrix, the new nail may grow, but in a distorted form. However, if the matrix gets destroyed, the new nail will not grow in any form.

In today's lifestyle, we expose our nails to many stresses, such as detergents and hot water, that damage the matrix, making nails thinner, weaker, and less able to grow. To better understand the condition of your nails, refer to the diagnostic chart on the following page.

Copper and Tin Peptides Renew and Beautify Nails and Hands

SRCPs not only renew damaged skin and hair. They also repair and strengthen nails while moisturizing dry hands. Copper and tin peptides enable your nails to grow faster and your hands to look younger than ever before. They fortify and thicken nails while smoothing out cuticles. At the same time, they drench hands in youthful suppleness.

Nail Diagnostic Chart

Use this diagnostic chart to look at and understand the condition of your nails:

DESCRIPTION	POSSIBLY Due To...
Splitting, Brittle Nails	Irritating substances used in such products as harsh detergents or nail polish removers, or silica deficiency
Longitudinal Nail Ridges	Aging, inadequate absorption of vitamins and minerals, kidney failure, or thyroid disease
Horizontal Nail Ridges	Nutrition problem, injury, or infection
Discoloration	May be an indicator of anemia
Purple or Black	Typically due to trauma, or may be sign of vitamin B12 deficiency. Also a streak (black or brown) from the base of the nail that extends all the way to the tip may be an indicator of melanoma. See your medical provider.
Yellow Color	Fungal infection, psoriasis, diabetes, heredity, or use of tetracycline
Red / Dark Pink	May indicate poor peripheral circulation
Half Pink and Half White	Fungal infection or kidney disease
Blue	May indicate that blood is not receiving enough oxygen due to a respiratory disorder, cardiovascular disease, or lupus erythematosus
Large Moons	Possible overactive thyroid, genetics, or trauma
No Moons	Possible underactive thyroid or genetics
Soft Nails	Malnutrition, contact with strong alkali substance, endochrine problem, or arthritis
White, Soft Nails	Fungal infection
Thick Nails	Poor circulation, fungal infection, or persistent nail trauma (which may cause hardening)
Loose Nail Plate	Injury, psoriasis, fungal or bacterial infection, side effects of medication, chemotherapy treatments, thyroid disease, Raynaud's Syndrome, or Lupus
"Pitted Nail" (Yellow/Brown spots)	Possible eczema, psoriasis, or hair loss condition
Spoon Shape	Possible thyroid disease or iron deficiency
Club Shape	Cirrhosis of the liver, or chronic respiratory or heart condition
Wasting Away of the Nail	Injury or disease
Infected Nail: Red/Tender/Swollen	Yeast infection or bacterial infection
Complete Loss of Nail	Trauma

SUPPLEMENTS FOR NAIL HEALTH

Biotin - Biotin can strengthen brittle nails and bring them back to health and luster. Take 2.5 mg a day if you are not pregnant. In one placebo-controlled, double-blind clinical study, 60 patients who had poor nail quality but had no overt biotin deficiency were treated for 6 months with 2.5 mg of biotin per day. The improvement in nail quality was measured by (1) the resistance of the nails to swelling after incubation with an alkaline agent (NaOH), (2) the rate of water loss through the fingernail (transonychial water loss), and (3) the separate judgments of nail health by the clinical investigator and by the patient. All measured parameters showed improved nail quality (Gehring 1996). A Swiss veterinary report study described the treatment of biotin for horses' cracked hooves, which are biochemically similar to fingernails (Scher 1994).

MSM - Supplements of 2-4 grams daily of sulfur-rich MSM (methylsulfonylmethane) have been shown to strengthen fragile nails. MSM also encourages your fingernails, toenails, and hair to grow faster because you have more sulfur in your fingernails and hair than any other cells of your body. Here's what an individual supplementing with MSM had to say:

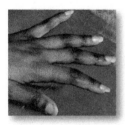

" I take MSM, 4-6 grams daily, and have noticed amazing improvements in my hair growth and nail growth. My nails are stronger, break much less often, and I can prove it!...I can tell how much faster they are growing because I have to cut/clip them so much more often!" —C.M.

Gelatin - Gelatin is a protein source of nine essential amino acids: histidine, lysine, leucine, tryptophan, valine, phenylalanine, methionine, threonine, and isoleucine—all building blocks of protein. The article "Gelatin-cystine, keratogenesis and structure of the hair" in *Boll Soc Ital Biol Sper* (Morganti et al 1983) states that the oral ingestion of gelatin significantly increases the degree of hardness of finger and toenails.

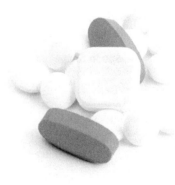

PROTECTING NAILS Like hair, nails are usually healthiest in their natural state. While nail polishes and cosmetic nails may improve your appearance, they tend to degrade nail health.

If you can avoid repeated wetting and drying of your nails, you will minimize brittle nails, chipping, splitting and breaking. Also try to avoid alkaline detergents, soaps, and cleaners. Instead, use cleansers with a slightly acidic pH to prevent loosening of the protein fibers that form the nail.

In recent years, more nail damage is caused by cosmetic/beautifying procedures than ever before. Cosmetics such as nail polishes, gel manicures, and artificial nails generally degrade nail health. Give your nails a break from cosmetic polishes and artificial nails for one to three months per year to allow the nails to recover. Treatments such as nail strengtheners and hardeners can help to protect nails from breakage, but polish removers weaken nails. When applying coatings of nail strengtheners and hardeners, apply them as subsequent layers over the previous treatments rather than removing earlier coatings.

Cotton lined rubber gloves are best for nails and should be used during household or job-related work that involves getting the hands wet. You can also minimize damage inflicted by environmental onslaughts and artificial treatments by applying a tin peptide-based moisturizing cream to restore the health of your nails.

Restoring Cuticle Health and Hangnails

Since the cuticle skin is especially thin, dermatologists recommend you take special care not to damage this sensitive area. Doctors recommend that you do not cut or nip the cuticle, since it acts as a protective barrier against bacteria. An intact cuticle helps to prevent infection of the nail. Ragged cuticles can deform the shape of the growing nail. Some people have found tin peptide hand creams and cuticle oils help to keep the cuticles soft, supple, and healthy.

Hangnails produce small tears or splits in the nail plate or surrounding tissue. They often result from dry skin or injury. When hangnails tear, they can cause chronic pain and infect the area. Hangnail problems respond well to tin peptide treatment.

Cosmetic Nails

In the late 20th century, a wide variety of artificial nails have increased in popularity. Women use them in conjunction with natural nails and not as a replacement.

They can elongate or beautify nails. They also camouflage discolored, thickened, or malformed fingernails. Unfortunately, the glues used to fasten the artificial nails may cause both allergic contact dermatitis and nail damage.

The pre-formed plastic nail is the most popular type of artificial nail. Some come pre-glued (as do press-on types), while others require one to apply glue separately. The acrylic glues typically contain methacrylate, a chemical which can cause allergic contact dermatitis. There are stronger adhesives that provide better bonding, but these can cause the nail plate to separate from the nail bed or cause the biological plate to split into layers. Pre-formed cosmetic nails are not recommended for people with weak nails.

Gel Manicures

Gel manicures can seem like nail heaven—especially if you're a nail-polish addict. These lacquers dry quickly and contain a chemical component that hardens under a UV light, delivering glossy color that lasts for several weeks without chipping or losing its shine.

This may sound like heaven. But gel manicures have a dark side: They can seriously damage your nails.

For starters, you have to soak them off with 100% pure acetone—which is even more damaging than traditional polish removers. The harsh solution can cause nails to weaken and, in some cases, cause an eczema-like rash on the skin around the nails.

But the worst damage comes after a few weeks, when the polish starts chipping. You may then decide to try peeling or filing the polish off. But the top layer of the nail often comes with it, leaving nails thin and susceptible to water damage. At that point, you have to wait until a new, healthy nail plate grows in, which could take months.

Sculpted Nails

These custom-made artificial nails are sculpted to fit exactly over your natural nails. Sculpted nails fit extremely well, and you may have a difficult time differentiating this custom nail from a natural nail. This nail sculpture, made from acrylic polymers, requires more care than natural fingernails.

Although they can look like art on your fingers, you may pay a cost for their enhancement. After two to four months of wear, the natural nail plate may turn yellow, dry out and thin.

For this reason, you should not wear sculptured nails for more than three consecutive months before allowing your natural nails a break of at least one month to improve their health. Sometimes silk or linen cloth wraps used together with nail sculptures can strengthen the artificial nail.

CONCLUSION Your nails emerge from your skin and are a part of it. To keep your nails strong, beautiful, and healthy, you need to follow the same rules as you do for skin.

Protect your delicate nails from environmental assaults, including self-inflicted damage from nail beauty treatments. When choosing products to beautify or transform your nails, select the ones that cause the least damage. If, as is often so, some damage is unavoidable, make sure you take time to baby your nails back to health afterwards.

Since nails, just like your skin, need to undergo constant renewal to stay strong and beautiful, skin regenerative ingredients such as SRCPs and tin peptides will help you maintain your nails in top condition even if you cannot imagine your hands without a sophisticated manicure, nail polish, or even artificial nails.

In short, taking care of your nails is in many ways similar to taking care of your beautiful skin. When you understand nail biology, it becomes very easy to select products that will keep your hands soft and smooth and your nails gleaming with health.

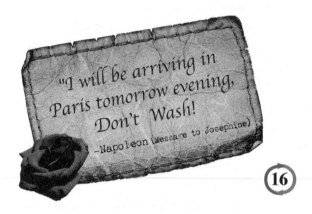

"I will be arriving in Paris tomorrow evening, Don't Wash!
—Napoleon (Message to Josephine)

(16)

FORMULE DE L'AMOUR
SPREAD THAT LOVING FEELING WITH FRAGRANT PHEROMONES

Do you feel love in the air? Picture yourself lapping through a field of lilacs with a fluttering heart as you gaze upon the sexiest person alive. What is the fragrant formula of love? Can we seek and sniff out Mr. or Ms. Right? Imagine yourself sipping an espresso at a local cafe, reading the paper, minding your own business. Suddenly, a strapping young man or lovely seductress enters the room, and you are immediately struck with Cupid's arrow. You not only sense a chemical attraction, you smell it! Cupid has just struck you with pheromones, the 'smellprints' that evoke the chemistry of attraction. The aroma of coffee fades as pheromones brew up the scent of passion. Such is the power of pheromones. These intoxicating chemicals are given off by humans, animals, and plants. They serve to attract and stimulate others. Research shows that human pheromones may stir up a host of behaviors, ranging from mothers kissing their children to men being attracted to large-breasted women.

Raging hormone and sizzling pheromone levels peak around age 18 and then slowly decline through the rest of our lives. When we enter a room at age 40, our pheromone signal no longer excites others as it did when we were 18. When we gaze amorously at a young beauty, we tend to assume that our eyes incite the chemical amalgam that causes our hearts to flutter. But we may fail to consider how scents also activate our senses. As we age, our lack of appeal may be in large part due to our drop in pheromones. As a result, the most effective way to attract others, as we grow older and wiser, is to enhance our signals with supplemental pheromones, just as we take supplements of antioxidants to keep healthy and ward off disease (Kohl & Francoeur 1995, Cutler 1996, Pickart 2005).

THE TWO TYPES OF PHEROMONES

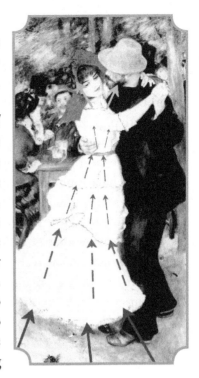

While pheromones produce less obvious reactions in humans than in other animals, they strongly shape our behavior. As pheromones move among us, they activate pre-coded genetic programs.

Pheromones fall into two categories (*signal* and *primer*) that attract us to each other in different ways. Signal pheromones move through the air. These airborne particles ascend on their airy journey after the body's heat evaporates them. When you wear clothes, your body heats the air, causing it to rise toward the highest opening. As the heated air rises, it picks up the pheromones secreted from your skin. When the air emerges around your face, it causes people to notice you. It takes about one second for smells from your face to reach someone 50 feet away in still air. In addition to making others aware of our presence, signal pheromones also cause immediate changes in behavior by activating certain areas of the brain.

The primer pheromone (a heavy protein) is passed directly by kissing or skin-to-skin contact. When a mother kisses her baby, it increases mother-baby bonding. And I'll bet we all can remember that first romantic kiss! This beautiful moment provided us with a perfect opportunity to check out pheromones. These bonding signals may explain why kissing occurs in all human cultures; it is a way of passing pheromones.

Priming pheromones increase the production of many hormones that affect development, metabolism, and mating behavior. These pheromones can take time to weave their special links. Consider how, at times, fertile women find it difficult to conceive. In married couples, it takes an average of six months to get pregnant. Perhaps the woman's body must slowly adjust to her husband's pheromones before becoming receptive to pregnancy. Women love to cuddle and snuggle—something that a new husband quickly learns will help him have a smooth relationship with his wife.

Why Women Call Men "Pigs"

In pigs, deer, goats, sheep, and some other animals, males compete for females on the basis of pheromone strength rather than physical strength or beauty. The animals with the strongest pheromones 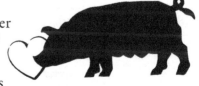 exude confidence and display threat without giving signals of fear. This reduces the incidence of actual physical combat for females, especially among deer and moose. The male pig that signals the strongest pheromones causes a psychological castration of his competition. It's the survival of the fittest pig!

Now does this make for a chauvinist pig, or is it just an animal driven by hormonal instinct? I'll let you decide.

This type of pheromone dominance may also apply to us. Many believe that the pheromone response in humans and pigs is similar. As hard as this may be on the ego, it's probably true! Before we protest with a squealing 'oink-oink', consider how truffles entice both pigs and humans—and no, I'm not talking about chocolate truffles releasing pleasure hormones in women. Chocolate truffles derived their name from the highly prized truffle mushroom, a fungus that grows underground near oak trees in France and Italy. These have long been prized as a human aphrodisiac. Pigs, too, passionately lust for truffles and are used to sniff out and locate this precious fungi. Now here is some more amusing food for thought: Why do women often call men pigs when men rarely use this term for women? Could it be that ever since wild pigs were domesticated 7,000 years ago, women intuitively knew that many male human hormones resemble those of pigs? Yes, if you are a man, your pheromone scent may affect females more strongly than your good looks, money, or wit.

QUOTABLE QUOTES: *The truffle is not exactly an aphrodisiac, but it tends to make women more tender and men more likeable.*
—*French gastronome Brillat-Savarin*

The key pheromone in pigs, androstenone, gives boar urine its characteristic odor and also accounts for some of the odor in human male urine. Both women and female pigs respond to the smell of androstenone in their male partners. Pig breeders spray androstenone from aerosol cans on the backs of female pigs to determine whether the female is ready for breeding; if the sow arches her back, she is sexually receptive.

Smells Stir Our Emotions Into a Sensual Broth

During the Middle Ages, a man would wipe his brow after dancing and present the cloth to his lady as a token of his love. He may not have consciously realized that his smell would remain with her as a momento. The wives of Welsh miners put their husband's nightshirts on their pillows in order to smell their men who spent nights away in the mines. Even today, a lady might wear her beau's unwashed T-shirt. Aah! The compelling force of pheromones.

QUOTABLE QUOTES: *The purest union that can exist between a man and a woman is that caused by the sense of smell and is sanctioned by the brain's normal assimilation of the animate molecules emitted by the secretions produced by two bodies in contact and sympathy, and in their subsequent evaporation.* —*Auguste Galopin*

How do pheromones evoke your emotions? Current theories postulate that smells affect the brain's emotional control areas by activating nerves in the vomeronasal organ (VMO) in the nasal septum. To understand how the sense of smell influences the brain, it helps to understand how the brain works. The brain consists of three areas. The lower part of the brain, the brain stem, controls functions such as breathing and heartbeat. The central area, called the limbic system, generates emotions. Some limbic areas promote feelings of peace, contentment, and attraction, while other areas cause feelings of anger, rage, hostility, loneliness, and so on. The conscious brain, where thinking occurs, occupies the topmost and outer area of the brain. However, the conscious mind does not emit emotions. The reason we love someone has more to do with how that one smells to the limbic system than what we consciously think. Smell signals are sent directly to the limbic system where emotions arise.

QUOTABLE QUOTES: *Her breasts, like lilies, 'ere their leaves be shed;*
Her nipples, like young blossomed jessamines;
Such fragrant flowers do give most odorous smell.
But her sweet odour did them all excel. –Edmund Spencer

Pheromones affect how we feel about and react to others from the moment we are born. Infants have an oral fixation as they cuddle their mother's breasts. Newborns follow the sweet breast scent emanating from the nipple/areola. The aroma evokes feelings of love, safety, and nurturing, which guide the infant to nurse. Within minutes of birth, the mother's breast fragrance exerts its pheromone effect, causing the baby's head to turn and helping to guide the baby to successful suckling of milk. These nipple pheromones may also explain men's irrational obsession with women's breasts (Winberg & Porter 1998, Porter & Winberg 1999, Schaal et al 2003).

Since smells have such a powerful impact on our emotions, it should come as no surprise that a lack of smell limits our ability to emotionally bond. Approximately 1.3% of the population is born with a total lack of smell, known as anosmia. Persons with anosmia often complain about a lack of libido. While they may marry, emotional distance remains a problem. Likewise, the decline in sex drive with aging coincides with the decline in smell.

PHEROMONES ACT EVEN IF YOU CAN'T SMELL THEM

While many pheromones give off distinctive scents that evoke emotion, they may be too weak to consciously detect. For example, a male dog can respond to pheromones from a female dog at a distance of up to three miles, at a concentration too faint to consciously smell. Humans also respond to pheromone levels that are too low to smell. At Stanford University, Sobel and colleagues found that an airborne fragrant pheromone (oestra- 1,3,5(10),16-tetraen-3yl acetate) activated brain centers even when present at concentrations below a threshold of conscious detection (Sobel et al 1999).

Bathing and the Decline of Bonding

As our culture advances, we tend to bathe more and bond less. This suggests that washing removes skin pheromones and weakens interpersonal bonding in families and between couples.

The tie between washing and the decline of chemical attraction is present throughout history, from ancient to modern times. In the Roman Republic, family ties were very strong. However, as this society evolved into the wealthy Roman Empire, with its adequate water supplies and free municipal baths, personal bonds grew weaker, divorce became common, and social disorganization increased. With the rise of early Christianity and its dislike of nudity and bathing, family ties began to strengthen.

In the USA, California led the way in personal cleanliness. By the 1940's, many Californians bathed or showered daily, washing away their personal pheromones in the process, while most of the United States stuck to weekly bathing. Soon, California also led the nation in divorce rates and family breakdown. At about the same time, Scandinavia led Europe as a hallmark for personal cleanliness, and soon it also experienced family breakdown. Swedes often complained that they felt cultural isolation. Both California and Scandinavia, with their immense social programs, prosperous economies, and basic friendliness have not solved these problems.

WHY EXPENSIVE PERFUMES DON'T WORK
Studies by Alan Hirsch and Jason Gruss (Smell and Taste Treatment Research Foundation, Chicago and University of Michigan) found that expensive perfumes are less effective than many essential oils and common foods. They studied the effects of several different scents on sexual arousal of men and women by comparing the subjects' blood flow in sexually aroused tissues (penile or clitoral blood flow) while wearing scented masks and while wearing non-odorized, blank masks. Expensive perfumes increased blood flow by only 3% in men. In contrast, the combined odor of lavender and pumpkin pie produced a 40% increase in men. Many other scents also worked better than the perfumes. While these results pertain to men, the researchers reported that women also responded poorly to expensive perfumes and positively to other smells.

Hirsch suggests that certain scents may increase sexual arousal by acting on the brain in three different ways: by reducing anxiety, which inhibits natural sexual desire; increasing alertness and awareness, making the subjects more aware of sexual cues in the environment around them; and acting directly to the septal nuclei, a portion of the brain that induces sexual arousal (Hirsch 1998).

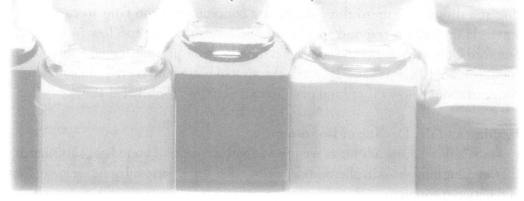

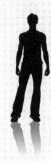

MEN: Effect of Perfumes and Scents on Blood Flow in Male Sexual Tissue

ITEM TESTED	Median % Increase in Penile Blood Flow
Lavender & Pumpkin Pie	40
Pumpkin Pie & Doughnut	20
Orange	19.5
Black Licorice & Cola	13
Black Licorice	3
Lily of the Valley	11
Vanilla	9
Pumpkin Pie	8.5
Lavender	8
Musk	7.5
Peppermint	6
Cheese Pizza	5
Roasting Meat	5
Rose	4
Strawberry	3.5
Oriental Spices	3.5
Expensive Perfumes	Averaged 3.0
Chocolate	2.8

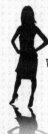

WOMEN: Effect of Perfumes & Scents on Enhancement of Clitoral Blood Flow

ITEM TESTED	Median % Increase
Cucumber and Licorice Candy	13
Baby Powder	13
Lavender & Pumpkin Pie	11
Charcoal Barbecued Meat	Inhibited: Anti-arousal
Cherries	Inhibited: Anti-arousal
Expensive Men's Colognes	Inhibited: Anti-arousal

Above Chart based on publications of Alan Hirsch and Jason Gruss

Social Pheromones — Calming Aphrodisiacs

Have you ever entered a crowded room and felt anxiety and agitation? Or how about road rage? You're stuck in traffic not going anywhere with drivers honking and cursing. What can you do?

Although most research has focused on sexual pheromones, there are aromatic oils that also boast harmonizing properties that change behavior patterns, reduce mental stress, and improve social interactions.

These "social pheromones" include many long established pure essential oils that have been used for thousands of years in social events, weddings, and spiritual gatherings. For example, sanatol (one of the active ingredients in sandalwood oil and Asian oud), has harmonizing and anti-conflict properties. When mice are caged together, this leads to conflict and fighting. Exposure to the smell of sanatol reduces the conflict among the mice. Ylang Ylang calms with similar anti-conflict properties.

Lavender oil reduces perinatal discomfort in women following childbirth and the pain of patients in intensive care units. Remaining still inside a cramped magnetic resonance scanner often causes anxiety and claustrophobia. Whiffs of heliotropin, a vanilla-like fragrance, before the procedure reduced patient anxiety 63 percent. Some aromatic oils known for their aphrodisiac qualities are jasmine, ylang-ylang, rose, sandalwood and vanilla, but this aphrodisiac effect may be due to how well they calm us and reduce stress . . . ahhh . . . nothing like calmness followed by sensuality!

Remember, these social pheromones can calm the worst of moods and decrease conflict in social situations. Ylang Ylang is just one of several pheromones that has been shown to lessen conflict and aggressive behavior. Sandalwood oil also has a calming affect by reducing anxiety. And if you are under mental stress at work or school, try lavender oil, which can calm you down so that you can focus and be more alert while having an uplifted, friendly attitude.

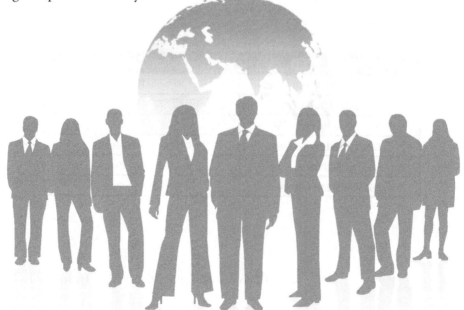

EFFORTS TO CREATE AN EFFECTIVE PERFUME Several companies have been set up to develop romantic pheromones for consumers, based on the human pheromone, but most have failed to deliver results.

For me, the use of aromatic plant oils as body perfumes was just an idea. Since women love irresistible perfumes to lure men, I became fascinated with pheromones that might trigger attraction even better than perfumes. I read everything I could as I delved in a fragrant web of research. My conclusions are as follows:

1. If pheromones are species-specific, humans shouldn't be able to detect animal-derived pheromones. But even if they could, what reactions might we expect? Taking into account that many animals become more dangerous during mating periods, humans shouldn't be attracted to the smell of a ready-to-mate boar; they should feel fear or aggression.

Androstenone triggers both sexual attraction and aggression in boars. In mice, certain pheromones cause male mice to kill other male mice (male odors increase attacks, female odors decrease attacks). Male lions and bears will, at times, kill the offspring of a female in order to mate with her. If purely sexual human pheromones (similar to pig androstenone) were discovered, they couldn't be used in a perfume. If humans followed the urge for pheromone-induced mating, people would get arrested!

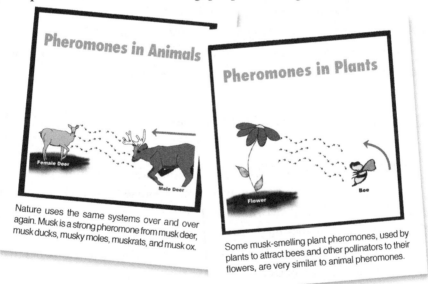

Nature uses the same systems over and over again. Musk is a strong pheromone from musk deer, musk ducks, musky moles, muskrats, and musk ox.

Some musk-smelling plant pheromones, used by plants to attract bees and other pollinators to their flowers, are very similar to animal pheromones.

2. Human interactions are complex, and the social element is very important. There could be 100 human pheromones that affect different aspects of behavior.

3. Some musk-smelling plant pheromones, used by plants to attract bees and other pollinators to the sweet smell of nectar, are very similar to animal pheromones. Nature uses the same systems over and over again. For example, musk is a strong pheromone from musk deer, musk ducks, musky moles, muskrats, musk ox, and musk beetles. However, similar pheromones exist in musk melons, musk hyacinths, musk cherries, musk thistle, musk rose, musk plums, and musk wood.

Brain research suggests that calming oils may enhance sexual pleasure. Neuroscientist Gert Holstege (University of Groningen), using positron-emission tomography, found that to achieve a sexual climax, the amygdala (the brain's center of vigilance and fear) is silenced while activity in brain areas that are involved in judgment and reflection are greatly reduced. This occurs in men and even more so in women. He commented, "Fear and anxiety need to be avoided at all costs if a woman wishes to have an orgasm" (Holstege 2005).

4. When creating pheromone perfumes, most companies just use the molecule with the chemical smell rather than the original essential oil. But we don't know which component of the complex mixture is able to communicate with our brain; it might even be an odorless component! By throwing away everything but the part that the nose can smell, these companies might also be throwing away the magic.

5. Historically, many of the traditional mood-altering essential oils have also been used for skin care. Patchouli has long soothed as an anti-inflammatory and aid for dry, cracked skin. The oil of lavender soothes skin and was applied to wounds in ancient Greece and Rome. It is still enjoyed today. Sandalwood can regenerate your skin while also treating acne, dry skin, rashes, chapped skin, eczema, itching, and sensitive skin. It also has anti-skin cancer actions (Kaur et al 2005, Dwivedi et al 2003, Dwivedi & Zhang 1999). You can dab on Ylang Ylang to treat eczema, acne, oily skin, and the irritation associated with insect stings or bites. With so many ways to benefit from essential oils, it is difficult to find a reason not to use them.

QUOTABLE QUOTES: *Thy God hath anointed you with the oil of gladness.*
—Saint Paul

FROM THEORY TO PRACTICE You are probably thinking that all of these pheromones sound enticing. But you may be asking yourself, "Which one should I use and how do I know it will really work?" I hear you! So after my preliminary research, I decided to put this sweet smelling theory into practice. I tested pheromones on some very enthusiastic perfume-lovers. These women wanted natural ingredients that could sensually and socially attract better than their expensive perfumes.

The volunteers were asked to wear each of the pheromones and record people's reactions. In every case, the test subjects found few positive responses to the human pheromones. Conversely, all of them reported positive responses to at least some of the plant pheromones! These women elicited affection, flirtation and socially uplifting interaction. People were so much more friendly and talkative both at home, work, and when they were out socializing. Based on their responses, the most effective plant pheromones were the essential oils of *jasmine, ylang ylang, nutmeg, sandalwood, Asian oud, patchouli,* and *lavender.*

BODY PERFUMES WITH PLANT DERIVED PHEROMONES

"Exactly which pheromones should I try?", you may ask. Based on my experiments, the following plant pheromones won rave reviews; you may want to experiment on yourself to see what you attract! Some of the most popular scents include: patchouli (good for attracting women), ylang ylang (good for attracting men), musk, sandalwood, and jasmine (these three are universal attractants). By using an appropriate version of perfume oils based on plant pheromones, you can strongly modify your personal "odor signature" in a positive way.

Think Torso and Legs, Not Wrists and Earlobes

For thousands of years, men and women applied perfumes to their torso and legs. Why was this the case? Well, the heat of your body evaporates pheromones and scents and blends them into your individual odor signature. This signature brew is made up of a complex mixture of pheromones, body oils, fatty acids, sweat, and hormones such as androsterone secreted onto the skin from the apocrine glands. In addition, the 40 million skin cells that you shed each day are combined to your odor signature.

However, the modern method of applying perfumes to the wrists and earlobes only reflects the ignorance of the modern cosmetic industry. It is best to apply body perfumes after a bath or shower. Dry yourself, and then apply pheromone products on your body, especially on large, heat-producing areas such as the chest, breasts, and legs. If you bathe at night, the oils should be applied to your dry skin in the morning.

Finding a perfume with plant derived pheromones that best complements your unique odor signature and attracts the type of people that you desire, may take some trial and error. Work your way through the oils one by one until you find the one that is most effective for you. Apply the oil, then dress normally and go about your daily routine.

If the oil is working, responsive people will unconsciously notice you from three-to-five feet away. Watch for those who unexpectedly turn and smile or extend conversations. Using plant-derived pheromones is a little like trolling for salmon while testing different lures; it takes some time, but keep trying and eventually you'll find the right lure (scent).

As you have fun testing pheromones, enjoy how the multitude of scents elicit feelings of one kind or another. Create an aura of power and confidence, or of capable competence, cool composure, warmth and friendship, empathy and compassion, and sexuality. Encourage a nesting vibe in men. Encourage peaceful interactions with your family members. These scents have been passed down through generations and evoke current cultural perceptions with sense memory. Pheromones can feel magical as you become the star of your own social interactions.

Plant Derived Pheromone Chart

Note: These are general comments from wearers of plant derived pheromone products. Responses may vary widely among individuals.

Mood Enhancer	Mood Effects	Effects on WOMEN	Effects on MEN	Traditional Uses
LAVENDER	Calming Relaxing Soothing	STRONG	STRONG	Skin healing, beneficial for acne, burns, wounds, rashes, psoriasis, PMS, stress, tension, and muscle cramps
JASMINE	Erotic Very Pleasant	STRONG	MODERATE	Aphrodisiac: Said to increase arousal, attractiveness, and appeal. Emotionally produces feelings of optimism, confidence, euphoria, reduces tension, anxiety and depression, relieves menstrual cramps and pain
ASIAN OUD	Calming Erotic	STRONG	STRONG	A historical favorite in Arab countries, produced by a fungus that lives on trees
YLANG YLANG	Erotic Relaxing	MODERATE	STRONG	Strong aphrodisiac: said to increase arousal and attachment. Traditionally spread on the marriage bed in Bali
SANDALWOOD	Erotic, Musk-like, Relaxing	MODERATE	STRONG	Scent is very similar to musks from animals such as deer musk, civitone musk from civit cats, and castorium from beavers which are traditional aphrodisidacs for both men and women
NUTMEG	Energizing	STRONG	STRONG	Very stimulating, helps with frigidity, impotence, neuralgia, and nervous fatigue. Used for better circulation, arthritis, gout, muscular aches and pains
PATCHOULI	Mildly Erotic	STRONG	LOW	A favorite of women: erotic for women, probably not for men

Questions? Email: ghkcopperpeptides@gmail.com

17

YOUR SKIN UNDER THE SUN
Better Protection, Less Damage, More Fun

Remember how at the end of a long, gloomy winter you experienced joy as the warm touch of golden sunrays finally touched your skin? How you felt your mood improve and your skin clear up as it glowed with good health?

Yet, now you have been told to stay away from sun. You have been advised to never leave home without sunscreen. You have been warned that even if you become vitamin D-deficient, because of lack of sunshine, you should keep using your sunscreens.

Now let me ask you a question: Do you believe that you should still trust your intuition? Well, I have good news for you—there is more about sun science than meets the eye. Let's explore how you can keep your skin young and healthy, while enjoying the sun at the same time.

FROM SUN WORSHIPPERS TO TAN JUNKIES

Hundreds of years ago, Copernicus proclaimed the sun to be the center of our universe. Throughout thousands of orbits, humans have worshipped the sun's warmth and power.

Primitive societies believed in a sun god that warmed their bodies, souls, and brought in the harvest. They praised the sun for its power to heal certain illnesses. In Ancient Greece, a lovely bronze tan was considered a symbol of good health and a vigorous spirit.

This all changed though during medieval times. If you remember Lady Rowena from Sir Walter Scott's *Ivanhoe*, you'll recall that in those times, "fair" was synonymous with "beautiful" and "noble". Consequently, ladies would go to great lengths to protect their skin from the sun by staying indoors and wearing hats and veils.

However, after the Great Industrial Revolution, pale skin became something you might have as a result of spending long hours inside a gloomy factory. In other words, it became the characteristic of a low social status and hard work. On the contrary, tanned skin then became a symbol of a leisure lifestyle. Even today, although we keep hearing about the dangers of UV-radiation, a deep bronze tan somehow makes us think of tanning salons, luxury yachts, lush golf courses, and tropical beaches.

In the early 20's, tanning became a fashion statement when Coco Chanel obtained a suntan while cruising from Paris to Cannes.

Soon, almost everyone wanted to have a good tan. For some people, it was easy—their skin would tan quickly and without a sunburn. Those less fortunate had to suffer through painful sunburns and have their skin peel many times before they managed to achieve the desired bronzed tint.

When the cosmetic industry came up with the idea of chemicals that could filter out a certain portion of UV-rays to prevent sunburns, those products immediately became wildly popular. Unfortunately, they were also very unsafe.

QUOTABLE QUOTES: *L'assaut au soleil des blancheurs des corps de femme...*
The assault on the sunlight by the whiteness of women's bodies...
—Arthur Rimbaud 1854-1891

Dangerous Protection

The first sunscreens contained a very harmful estrogenic chemical called PABA (para-aminobenzoic acid), which filtered a portion of sunlight responsible for sunburns. This particular part of sunlight is called **UV-B radiation**, and it is primarily responsible for suntans, sunburns, and vitamin D synthesis. By blocking UV-B rays, sunscreens allowed people to stay under the sun much longer than they normally would.

Circa 1970, the FDA began advising people to use sunscreens to prevent skin cancer. So you'd think the rate of skin cancer went down. Hardly!

In the early 1970's, there were 6 cases of melanoma for every 10,000 people in the United States. But by the beginning of the 2000's, the numbers nearly tripled despite growing sun awareness and increased use of sunscreens among Americans.

To understand why the rate of melanoma in the U.S. climbs despite widespread use of sunscreens, we must take a closer look at UV-radiation and its effects.

THE HIGH PRICE OF A "SUNBURN-FREE" TAN

The term **ultraviolet radiation** refers to everything that falls within the category between X-rays and visible light spectrum. Although it has a shorter wavelength than visible light (our eyes cannot see it), we can feel its effects through a painful sunburn or see its results in a beautiful tan.

There are three distinct diapasons of UV-radiation: *UVC-R*, *UVB-R*, and *UVA-R*. These differ in energy level and ability to induce a tan or burn the skin. They

also produce other biological effects. It is interesting to note that 98.7% of all UV-radiation that reaches the Earth is actually UVA-radiation. You could call it "the most aesthetically appealing" type of UV-radiation because exposure to it can result in beautiful, long-lasting tans.

UVC-R or germicidal light has a 280-100 nm wavelength. It carries high energy and is very damaging to living tissue; however, it does not penetrate the Earth's atmosphere. This type of UV-radiation can be found in germicidal UV wands and disinfecting blue lamps in hospitals.

UVB-R (315-280 nm wavelength). Its energy is lower than that of UVC, but is still enough to induce a suntan and sunburn as well as stimulate vitamin D production. It can also damage cell DNA; however, its penetrating ability is limited to the upper skin layers, which undergo rapid renewal and can easily get rid of the damage.

UVA-R (410- 315 nm). The most dangerous type of UV-radiation. Although it has low energy and never burns the skin, it can penetrate much deeper than any other UV-radiation, and therefore can damage skin collagen and cell DNA, causing premature aging, immunosuppression and in some cases, skin cancer. But it does induce a nice, long-lasting tan.

According to researchers, this type of tan is different from UVB-induced tanning and results from a darkening of existing skin pigment, rather than an increase of melanin production. Therefore, it is less protective than UVB-induced pigmentation. Additionally, recent studies have found that this kind of radiation can penetrate deep into skin and (if given enough time) ravage proteins and DNA, accelerating skin aging.

Next, there's UVB—the kind of UV that gives fair-skinned beauties a much desired tan, or a sunburn if not careful. It can damage the skin but doesn't penetrate into the deeper layers. UVB is essential for vitamin D synthesis in the skin.

Finally, UVC is a germicidal, ozone-producing radiation. Very little UVC reaches our skin except in high altitudes.

Nobody likes red, swollen, peeling skin and due to the fact that UVB can cause a sunburn, it has long been considered the most harmful type of radiation. Nevertheless, a sunburn (albeit painful and uncomfortable) does serve important biological functions.

In short, it ensures that your skin stays protected from too much UVA as well as helps clear off any damage.

How so? First, a sunburn will naturally limit sun exposure for those with fair skin and insufficient melanin production. No matter how badly a fair-skinned lady may want her tan, the red and swollen back and shoulders (not to mention a red and peeling nose!) soon forces her to flee to more shaded areas.

> You might be tempted to reach for any old bottle of sunscreen on the grocery store shelf to protect yourself from the sun. DON'T! Chemical sunscreens contain oily chemicals that strongly absorb the energy in light photons and can cause more harm than good.

QUOTABLE QUOTES: *Estrogenic sunscreen chemicals might explain most of the social changes in California over the past 30 years.*
—A California customer

After a sunburn, the damaged skin quickly peels off together with the newly acquired tan. Today, scientists have discovered that not only does the skin peel after the sunburn, it also frantically renovates and remodels itself, pushing out damaged cells—or forcing them to commit suicide—thereby entering a state of programmed death. So even when UVB damages skin, this damage rarely accumulates.

Furthermore, since a UVB-induced sunburn naturally limits the amount of time one can stay out in the sun, there is less time for UVA to do its damaging work. If you do not burn, it just means you have enough melanin in your skin and may not worry about sun damage (unless you're exposed for a very long period of time). Dark skin is naturally more resilient to UV-radiation because it evolved in the abundance of sun. But it still needs plentiful sunlight, since it is more prone to vitamin D deficiency. Today, in addition to old-fashioned UVB sunscreens, there is now an array of UVA/UVB options that claim broad-spectrum protection. However, not every consumer knows that SPF (sun protection factor), a familiar indicator of the product's efficiency, really only refers to protection from UVB rays and tells us nothing about the level of UVA protection.

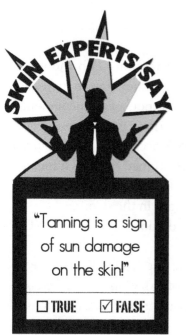

"Tanning is a sign of sun damage on the skin!"

☐ TRUE   ☑ FALSE

Should You Avoid the Sun?

Today, the media hypes the dangers of tanning and encourages you to slather on tons of sunscreen, even if you are only in the sun for a short period of time.

But is it really healthy to avoid the sun altogether? Consider the following: Humans evolved in the presence of abundant sunlight. Geneticists and archaeologists calculate that our ancestors lost their body hair 1.2 million years ago but only started wearing clothes 72,000 years ago. So for more than 1,128,000 years, our forbearers lived in splendid nudity and flourished.

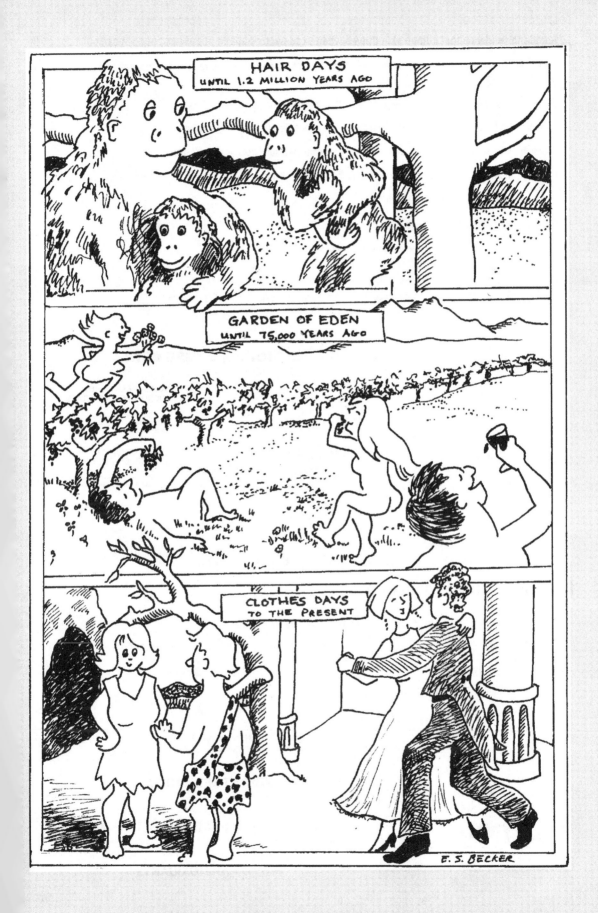

Additional evidence that human skin thrives when exposed to sunlight (Hobday 2000, Holick 2003).

• In the United States, people in professions with high sunlight exposure (such as farmers and mail carriers) live the longest.

• Cancer rates are the highest in northern states with the least sunshine.

• Rates of the major lethal cancers are drastically lower in people who get more sunshine.

• Sunlight-associated cancers increased most in locations where sunscreen was most heavily promoted.

• Sunlight improves the moods of those with seasonal affective disorder (SAD).

• Psoriatic skin lesions are reduced by sunlight.

• Sunlight raises testosterone levels in males.

• Sunlight exposure may reduce the incidence of schizophrenia.

• Sunlight improves bone health.

• Sunlight decreases auto-immune diseases such as multiple sclerosis, Type 1 diabetes, and rheumatoid arthritis.

Old Fashioned Sunscreens

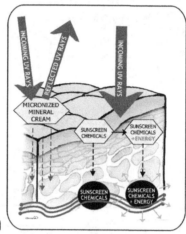

SUN SCREENS with MICRONIZED MINERALS

Can penetrate and accumulate in lower layer of skin

UV ABSORBING SUNSCREEN CHEMICALS:

As much as 35% of sunscreen chemicals enter the blood stream

SUNSCREEN CHEMICALS + ENERGY:

Once sunscreen chemicals combine with energy, they can enter the blood stream and damage the DNA

Healthier Sun Protection

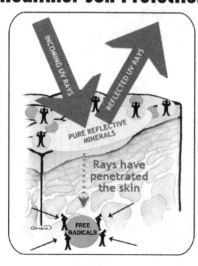

PROTECTIVE CREAM on skin
ANTIOXIDANTS & Pure Reflective Minerals
Topically protect skin from Free Radical formation:

SRCPs
Vitamin E Family
Tocotrienol Family
CoQ10
Lycopene
Lutein

= PROTECT

= BREAK DOWN

PROTECTIVE ANTIOXIDANTS within SKIN
Fight off Free Radical formation:

Superoxide Dismutase
Vitamin E Family
Tocotrienol Family
CoQ10
Lycopene
Lutein
Vitamin C

= FREE RADICALS

= PURE REFLECTIVE MINERALS

= ANTIOXIDANTS

SUNLIGHT AND GOOD HEALTH

A certain amount of sunlight is necessary for good health. Sunshine activates a gene called pom-C, which in turn helps create melanin that determines skin color. This beneficial gene enhances sex drive, the endorphins or "happiness hormones", as well as leptin, which helps burn fat and keep you thin.

The sun also promotes health and beauty by triggering the skin to produce vitamin D. Vitamin D refers to two very similar molecules: vitamin D3 named cholecalciferol, created in the outer skin's keratinocytes (remember that GHK-Cu increases keratinocyte proliferation) in response to UVB light and vitamin D2 called ergocalciferol, produced in plants. Then, within the body, both of these types are converted into vitamin 1,25D, the active form of vitamin D.

This essential nutrient helps build strong bones and muscles that may contribute to beautiful smiles and sculpted bodies. Furthermore, vitamin D strengthens immunity and reduces breast cancer which can promote longevity. Deficiencies of vitamin D increase bone fractures, susceptibility to infection, and auto-immune diseases.

When a bikini-clad woman with a white complexion basks in the summer sun, her skin generates 10,000 units of vitamin D in as little as 10 to 15 minutes! However, less is more since exposure over that amount does not increase vitamin D. During winters in Northern Europe, where sunlight is sparse, 92% of adolescent girls and 37% of older women were found to be vitamin D deficient.

Conversely, in climates with long, sunny seasons, skin with higher levels of melanin synthesizes much less vitamin D. Caucasian skin absorbs approximately twice as much vitamin D as African skin. Those with darker complexions are at serious risk for vitamin D deficiencies. Topical sunscreens can reduce vitamin D production by more than 98%.

Persons who have more sun exposure have much lower rates (reductions of 40 to 80%) of major internal cancers that cause 99% of cancer deaths (breast, colon, prostate, ovarian). This appears to be linked to low vitamin D. A three-year study of 1,179 women in Nebraska found daily supplementation of 1,100 units of vitamin D3 and 1,400 mgs of calcium lowered cancer risk 77%.

While many of the sun's healing benefits are attributed to an increased production of vitamin D, the sun's actions are likely to be far more complex. Sunlight generates many other molecules in the skin, perhaps dozens or hundreds more. Some individuals who suffered from seasonal affective disorder (SAD) during dark winter months have told me that extra vitamin D (400 to 1,000 units per day) failed to alleviate their depression, whereas a brief sojourn in a UV tanning booth every week did relieve their mid-winter depression.

Your skin maintains UV anti-oxidant protection under full sunlight for approximately 45 minutes, but ultraviolet tanning booths produce 10 times the UV intensity of full sunlight. So the time spent using tanning booths should be quite brief—2 to 4 minutes.

As for the mixture of vitamin D and sunlight, the best answer may be to take vitamin D supplements (1,000-2,000 units daily, there is no consensus about the optimal dosage) combined with 10 to 15 minutes of moderate sunlight several times weekly on areas of your body that rarely are exposed to sunlight.

Sensible Suntanning

Does the idea of obtaining a healthy tan sound like an oxymoron? It may, if you have spent years avoiding the sun. While too much sun can damage the skin, a low dose of golden rays can enhance your mood and health. Now that's good news, isn't it? You can obtain the life-enhancing effects of sunlight and still keep your skin healthy and attractive.

The basic strategy is to increase melanin production. Melanin, your brown and black pigment, not only shields the skin from excessive UV-radiation, but it also helps block UV damage by serving as a free radical scavenger. Sensible suntanning is a balancing act since too much sun can damage the skin. Keep in mind that sun-induced skin damage and tanning (melanin production) are two *separate* biochemical processes and are not linked.

Sunless Production of Melanin

After topical SRCPs were sealed on the leg for a week, the cup was removed leaving the skin tanner by naturally increasing the production of melanin.

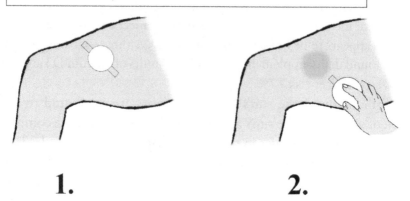

1.   2.

In spite of what you may have heard, a tan does not damage your skin. In human safety studies of SRCPs, the testing lab observed strong melanin production in human skin in the total absence of light when small cups of strong SRCP creams were taped to volunteers' skin for 5 days.

So go ahead! Have fun in the sun. Just go slow. Your key for achieving a fabulous tan is to sunbathe sensibly in stages and not overdo it. For most, I recommend suntanning a maximum of 20 to 30 minutes a day to produce the best results.

Whole-body suntanning (the most efficient and safest method) permits maximum sunlight exposure in the shortest amount of time since the sun reaches a larger area of the body. On the other hand, children generally need less sun than adults; most have thin skin that burns quickly and should not be exposed to sunlight for more than 5 to 10 minutes at a time. Infants under age 1 should be protected from intense sunlight at all times.

When you tan sensibly, your skin's natural protective system can defend you. This protective system includes defenses against oxygen radicals, such as vitamin E and beta-carotene, as well as copper-zinc superoxide dismutase, which detoxifies oxygen radicals and reduces skin damage.

In addition to monitoring how much time you bask in the sun, you may want to adopt protective measures when you take tropical vacations or spend longer periods enjoying the sunshine. Take the following steps before sun exposure:

YOUR GUIDE

HOW TO GET A BETTER TAN WITH LESS SKIN DAMAGE

3 Days Before	Take supplemental anti-oxidants: vitamin C, Co-Q10, alpha lipoic acid, vitamin E, beta carotene, or antioxidant loaded whole vegetables.
BEFORE Sunning	Apply a **copper peptide lotion fortified with titanium dioxide**: Helps moderate UV rays and diffuses light, supplies copper to assist melanin production for a natural, perfect tan
Tanning Times	Mid Morning (around 10:30 am) or Afternoon (around 3:00 pm) Tan in natural sunlight for 20-30 minutes
AFTER Sunning	Apply a **copper peptide lotion with antioxidants**: Helps to repair possible skin damage from exposure

MELANIN = GOOD

DAMAGE = BAD

1. Prior to suntanning, apply a thin coat of a copper peptide lotion fortified with titanium dioxide to remodel skin. The inclusion of titanium dioxide scatters UV light and should be accompanied by high levels of anti-oxidants. A small amount of water may be used to help spread thick creams. Recent studies suggest that GHK, my earlier generation SRCP, may prevent UV damage. However, further studies will be needed before making absolute claims. This exciting new research will be discussed later in the chapter.

2. If you burn easily or plan to extend your stay in the sun, apply a natural mineral sunscreen over copper peptide creams. Read more about natural sunscreens in the following pages.

3. After suntanning, apply a second-generation copper peptide product fortified with antioxidants. Suntanning produces damage to the skin barrier that must be promptly repaired to reduce peeling. SRCP creams help the process of remodeling the skin barrier.

4. Three days prior to tanning, take a daily supplement of Vitamin C (1 g), Co-Q10 (30 mgs), alpha lipoic acid (100 mgs), Vitamin E (400 units), and tocotrienols (35 mgs). Several skin researchers have recommended beta carotene (30 mg), mixed carotenoids from algae (50 mg), Vitamin E (400 units), and Vitamin C (1 g). Also, consume many antioxidant-loaded whole vegetables.

5. Wear UV sunglasses that absorb ultraviolet light to protect your eyes. Also, wear large hats and protective clothing during times of prolonged sun exposure.

6. When you sunbathe in a swimsuit, or better yet in the nude (as did our ancestors for millions of years), you obtain the maximum sunlight benefits with minimum skin damage.

But for how long per day should you expose your nude or semi-nude body to sunlight? The answer may lie in our special tie to the sun which spans thousands of years. Given the life-giving force of the sun, it is not surprising that our ancestors soaked up healing rays to reap its medicinal powers.

Greeks believed that the therapy of sunbathing called heliotherapy could cure certain illnesses. And medical literature dating back to 1500 B.C. from India mentions treatments of natural sunlight for skin conditions.

During the past century, many European clinics nestled in mountain regions offered whole-body sunlight treatments to heal skin wounds and infections. Physicians prescribed 15 to 30 minutes of sunlight twice daily and were warned not to start sunlight exposure too rapidly.

Wrinkle-Free Sunshine

Perhaps, like many of us, you relish the sun as it warms your skin and nurtures your senses. Yet you fear that a blazing sun will sizzle your skin, turning you into a wrinkled prune!

So what is the key to wrinkle-free sunshine? Moderation and enjoyment is the key. Reduce exposure to no more than 10 to 15 minutes a day, in the morning or afternoon sun when UV rays are less damaging. However, enjoy yourself while basking in the beauty of your favorite landscape—perhaps at sea or pruning your rose garden. The secret is to wear minimal clothing, so you can expose most of your body to the healing rays.

However, you will want to wear a sunblock on more wrinkle-prone areas such as the face, neck, hands, and chest. After 15 minutes, apply sunblock to the rest of your body—then continue to reflect on nature as reflective sunscreens protect your wrinkle-free skin.

Note: Although the FDA attests that the use of the word "sunblock" is misleading, in this publication from time to time, we may still use this word since the vast majority understand its meaning. However, "reflective minerals" is a more accurate term.

SPF is measured by evaluating skin redness after UV-radiation with and without a sunscreen. But UVA rays do not cause skin reddening and sunburn, and therefore UVA protection cannot be measured this way. Even though there is a special test that can be used to measure UVA protection (a pigment darkening test or PDT), sunscreen manufacturers were not required to perform this testing until recently.

Too Much of a Good Thing

While moderate sun exposure benefits the skin, too much of a good thing can overwhelm the skin's protective system. Lester Packer (University of California, Berkeley) found that as the dosage of UV-radiation increases, the skin's antioxidant defenses get overwhelmed.

As a result, free radicals form and cause cellular damage, such as lipid peroxidation and oxidative modification of proteins and cellular DNA. As little as 45 minutes of noon-day exposure can reduce the skin's protective vitamin C levels by 80% and lower other skin antioxidants. It takes the skin's melanocytes 2 to 5 days to produce protective melanin. In contrast, a severe burn can occur in just a few hours (Podda et al 1998).

The bottom line is: You can't rush a sensible suntan. It takes a minimum of 1 to 2 weeks to develop a healthy tan. As you expose your body to the sun, the skin thickens and increases your resistance to burning.

Be careful about sun exposure if you take medications such as tetracycline, antihistamines, "sulfa" drugs, diuretics, and some oral contraceptives that can make your skin more sensitive to light.

Recent studies have found that many so-called broad-spectrum sunscreens provide only minimal UVA protection.

The only type of sunscreens that provide balanced UVB/UVA protection are natural reflective minerals such as titanium dioxide. However, chemical corporations try to convince consumers that natural sunscreens (as well as our skin's own melanin) do not provide enough UV protection.

At the same time, sunscreen manufacturers push products with higher and higher SPF ratings that are loaded with alien chemicals. To promote such products, they promise such things as "all day protection" and "more time under the sun".

High SPF sunscreens (only achieved by the use of alien chemicals) give the illusion of protection by preventing sunburn and peeling. **Truthfully, there is no sunscreen that provides 100% protection.** Fooled by such an illusion, many beachgoers happily bask under the sun for hours without much burning or skin peeling. So now, while their skin still becomes severely damaged, the injured cells cannot peel off and may remain in the skin for decades as slow, ticking time bombs until they turn cancerous.

Chemical Sunscreens Aren't the Answer

Chemical sunscreens strongly absorb UV-radiation; however, they also have a dark side... and no, I'm not talking about blocking the dark side of shade! UV absorbers should never have been used for sunscreen protection.

When I was a college student performing chemical syntheses, we would mix UV-absorbing oils into batches of chemicals that needed free radicals to start the chemical reaction. We would then flash the mixture with a UV light, and the reaction would commence—sort of like putting a match to paper. For fifty years, chemists have known that UV-absorbing oils and UV-radiation generate a huge number of free radicals.

The same free radical damage occurs within human skin. The sunscreen oils do not just sit on the skin's surface and stop UV-radiation. As much as 35 % of a sunscreen chemical can pass through the skin. But the story is more complicated. Sunscreen chemicals, even so-called stable ones, breakdown after absorbing UV energy.

These rarely studied breakdown products, which are toxic to cultured cells, then penetrate the skin. The toxic chemicals and their breakdown products are then able to pass the outer layer of dead skin and come into contact with living tissue.

QUOTABLE QUOTES: *Safety of sunscreens is a concern, and sunscreen companies have emotionally and inaccurately promoted the use of sunscreens.*
— Berwick M. Clin Pharmacol Ther. 2011;89(1):31-3

Recent studies led by Kerry Hanson from the University of California Riverside found that when UV-radiation hits the sunscreen chemicals (such as octylmethoxycinnamate, benzophenone-3, and octocrylene) within the skin, these oils generate copious amounts of free radicals that injure cell walls, lipid membranes, mitochrondria, and DNA which produce skin damage and visible signs of aging.

The authors state that, under some conditions, "the UV filters in sunscreens that have penetrated into the epidermis can potentially do more harm than good." (Hanson et al 2006).

Terge Christensen, a biophysicist at the Norwegian Radiation Protection Authority, found octyl methoxycinnamate (OMC), a major sunscreen chemical, to kill 50% of cultured mouse cells at 5 parts per million, a dose far lower than the level used in sunscreen products.

If the cells were also exposed for 2 hours with simulated daylight, the OMC and light doubled the toxic actions.

So such "protective" chemicals may actually increase your risk of sun damage. As another example of a harmful sunscreen chemical, consider psoralen used with UV light to treat psoriasis. Psoralen is similar to sunscreen chemicals, and the rate of skin cancer in patients treated with psoralen is 83 times higher than among the general population (Stern & Laird 1994).

Many sunscreen chemicals also have strong estrogenic (estrogen-like) actions that may cause problems in sexual development and adult sexual function. These include an increased rate of cancer, an elevated rate of birth defects in children, a lower sperm count and smaller penis size in men, and a plethora of other medical problems. The effects are similar to those of many banned chemicals, such as DDT, dioxin, and PCBs.

Margaret Schlumpf and her colleagues (Institute of Pharmacology and Toxicology, University of Zurich, Switzerland) have found that many widely used sunscreen chemicals mimic the effects of estrogen and trigger developmental abnormalities in rats (Schlumpf et al 2001).

Expected Effects of Estrogenic Chemicals in Humans

In Women	Endometriosis
	Migraines
	Severe PMS
	Erratic Periods
	Increases in Breast and Uterine Cancer
	Fibrocystic Breast Disease
	Uterine Cysts
In Men	Lowered Sperm Count
	Breast Enlargement
	Smaller Than Normal Penis Size
	More Testicular Cancer
	Undescended Testicles
	Loss of Libido

What About Micronized Sunscreens with Nanoparticles?

In an effort to avoid the pasty white look of sunscreens containing large particles of zinc oxide or titanium dioxide, sunscreen manufacturers have reduced the particle size of these UV-absorbing molecules to the nanoscale (meaning that the lotion or cream is more transparent and cosmetically appealing).

Manufacturers know that today's consumers prefer invisible sunscreens and would be more likely to apply such a product multiple times during the day, resulting in big profits for cosmetic companies. But does this nano-technology used in the development of these sunscreens mean that they are safe?

A recent study performed on a lotion containing nanoscale zinc oxide isotope particles applied twice daily for a 5 day period found very interesting results. Participants had their skin studied and their urine and blood samples collected. Upon examination, the team detected the isotope in ALL of the participants' samples. Although the person who conducted the study added, "I've tried to make the point that the amount we actually saw in the blood was quite tiny", the point is that it was found in ALL the volunteers' samples, indicating that it was absorbed into the skin. The real question is: If this is what was found after only 5 days of usage, what would have been discovered after 100 days? Or after years of usage?

A safety study in rats found that zinc oxide nanoparticles (in levels used in sunscreens) applied over a period of 28 days, resulted in skin collagen loss.

Along the same line of thought, scientists at the University of California at Los Angeles also found that nanoparticles in sunscreens can enter and "wander throughout the body, potentially disrupting body functions on a sub-cellular level".

The University Women's Hospital in Basel, Switzerland investigated this phenomenon by testing the breast milk of mothers twice a year for three consecutive years (Schlumpf et al 2010). The participants' usage of various sunscreens were carefully logged. What did they find? That 85% of the human milk samples that were tested contained UV filters! Although very little is known about the significance of infants taking in milk contaminated with UV filters, the team leader confirmed that "human milk was chosen because it provides direct information on exposure of the suckling infant and indirect information on exposure of the mother during pregnancy".

There is no denying that sunscreen chemicals can be absorbed into the body. This underscores the importance of carefully reviewing the types of products we use. Using certain products simply because they are more "aesthetically appealing" (such as sunscreen oils or clear sunscreen products) does not mean that it is the healthiest option for our skin. It is the potential issues that may arise after long term use of such products that should be of concern to all of us.

How Natural Sunscreens Are Different

What makes a good sunscreen? It's very simple. It should not penetrate the skin and should never reach the bloodstream. We want sunscreens on our skin, not inside our bodies. A good sunscreen should be non-toxic and non-irritating. We want protection, not additional damage. It should protect the skin from both UVA and UVB radiation. Even though it is UVB that causes sunburn, we want our skin to be protected from UVA that can give us wrinkles and skin cancer.

Do such sunscreens exist? Yes. You will find all those qualities in pure mineral sunscreens containing titanium dioxide and zinc oxide. These old fashioned sunscreens may leave a whitish tint on your skin, but this is how you know they are protecting you. However, even if you use natural sunscreen minerals, never overexpose your skin to the sun. Remember, sensible tanning is your best way to glowing beauty.

AVOID SUNSCREENS THAT CONTAIN THE FOLLOWING CHEMICALS:

Para-aminobenzoic acid

Octyl salicylate

Avobenzone

Oxybenzone
(or benzophenone-3)

Cinoxate

Padimate O

Dioxybenzone

Phenylbenzimidazole

Homosalate

Sulisobenzone

Menthyl anthranilate

Trolamine salicylate

Octocrylene

Octyl methoxycinnamate
(or octinoxate)

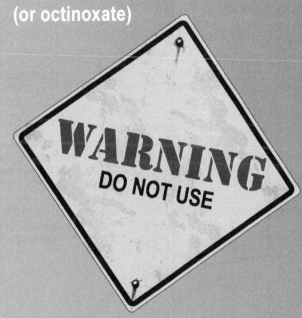

Sunscreen Chemicals Have 3 Primary Defects

They are powerful free radical generators	Their free radical generation increases cellular damage and changes that lead to cancer
They often have strong estrogenic activity	They increase risk of cancer and other medical problems
They are synthetic chemicals that are alien to the human body and accumulate in body fat stores	The human body is well adapted to detoxify biologicals that it has been exposed to over tens of millions of years. But it has often had difficulty removing non-biological compounds such as DDT, Dioxin, PCBs, and chemical sunscreens

How Chemical Sunscreen Oils Damage Skin

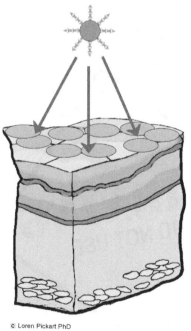

Sunscreen Oils on top of skin absorb UV rays and protect.

However, when they enter the skin it causes damage.

Up to 35% of applied sunscreen enters the skin.

© Loren Pickart PhD

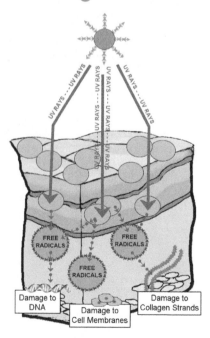

FREE RADICALS

FREE RADICALS

FREE RADICALS

Damage to DNA

Damage to Cell Membranes

Damage to Collagen Strands

APPRECIATING YOUR NATURAL SKIN COLOR

Today's media tries to convince women that their natural skin color is not fashionable. Dark-skinned women are urged to use skin lightening cosmetics, while fair-skinned women are pressured to tan. This can be very dangerous.

The beauty of dark skin lies in its ability to produce abundant melanin, which gives it an excellent, natural defense. Darker skin tones are more resilient and are able to withstand intensive UV-radiation for longer periods of time. When we try to prevent this lovely skin type from producing melanin, in essence we violate it, destroying its fortress of protection.

On the other hand, fair skin often produces little melanin. It evolved in Northern areas where the most important task for skin health was to ensure vitamin D production; UV light defense was not as much of an issue.

So this type of skin should not be pushed or forced into wild melanin production. It should naturally be kept fair and exposed to sun only during morning hours for a limited period of time. Light tanning with a titanium dioxide sunscreen is best, whereas attempts to achieve an unnatural darker tan can prove quite dangerous.

My best advice would be: **Treasure and love the skin you have.** Refuse to damage it with unnatural bleaching or tanning methods. Remember, beautiful skin is skin that is healthy and youthful *regardless* of its color! Being smart about sun means avoiding trends pushed upon us by the media. Find beauty in your skin by refusing to alter your natural skin type and color.

MY NOTE TO HAPPY SUN WORSHIPERS:
To all of you sun worshipers who revere the sun...go out and bask slowly. Relish the sunrise and sunset and the healing power of sunlight...in small cozy doses to warm your sun senses.

YOUR GUIDE

HOW TO CHOOSE SAFER & HEALTHIER SUN PROTECTION

PHYSICAL SUNSCREENS	Physical reflective sunblockers contain inert minerals such as titanium dioxide and work by reflecting the ultraviolet (UVA and UVB) rays away from the skin. 👍
CHEMICAL SUNSCREENS	Chemical sunscreens prevent sunburn by absorbing the ultraviolet (UVB) rays but may increase your risk of cancers of the breast, ovaries, prostate, and colon. Chemicals such as avobenzone, benzophenone, ethylhexyl p-methoxycinnimate, 2-ethylhexyl salicylate, homosalate, octyl methoxycinnamate, oxybenzone (benzophenone-3) are used as the active ingredients. 👎
MICRONIZED SILICONIZED PHYSICAL SUNSCREENS	Micronized or encapsulated physical sunblockers penetrate into the skin while pure titanium dioxide remains on the skin's surface—where you really want it to stay. 👎
UN-MICRONIZED PHYSICAL SUNSCREENS	Pure, non-micronized (and often pasty) minerals are better reflectors of ultraviolet light. 👍

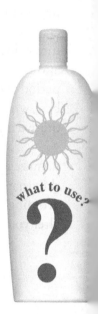

what to use?

?

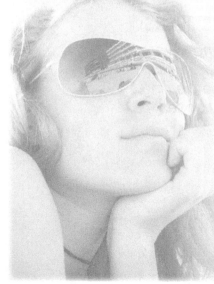

"Friendship is precious, not only in the shade, but in the sunshine of life; and thanks to a benevolent arrangement of things, the greater part of life is sunshine." —Thomas Jefferson

"Live in the sunshine, swim the sea, drink the wild air." —Ralph Waldo Emerson

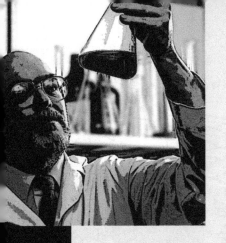

ANTIOXIDANT DISCOVERY In 1984, I observed that GHK-Cu possesses a mild antioxidant activity similar to the enzyme superoxide dismutase, which manifests itself as a calming of red and irritated skin. Steve Aust's lab at *Utah State University* discovered that GHK-Cu blocks the damage-induced release of oxidizing iron molecules from ferritin. Further discoveries followed. Vinci et al at the *University of Catalina* in Italy reported that GHK-Cu blocks tissue damage by interleukin-1.

Vinci C, Caltabiano V, Santoro AM, Rabuazzo AM, Buscema M, Purrello R, Rizzarelli E. Copper addition prevents the inhibitory effects of interleukin 1-beta on rat pancreatic islets, Diabetologia, 1995; 38:39-45

Soon after, Robert Koch's lab at *Stanford University* reported that GHK-Cu shuts down the production of the scar-forming protein TGF-ß-1 by normal and keloid fibroblasts. Interestingly, they also found that retinoic acid, thought to trigger remodeling, actually increases this scar-forming factor.

McCormack MC, Nowak KC, Koch RJ. The effect of copper tripeptide and tretinoin on growth factor production in a serum-free fibroblast model, Arch. Facial. Plast Surg 2001;3:28-32

Canapp et al found that GHK-Cu suppresses the tissue damaging cytokine TNF-alpha (tumor necrosis factor-alpha) and shifts the balance of proteases that dissolve proteins and anti-proteases toward more anti-protease activity.

Canapp SO Jr, Farese JP, Schultz GS, Gowda S, Ishak AM, Swaim SF, Vangilder J, Lee-Ambrose L, Martin FG. The effect of topical tripeptide-copper complex on healing of ischemic open wounds. Vet Surg. 2003;32(6):515-23.

In wound healing models, biotinylated GHK increases the production of anti-inflammatory proteins, such as copper, zinc-superoxide dismutase, that detoxify oxygen radicals. GHK-Cu also acts to detoxify some dangerous products of free radical reactions. Beretta et al discovered these effects of GHK-Cu and proposed that this molecule may be useful in preventing many degenerative diseases of aging such as Alzheimer's disease, neuropathy, retinopathy, atherosclerosis, and diabetes. They demonstrated that GHK binds alpha,beta-4-hydroxy-trans-2-nonenal—a toxic product created from the lipid peroxidation of fatty acids that plays an important role in the pathogenesis of several age related conditions.

Beretta G, Artali R, Regazzoni L, Panigati M, Facino RM. Glycyl-histidyl-lysine (GHK) is a quencher of alpha,beta-4-hydroxy-trans-2-nonenal: a comparison with carnosine. insights into the mechanism of reaction by electrospray ionization mass spectrometry, 1H NMR, and computational techniques. Chem Res Toxicol. 2007 Sep;20(9):1309-14.

ARE SRCPs THE ANSWER? As I mentioned in other chapters, GHK was my first SRCP, the original skin remodeling copper peptide. GHK can provide a way to protect our skin from UV-free radicals. It may provide the answer to a nagging question: How can we protect our skin without applying harmful chemicals?

UV damage is mediated through molecules called Reactive Carbon Species (RCS)—a carbon equivalent of oxygen free radicals. When the UV energy transfers to the RCS molecules, they damage the components and cells of the skin.

Recent studies from Lipotec, the *Barcelona Bioinorganic Chemistry Department*, and the *University of Milan*, found that GHK would protect skin keratinocytes (the outer skin cells) from lethal doses of UV light. **See photographs below.** The GHK binds to the RCS molecules and inactivates them. They also found that GHK reduces the damaging glycation of proteins such as superoxide dismutase. The authors write: "Gly-His-Lys is able to help the natural protection of cells (Glutathione) to prevent the damage of RCS and UVB radiation and acts as a scavenger of specific RCS (HNE, acrolein) and prevents glycation of protein."

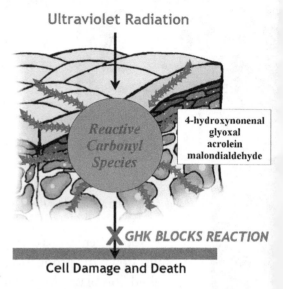

Lipotec (www.lipotec.com) sells products for cosmetic use that uses this technology.

Photographs of skin cell protection by GHK. Courtesy of Lipotec.

It must be emphasized that these results do not directly prove that GHK protects skin from UV damage. We performed a few uncontrolled studies with persons who had very fair complexions and sun-sensitive skin. Most reported that the SRCP creams made it easier for them to suntan and to tolerate sunlight when at the beach or skiing.

The methods that we used are detailed in the US Patent 5,698,184 by Pickart. However, given the current negative Zeitgeist concerning sunlight and skin protection, it has proven impossible to secure support to develop these observations into protective products.

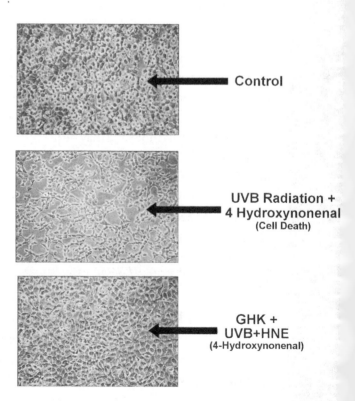

REDUCTION OF SUN DAMAGE Sun damage can be markedly reduced or removed by using a combination of SRCPs and beta hydroxy products and/or retinol. After about a month of treatment, the lesions should appear less noticeable as they diminish in size and thickness. After a week, you may notice a slight flaking of the skin around the periphery of the damage. This is usually followed by a shrinking and thinning of the lesion.

The following regimen has been found effective by many individuals:

1. In the morning, apply a light amount of a copper peptide serum to the sun-damage mark. If you have sensitive skin, start with GHK copper which is very gentle on sun-damaged skin.

2. In the evening, apply a hydroxy acid cream lightly on the sun-damaged area.

3. On alternative evenings, you may want to apply a moderate-to-very strong copper peptide cream on the area of sun damage. Start with a light application. For the sensitive breast and décolletage area, use a milder copper peptide product designed for this area.

A SUNSET CONCLUSION When you experience the joy that comes from the warm touch of sunrays against your skin or admire your own sun-kissed look in the mirror, trust your intuition! Your skin evolved in the abundance of sunshine, and it still has many biochemical pathways that are absolutely dependent on sunlight.

Yes, you should avoid overexposure to UV-radiation, which can damage your skin and accelerate aging. However, you should also make sure to enjoy a moderate dose of sunlight, which can help eliminate vitamin D deficiency, activate important enzymes, improve your mood, and make your healthy skin glow.

To avoid damage from too much sun, sunbathe in moderation, use pure mineral sunscreens, make sure your skin has enough antioxidants, and use SRCPs to further strengthen protection and stimulate repair.

Questions? Email: ghkcopperpeptides@gmail.com

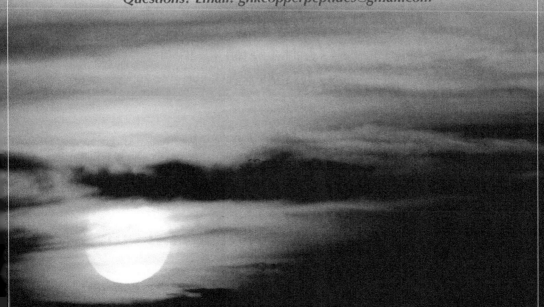

18

AFTER 50 YEARS OF DIETARY FRAUD,
WHAT FOODS ARE HEALTHY FOR YOUR SKIN AND HAIR?

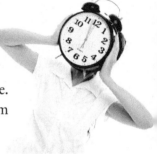

It may shock you to learn that the major dietary recommendations over the past 50 years have probably killed more people than they helped. I am not anti-government, and I am not anti-medicine. Moreover, I will be the first to admit that the great medical care from the University of Washington in Seattle has kept me in good health for many years despite serious heart problems. But the facts cannot be ignored.

Medical and US Government advice over the past 50 years has recommended the following:

1. SALT
Recommendations: Do not use more than 5.84 grams salt (2.3 grams sodium) daily.
Fact: Low salt intake is associated with higher death and cardiovascular disease rates.

2. SATURATED FAT
Recommendations: Avoid saturated fat.
Fact: Saturated fat intake is not correlated with heart diseases. The body needs a certain amount of saturated fat.

3. CHOLESTEROL
Recommendations: Keep your cholesterol below 100 mg/dL.
Fact: People with low cholesterol have lower life expectancy.

4. ALCOHOLIC DRINKS
Recommendations: Don't drink alcohol. It will ruin your brain.
Facts: Moderate drinking (3 to 6 drinks daily) improves the brain's cognitive abilities and reduces dementia in the elderly.

2014   2013   2012   2011   2010   2009   2008   2007   2006   2005   2004   200

My Diet Health Story

Almost all the men in the Pickart family died of heart attacks (myocardial infarction). My turn came in 1989 while on a trip to Europe, where we performed collaborative research studies on human wound healing and bone repair.

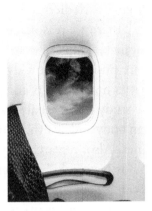

The first leg of the trip from Seattle to Detroit was difficult as the plane tried to avoid a thunderstorm over the airport, but finally the pilot said that we were running out of gas and would have to land. This led to my nervousness, since I remembered a previous accident at this airport two years previous in which 148 people died. The pilot did land —roughly but safely. I was an hour late for my flight to Frankfurt, Germany.

I was also carrying my suitcase by hand along with a bag containing analyzed clinical studies. As my plane was due for takeoff in 15 minutes, I hurried through the airport terminal when I had a sudden chest pain and wondered if it was a heart attack. There was little pain and no nausea except when I ran. I concluded that I had pulled a chest muscle.

So I went off to Frankfurt and Basel for 8 days, then returned home for a week, and finally returned to Europe, specifically to Reims, France and Prague, for another 10 days.

In Prague, a college professor named Milan Adam, who in 1990 became the Minister of Education in Czechoslovakia, took me to explore a mountain fortress built by the early Protestant Taborites. As we walked the grounds, I realized that something in my body was wrong as my chest pain began to increase.

After returning to Seattle, heart scans found that the main artery to my heart had been clotted off. My survival was due to running two miles a day in our hilly Bellevue, Washington neighborhood as this caused my body to develop an extensive collateral blood system that saved my life.

After subsequent heart bypass surgery at the University of Washington, I was put on a "heart healthy" diet with a total cholesterol goal of 100 mg/dL. For the past 28 years, the physicians at UW Medicine have kept me in reasonably good health, and I have been able to pursue my research.

Then suddenly, in 2016, my goal was raised to 172 mg/dL. So what happened to change my desired cholesterol number from 100 to 172?

Why Is There So Much Confusion Over Diets and Nutrients?

Over the past thirty years, advances in nutrition seemed to explode on the front pages of health magazines, in research journals, and in numerous nutrition books. In spite of all these advances, an ongoing debate ensues over what foods make up the optimal diet. Theories abound and often conflict from high carb to low carb diets to high fat and low fat to Vegan vs Paleo.

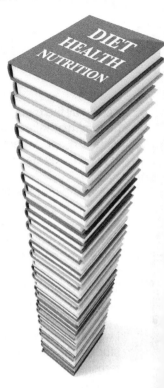

There are reasons for the confusion. First, there are too many quick, sloppy, or even false studies by academic researchers who are pushed to quickly publish large numbers of articles; quality is not a serious concern. It is much easier to make up a false study than actually do the work to help understand the human body and health. Look up "false medical studies" on the Internet. Also, research funding is increasingly controlled by "Old Boy Networks", and new ideas that contradict established ideas cannot get support. This control has made it increasingly difficult for young scientists, who develop virtually all new ideas, to obtain independent funding. Medical exploration would proceed faster if all the research money was given to the young people, and we let the "Old Guys" work for the young.

Can Food Fight Wrinkles?

There are few studies on this important question, but a study from Monash University of Australians over age 70 (177 Greek-born persons living in Australia, 69 Greeks living in rural Greece, 48 Anglo-Celtic Australians elderly living in Australia and 159 Swedes living in Sweden) found a decreased level of actinic sun damage with a diet high in vegetables (best), olive oil (second best), fish, legumes and fruit and low in butter, margarine, sugar, and whole milk products.

Ethnic Greek skin remained younger on a high intake of green leafy vegetables, broad beans, cheese, moussaka, eggplant dip, garlic, low fat yogurt, polyunsaturated oil and a low intake of milk, coffee, meat, pudding, butter and dessert. Swedes did best with a high intake of egg, skimmed milk, yogurt, lima bean and spinach pie and a low intake of roast beef, meat soup, fried potato, cantaloupe, grapes, canned fruit, ice cream, cakes and pastries, jam and soft drinks.

Anglo-Celtic Australians did best on a high intake of sardines, cheese, asparagus, celery, vegetable juice, cherries, grapes, melon, apple, fruit salad, jam, multigrain bread, prunes and tea (Purba et al B 2001). This study also found those with the least skin wrinkling had the highest blood levels of DHEA (dehydroepiandrosterone) (Purba et al A 2001).

MORE ON FOOD & HUMANS: 50,000 YEARS OF DIETARY CHANGES

Perhaps we should take a breath, step back, and consider how human nutrition has evolved since the time of our earliest ancestors. Scientists classify humans as omnivores, who are basically "opportunistic" feeders (survive by eating what is available) with anatomical and physiological traits designed to utilize a diverse diet from both animal and vegetable sources.

Pure plant-eaters, such as cattle and horses, have large intestines with a large surface area designed for the extraction of energy from grasses and leaves while carnivores (who often eat significant amounts of grass), such as lions and wolves, have short intestines that extract nutrients from easily digestible meats. But omnivorous humans have an intestine similar to omnivores, one that is able to digest both plants and meats. Humans descended from plant-eating primates that subsisted on a diet consisting mainly of plant sources (97%), especially fruits, vegetables, nuts, and roots plus about 3% meat.

Dietary Changes Since the Stone Age

DIET	Stone Age	Present Day Americans	EFFECT OF CHANGE
Simple Sugars	2 lbs / year	130 lbs / year	Diabetes, tooth decay
Essential Fatty Acids	Omega-6 is about equal to Omega-3	About 14 times more Omega-6 than Omega-3	More cancer, blood clots, auto-immune disease, depression
Trans-fats Hydrogenated Fats	Very little	High in many processed foods	Damage to cell membranes, more cancer and immunological diseases
Minerals	High in mountain areas with long lifespan	Lower because of processed foods	More heart disease, cancer, and arthritis
Meat	Hunted animals were low in fat: 3% fat	Farmed animals high in fat	Heart disease, diabetes, obesity
Soluble Fiber	High vegetable fiber diet	Low fiber diet	Intestinal problems

GENERAL DIETARY CHANGES

First Human Diets

Then, about 50,000 years ago, humans honed their hunting and fishing skills, adding large amounts of animal proteins and fats to their ration. During this time, diets were high in saturated fat as found in certain tribal peoples still living in more ancient ways (Data from Mercola.com).

TRIBE	PRIMARY DIET	CALORIES FROM FAT
Maasai tribe in Kenya/Tanzania	Meat, milk, cattle blood	66%
Inuit Eskimos in the Arctic	Whale meat and blubber	75%
Rendille tribe in NE Kenya	Camel milk, meat, blood	63%
Tokelau, Atoll islands in New Zealand territory	Fish and coconuts	60%

Human breast milk contains 54 percent of calories from fat.

These early diets may have been the "Most Natural Diets" for humans. In the early 1800s, the people of the Native American horse tribes west of the Mississippi River had a very high meat diet obtained from the American Buffalo. At this time, they were the tallest measured people in the world. Other studies may report somewhat different results, but the high dependence on saturated fat is still found.

Farming, Diets, and Carbohydrates

A second major change came about 10,000 years ago when grains were cultivated by early hunter-farmers. A new grain-heavy carbohydrate diet was born. This provided a more dependable source of food which supported an increased population. However, humans became shorter and smaller.

Sugar Arrives and Alcohol Increases

But perhaps the most deleterious change within the last 400 years was the arrival of cheap, refined sugar from slave plantations. The consumption of sugar dramatically increased, from about two pounds a year during the Stone Age to about 130 pounds a year today (in the USA). In the past, tooth decay was rare since simple sugars were hard to come by.

Alcoholic beverages, often made from sugar or molasses, became more readily available in the last 400 years. Alcohol consumption increased by a factor of 10- to 20-fold in Europe and was associated with social problems but also with an immense heightening of knowledge and civilization.

Modern Diet

The effect of the modern diet on health is very complex. Smoking and prior use of hydrogenated trans-fats complicate the picture. Many think the modern diet has produced or increased many degenerative diseases. Diabetes and cardiovascular disease were rare in the past. Many medical historians insist that modern epidemic of heart disease only developed after approximately 1820. Ancient medical writings from China, Europe, and the Middle East, going back over 2,500 years, do not report the incidence.

FOOD, SALT, SKIN, & HAIR So how does what we eat affect our skin and hair? What about nutritional supplements? In truth, there are very few studies on diet and the quality and youthfulness of your skin. "Scientific" needs for nutrients were originally derived from studies on the type of foods that would enable young rats to breed and have offspring. This was then applied to humans with a few modifications. There is less known, and more confusion, about dietary needs as we age than is generally realized. "Great dietary discoveries" almost always fail in larger, controlled studies. For 40 years, the dominant theories of cardiovascular disease and cancer insisted that excessive dietary fat was a major causative factor. But the largest study ever to ask whether a low-fat diet reduces the risk of getting cancer or heart disease, the *Women's Health Initiative*, found that a low-fat diet has no effect. The $415 million US federal study involved nearly 49,000 women, ages 50 to 79, who were followed for eight years. In the end, those assigned to a low-fat diet had the same rates of breast cancer, colon cancer, heart attacks and strokes as those who ate whatever they pleased (Howard et al 2006, Beresford et al 2006).

For all of today's focus on salt (sodium chloride) intake, which everyone knows is bad, many scientists have questioned this advice. One recent seven year study of 3,861 healthy people free of cardiovascular disease, measured 24-hour sodium in urine (more accurate than a diet survey). It was found that the lowest sodium intake was associated with higher cardiovascular disease mortality. The death rate in the low salt group was five times the rate in the high salt group (Stolarz-Skrzypek et al 2011).

Another analysis of seven studies of 6,250 persons with cardiovascular disease, of whom 665 died during the studies, found no evidence that salt restriction improved survival. But in patients with heart failure, salt restriction increased the death rate (Taylor et al 2011). In studies going back 30 years, 20 grams of salt daily given to pregnant women reduced pre-eclampsia hypertension and resulted in more successful pregnancies (Farese et al 2006).

For 50 years, every medical school taught about the dangers of excess vitamin D. Students were taught that ingesting more than 400 Units of vitamin D per day would cause serious health problems. But today, physicians prescribe up to 50,000 units a day for designated periods to raise blood vitamin D levels, without any ill effects. Once vitamin D levels are reached, many can continue to take 5,000 to 10,000 units to maintain optimum vitamin D levels. Before supplementing with 50,000 units, have your blood tested and retested according to your doctor's advice.

Food Wars—Veggies vs Paleolithic Diets

Vegetarians argue that a meatless or nearly meatless diet is the most healthy. At the other end of the spectrum is the Paleo Diet that emphasizes a version of the ancient diet of wild plants and some meats from animals that the human species consumed during the Paleolithic era—a period of about 2.5 million years that ended around 10,000 years ago with the development of agriculture.

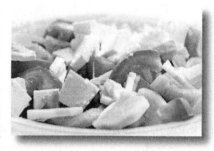

The Paleo diet's intellectual argument is that the human genome adjusted to such a diet during the 2.5 million year Paleolithic period but has not yet adjusted to more modern foods such as grains. The recommended Paleolithic diet consists mainly of grass-fed, pasture raised meats, fish, vegetables, fruits, roots, and nuts, and excludes grains, legumes, dairy products, salt, refined sugar, and processed oils.

As for which is best, there is little evidence. A 21-year follow-up study from the German Cancer Research Center (Heidelberg, Germany) of 1,225 vegetarians and 679 health-conscious non-vegetarians found no difference in overall mortality, although both groups had 41% lower death rates than the general German population. Meat eaters had twice the rates of smoking as the vegetarians. In both groups, smoking increased mortality while moderate to high physical exercise reduced mortality (Chang-Claude et al 2005).

It may be that just being careful about one's diet is the most important. An 80-year study from University of California Riverside of 1,500 people found that the best predictor of longevity was conscientiousness, forethought, planning, and perseverance in one's professional and personal life (Friedman & Martin 2011). Other studies have found the similar longevity benefits of conscientiousness (Hill et al 2011). The fact that you are reading this book means you are already high on the conscientiousness score.

Saturated Fat and Cholesterol

I was at the University of Minnesota in the 1960s where Ancel Keys fabricated the link between saturated fat, cholesterol and heart disease. In addition, the sugar industry funded research supporting this idea to avoid a focus on possible health effects of eating large amounts of simple sugars. The serious question is "Why was this trash supported by the medical establishment for 50 years despite literally billions of $$$ spent on cardiovascular research during that time?"

If you want more on this, get *Doctoring Data: How To Sort Out Medical Advice From Medical Nonsense* by British cardiologist Malcolm Kendrick. Also, Dr. Joseph Mercola has many articles on this on his website, www.mercola.com.

HEALTHY FATS We are often barraged with differing views for what makes up good vs bad fats. To decipher the confusion, we only need take a peek into fats consumed by our ancestors. Today's diet now differs from that of our predecessors who hunted wild game, fished and gathered their food. They consumed a diet low in saturated fat and high in essential fatty acids (EFAs). The foods of early humans contained omega-6s and omega-3s in a ratio of about 2:1. Today, people eat about 14 times more omega-6 fats (mostly from vegetable oils) than omega-3 EFAs. This imbalanced ratio makes our skin more prone to inflammation.

> *Flaxseed oil, an omega-3 fat called AHA, offers health and beauty benefits while maintaining the recommended ratio between omega-6 GLA fats and omega-3 fats.*

A study at Heinrich-Heine-University Dusseldorf in Germany found that daily supplements of 2.2 grams of borage oil or flaxseed oil for 12 weeks improved skin quality in women. Skin hydration increased, and the skin was less prone to irritations. A surface evaluation of living skin revealed that roughness and scaling of the skin were significantly decreased. (De Spirt et al 2009)

Cold water fish (salmon, sardines, herring and mackerel) provide excellent sources of omega-3 fatty acids that are found mostly in fish and seafoods. You need about 300 to 600 mgs daily of the omega-3s which are composed of DHA (docosahexaenoic acid), and EPA (eicosapentaenoic acid). Seafood, grass fed animals, and alpha- linoleic fat, found in many vegetable oils, provide excellent sources of these beneficial fats. Or just take a few grams of salmon oil and krill oil each day.

Omega-6 Fats May Improve Skin But Be Careful

In general, we have too much omega-6 in our bodies. But in many people, the omega-6 fats such as primrose oil, borage oil, and flaxseed oil can improve skin health and beauty. You can take 2 to 3 grams daily of such fats to alleviate skin irritating conditions. However, once the condition clears up, greatly reduce their use.

Saturated Fat and Coconut Oil

I started my research in 1962 at the University of Minnesota where the dishonest anti-saturated fat theory was started. There was a huge fight over coconut oil. Many researchers had found that the peoples in Asia who ingested high amounts of coconut oil had very little cardiovascular disease. But this was dismissed as poor quality Asian research, and coconut oil was banned from recommended food lists.

However, today coconut oils are considered healthy and medium-chain triglycerides (MCTs) have become a popular source of coconut oil benefits. My personal preference is oils which are 93% MCTs as they are easy on the stomach. Coconut oil may make you sleepy, so take it before bed.

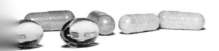

42   1941   1940   1939   1938   1937   1936   1935   1934   1933   1932   1931

MCT benefits are said to include:
- Appetite reduction and weight loss
- Improved cognitive and neurological function with possible implications in neurodegenerative diseases
- Increased energy levels and improved athletic performance
- Improved mitochondrial function and subsequent reduced risk for diseases such as atherosclerosis, diabetes, cancer, cardiovascular disease, autoimmune diseases and epilepsy

THE MEDITERRANEAN DIET: A VERY HEALTHY HIGH FAT DIET

If you want a healthy heart, take heed of the Lyon Heart Diet Study. This small, but influential study was based on the Mediterranean Diet. This diet is based on Cretan diets where men had exceptionally low death rates from heart disease despite moderate to high intake of fat. The primary foods diet included a high consumption of olive oil, legumes (such as peas, beans, lentils), unrefined cereals and bread, moderate to high consumption of fish, moderate consumption of dairy products (mostly as cheese and yogurt), and moderate portions of poultry. Fruit, roots, and green vegetables were consumed daily, while dieters ate less beef, lamb and pork, and butter and cream were replaced with margarine high in α-linoleic acid. The Mediterranean diet is high in salt from foods such as olives, salt-cured cheeses, anchovies, capers, salted fish roe, and salads dressed with olive oil.

The trial consisted of more than 600 patients who had recovered from a first heart attack. They were randomly selected to either continue their present diet or eat a Mediterranean-style diet. Although the Lyon Heart Diet did not reduce blood lipids, it did lower cardiac deaths and coronary events by 70 percent within one year (rising to 76 percent reduction after two years). These results correlated with the combination of monosaturates and omega-3 content of the diet. Blood samples found that the diet increased blood antioxidants (vitamins E and C) and omega-3 fats while reducing omega-6 fats. Surprisingly, those on the Lyon Heart Diet experienced no change in blood pressure or cholesterol as compared to the control (normal diet) patients. The diet also reduced cancer by 61 percent after four years, perhaps due to not only the anti-cancer actions in olive oil but to the variety of fruits, vegetables and omega-3 fats (de Lorgeril et al 1998).

Sugars and Carbohydrate

Be aware that FDA regulations only label sucrose as sugar. However, there are many other types of sugar molecules not identified as sugar on packages of white bread and other non-sweet foods. These other sugars are labeled fructose, glucose, high fructose corn syrup and maltose, fruit juice concentrates, honey, dextrose, lactose, maltose, and molasses, all of which are sugars that are no better than sucrose.

1930   1929   1928   1927   1926   1925   1924   1923   1922   1921   1920   191

Excess sugar damages the skin by increasing **'AGE'** (**advanced glycosylation end-products**). These substances form a harmful waste that can prematurely age skin. They attach to your collagen and break it down which increases wrinkles. Whole fruits, vegetables and unprocessed grains provide essential sugars from complex carbohydrates without affecting blood sugar levels and increasing the need for insulin. But processed carbohydrates such as white bread, cake, potatoes and pasta are quickly broken down and raise blood sugar levels (Bruce et al 2000). When you overproduce insulin after eating too much sugar, your blood sugar falls, and your energy level plummets. As a result, you crave more processed carbs, and the cycle begins anew. Thus, the more sugar you eat, the more you crave as you ride the blood sugar roller coaster.

Sugar May Increase Cancer Growth: The Warburg Effect

In the 1930s, Dr. Otto Warburg, while working in Germany, wrote: "Cancer, above all other diseases, has countless secondary causes. But, even for cancer, there is only one prime cause. Summarized in a few words, the prime cause of cancer is the replacement of the respiration of oxygen in normal body cells by a fermentation of sugar." He discovered that cancer cells have a fundamentally different energy metabolism compared to healthy cells and that simply giving too much sugar to a cell will provoke it to start exhibiting all the phenotypes of cancer.

To sum this up simply: cancer cells grow more rapidly when a person uses more sugar and carbohydrates which are converted into sugars. Cancer growth is complicated, but keeping sugar and carbohydrate intake low may be wise.

Human Blood Oxidations Increase With Age as Anti-Oxidant Defenses Collapse

Fatty acid oxidation products increase as two key antioxidants (superoxide dismutase and melatonin) decrease.

FRUITS & VEGETABLES We should emphasize diets rich in fruits and vegetables. This gourmet garden of delicacies provides our bodies with many vitamins, valuable phytonutrients and antioxidants. A fundamental change in the human diet over the centuries has been the diminished intake of low-calorie plant foods. The colorful fruits and vegetables sold at your neighborhood grocery store provide a wide variety of more than 600 phytonutrients that benefit our health, including terpenes, organosulfides, isothiocyanates, indoles, dithiolthiones, polyphenols, flavones, tannins, and protease inhibitors. Fruits and vegetables also contain carotenoids, a rich source of vitamin A and antioxidants.

918   1917   1916   1915   1914   1913   1912   1911   1910   1909   1908   1907

Dried Extracts of Fruits & Vegetables: Powerful Antioxidants

Decrease in Damaging Oxidations of Body Fats

Alpha-Tocophenol

Lycopene

Damaged Peroxide Fats

Days on Supplementation with Dehydrated Fruit and Vegetable Powders

Decrease in Damaging Oxidations of Body Fats (Based on: Wise et al)[2]

While processed juice contains health benefits, many say that freshly squeezed or extracted juice is better. Fresh juice also contains a significant level of hydrogen peroxide, which some scientists say serves as a natural stimulant to the immune system.

But even dried extracts of fruits and vegetables can reduce damaging lipid peroxidation products in the blood by as much as 75% within one week. Wise and colleagues reported that the daily supplement of 1.5 grams of dried extracts of fruits and vegetables reduced damaging lipid peroxidation products in the blood by 75 percent within one week. Lipid peroxidation products provide an excellent measure of the rate of damaging oxidations within the body. Conversely, protective antioxidants such as alpha-tocopherol and lycopene sharply rose. The fruit and vegetable supplements consisted of dried fruit and vegetable powders obtained by drying juices from apples, oranges, pineapples, papaya, cranberries, peaches, carrots, parsley, beets, broccoli, kale, cabbage, spinach, and tomatoes (see figure to the left) (Wise et al 1996).

Level of Oxidative Damage with Age

Activity by Percent

AGE

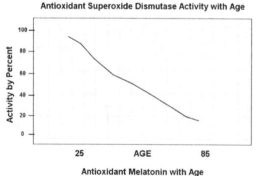

Antioxidant Superoxide Dismutase Activity with Age

Activity by Percent

AGE

Antioxidant Melatonin with Age

Melatonin Percent (100% = 25 year level)

AGE

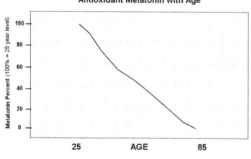

Charts Based on: Linnane A.W. et al

Extracts of fruits and vegetables can reduce damaging lipid peroxidation products in the blood by as much as **75%** within one week.

1906   1905   1904   1903   1902   1901   1900   1899   1898   1897   1896   1895

The carotenoids lutein (abundant in spinach and other green leafy vegetables) and lycopene (found in tomatoes) possess particularly strong antioxidant activity. Another powerful group of antioxidants are proanthocyanidins that are present in blueberries, red grapes, and many other deep colored fruits and berries. This is important because as we age, our antioxidant defenses decline and must be enhanced to reduce free radical damage.

Dietary Fiber

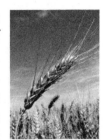

Are you ready for yet another reason to indulge in succulent plant foods? Plants contain an abundance of healthy fiber. One advantage of fiber is that it makes you feel full and does not raise your blood sugar. Most Americans do not eat enough fiber; some nutritionists recommend that we consume 40 to 50 grams a day, but the average American gets only 12 grams. Dietary fiber comes in two forms which provide different benefits: soluble, the type in oatmeal that gets sticky when wet, and insoluble, the sponge-like version in bran, fruit and vegetables that absorbs water and helps to prevent constipation.

Insoluble fiber improves digestion and is predominant in plant skins, husks, and the tough part of plants. Soluble fiber helps reduce blood cholesterol and the risk of heart disease and is found in pectin, guar, barley, and oat bran.

Even though fiber is so beneficial, it doesn't mean you have to run to the store and buy one of the many kinds of dietary fiber sold in a health supplement section. It is much better to take care of both insoluble and soluble fiber by eating more whole-grain foods, cereal products, fruits, and vegetables. As recent studies show, whole grains (such as oats) have much more to add to our healthy diet than just fiber, so the benefits of refined and processed fiber may not be the same.

SUPPLEMENTS: ARE THEY HELPFUL OR NOT? At meetings of scientists who study aging, virtually every meal was started by each person taking out a bag of supplements to add to the food. The best that I can say is that such people do live a long time. Also, supplements such as methylsulfonylmethane (MSM) has long been used to speed hair growth in horses while vitamin C helps synthesize collagen needed for contracting and tightening skin.

Roger Williams opened the door to modern nutritional supplements with his book in 1956, *Biochemical Individuality: The Basis for the Genetotrophic Concept.* Based on his studies on vitamins, he proposed that individuals varied widely in their nutritional needs for optimal function. For example, identical twins share the same genes, but their differing

> **NOTE:** Some supplements can affect the action of pharmaceutical drugs, so always inform your health care provider of your supplements.

894   1893   1892   1891   1890   1889   1888   1887   1886   1885   1884

environments can result in different nutritional needs as they grow older. Some people may require 1,000 times more intake than normal of a particular vitamin to maintain their health (Williams 1956).

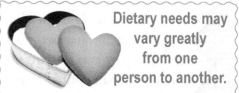

Dietary needs may vary greatly from one person to another.

There is no cookie cutter formula that will work equally well for all.

The great Linus Pauling, who created modern chemistry and stopped nuclear testing in the atmosphere, was heavily criticized for his advice on antioxidants, but worked actively and published research articles throughout his entire life. The first time I met him was in 1965 when his group would hold "Stop Nuclear Testing" banners in front of the Santa Barbara Library every Wednesday. The last time I talked with him, he was taking 17 grams of vitamin C daily. It must have helped; he lived and worked to the age of 93.

Pauling later extended William's ideas with "orthomolecular medicine", that is, the need for the right molecules in the right concentration to maintain health. The key idea is that genetic factors affect not only the physical characteristics of individuals, but also influence their biochemical milieu. Biochemical pathways present significant genetic variability, increasing susceptibility to various diseases such as atherosclerosis, cancer, schizophrenia or depression. These diseases are associated with specific biochemical abnormalities which are causal or contributing factors of the illness (Pauling 1968).

Cassia enjoying her daily dose of nutritional supplements

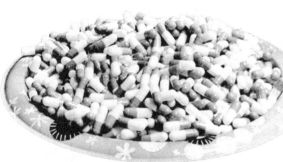

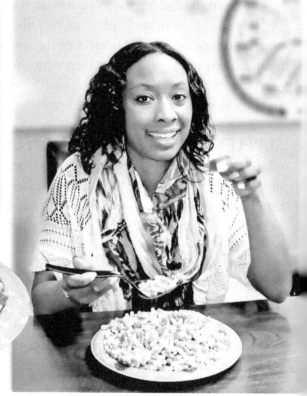

1882   1881   1880   1879   1878   1877   1876   1875   1874   1873   1872   187

RDA (Recommended Daily Allowance) is Not Adequate for Older Humans

The Recommended Daily Allowance (RDA) listed on the labels of processed foods and vitamin products provide the percentage of each of 19 essential nutrients you get per serving or dose. However, most people do not realize that the RDA was originally developed as the minimum nutrients required for young rats to successfully breed. The labeling fails to consider the changing nutritional needs of seniors and those with special diseases such as diabetes and heart disease.

While slight adjustments in the RDA have been introduced to reduce birth defects and heart disease, these underestimate your needs as you grow older. Many vital biochemicals, such as DHEA and alpha lipoic acid, decline dramatically with age. Also, our antioxidant defenses greatly weaken, and cells are more easily damaged by various types of molecules that cause oxidative damage to cells and tissues. As a result, the biochemical balances that produced a youthful body weaken, and this accelerates aging.

The chart on the previous page provides some supplements recommended by experts on human aging. However, take note, that we are all unique with individual dietary requirements. Depending on your health, you may only need a few of these supplements. For example, a person with cardiovascular disease may benefit more from omega-3 fats than the average person. Above all, please keep in mind that supplements do not substitute for high quality foods that contain a wide range of helpful nutrients, some of which science has not yet discovered. It's all a balancing act to find what works best for ourselves.

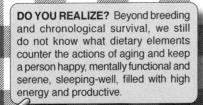

DO YOU REALIZE? Beyond breeding and chronological survival, we still do not know what dietary elements counter the actions of aging and keep a person happy, mentally functional and serene, sleeping-well, filled with high energy and productive.

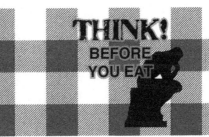

THINK! BEFORE YOU EAT

Not Vitamins, but Vitamin Families

Vitamins are natural substances necessary in small amounts in the diet for the normal growth and maintenance of our bodies. Each of the six main vitamins (A, B, C, D, E and K) has its own vitamin family. For example, the vitamin C family consists of at least seven forms of vitamin C, while vitamin E has four forms plus its closely associated tocotrienol cousins. Vitamin A and beta-carotene are part of a family of at least 400 members. According to recent research, mixtures of vitamins may provide more health benefits than the use of a pure vitamin.

The Sunshine Vitamin—Vitamin D

Make no bones about it: Vitamin D strengthens bones. But there's more to vitamin D than building 'dem bones.' This sunshine vitamin boasts many health claims–some may even sound contradictory. You've probably heard that sunlight may prevent cancer. How can that be when we also hear that sun exposure causes cancer?

The answer may lie with the power of vitamin D. A small amount of sun exposure, which produces vitamin D in the body, can reduce the risk of certain cancers while keeping bones strong. And a slew of new studies suggest that the vitamin offers a lot of other benefits: Diets high in D may ward off diabetes, gum disease, multiple sclerosis and auto-immune diseases. Vitamin D is a powerful weapon aiding the immune system to defend cells, the brain, liver, nerves, intestines, kidneys, pancreas, and skin keratinocytes.

So what is the best way to enjoy the sunshine vitamin? The best source is full body exposure to sunlight for 15-20 minutes a day which produces about 10,000 units of the vitamin. Many researchers recommend taking 5,000 units of supplemental vitamin D daily.

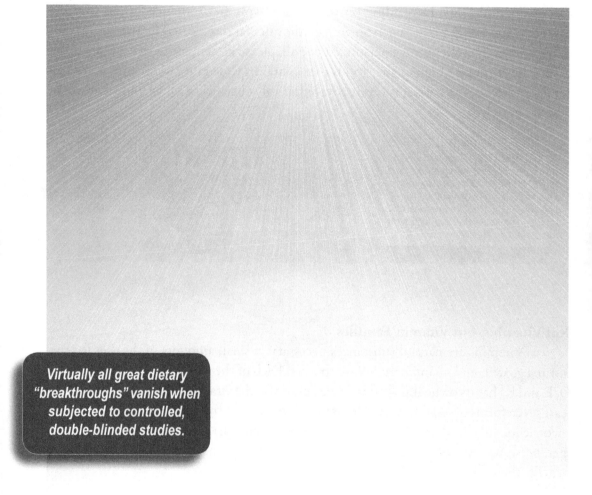

Virtually all great dietary "breakthroughs" vanish when subjected to controlled, double-blinded studies.

Examples of Supplements & Vitamins Recommended by Many Anti-Aging Scientists

This information is to illustrate important supplements used to restore internal biochemical balance. You may not need these supplements. (g=gram, mg=milligram)

	Vitamins & Supplements	Recommended per Day	PRINCIPAL ACTION
PROTECTIVE ANTIOXIDANTS	Alpha Lipoic Acid	30-200 mg	Recycles other antioxidants
	Vitamin C	0.5 to 1 gram	General antioxidant
	Coenzyme Q-10	30-200 mg	•
	Vitamin E family (all isomers)	400 mg	•
	Tocotrienols family	35-75 mg	•
	Lutein	20 mg	•
	Lycopene	5 mg	•
	Grape Seed Extract	50 mg	•
	Vegetable Extracts	1000-2000 mg	Mixture of antioxidants
	Melatonin	1-3 mg at bedtime	Helps sleep, protects brain
ESSENTIAL OILS	Omega-3 Oils	1-5 grams Salmon Oil Flaxseed Oil	See chapter text
	Omega-6 Oil Gamma Linolenic Acid	1-3 grams Borage Oil / Primrose Oil	Anti-inflammatory Omega-6 fat helps skin integrity, joint lubrication
BRAIN AND NERVES	Ginkgo Biloba	60 mg	Improves brain function
	N-acetyl-carnitine	0.5 to 1 gram	
	Choline / Inositol	1-2 grams	
MINERALS	Calcium	1-2 grams	For bone health and biochemical reactions
	Magnesium	500 mg	
	Zinc	7-15 mg	
	Copper	2-4 mg	
HAIR	Saw Palmetto Oil	80-160 mg	Reduces DHT
	Soy Flavonoids	30-300 mg	Estrogen effects
Elements of Collagen and Extracellular Matrix Proteins	MSM	0.5 to 1 gram	For joints and hair
	Vitamin C	500-1000 mg	For collagen
	Glucosamine	0.5 to 1.5 grams	For skin extracellular matrix and joints
	Chondroitin Sulfate	0.4 to 1.2 grams	For skin extracellular matrix and joints
Nitric Oxide Releasers	Arginine / Ornithine / Citrulline	1-6 grams	Vasodilator
OTHER	Extra Soluble Fiber	5-20 grams	Intestinal motility
	Red Wine	5-15 oz	Increases happiness, reduces illness
	Folic Acid	400 mg	Reduces illness
	DHEA	25-100 mg	Increases sexual and metabolic hormones and blocks cortisone damage

1966   1965   1964   1963   1962   1961   1960   1959   1958   1957   1956   1955

Drinking Alcohol May Improve Brain Function As We Age

I never had a drink until at age 18, and in the US Army, I was awakened at 2 AM by a group of drunken, but friendly soldiers who wanted me to taste the Georgia moonshine in fruit canning jars. One does not say "No" in such circumstances. Later, in graduate school at UCSF, I was surprised at the very bright biochemical professors who seemed to live on red wine. They knew something.

Studies in this area are blighted by religious and personal emotional issues. The two best, long-term studies have provided some unexpected results that indicate that alcohol has health positive effects. The Framingham Study in Massachusetts found in 1,053 women and 733 men of ages 55-88, the highest cognitive ability (verbal memory, learning, visual organization and memory, attention, abstract reasoning, and concept formation) occurred in men who drank four to eight drinks daily and women who had two to four (Elias et al 1999).

The Whitehall II study of British Civil Servants found in 4,272 men and 1,761 women of ages 46-68, the highest cognitive ability (five standard tests of short term memory, verbal and mathematical reasoning, inductive reasoning, and verbal fluency) were found in those drinking at the highest weekly levels (men > 241 grams of alcohol, women >161 grams). In men, this corresponded to over 30 drinks weekly (Britton et al 2004).

We do not recommend you drink such amounts, but as you grow older, you may have to choose whether you desire a functioning mind or a functioning body. It is best to drink alcohol slowly. When we rapidly down alcohol, blood can sludge in the smaller vessels due to rouleaux formation as red blood cells bind to each other and form stacks of cells. This stops oxygen and nutrients from flowing to the affected tissues and can produce a rupture of the blood vessels.

Use Moderation to Avoid Excessive Ethyl Alcohol

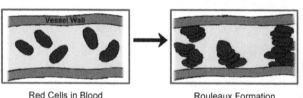

Red Cells in Blood

Rouleaux Formation
Blocks Small Vessels

The best advice is to spread drinks out. And drink some water before and while imbibing. If you are thirsty, it is very easy to drink much, too fast. Sipping drinks intermingled with a glass of water or two slows alcohol absorption.

Luigi Cornaro

But perhaps any advice on diet and health is no better than that from Luigi Cornaro (1467–1566) who was a Venetian nobleman near death at the age of 35 as a result of his dissolute way of life. He modified his eating habits and wrote *The Sure and Certain Method of Attaining a Long and Healthful Life*, which went through numerous editions; this was followed by three volumes on the same subject, composed at the ages of eighty-six, ninety-one and ninety-five respectively. He died in Padua at the age of 98.

1846   1845   1844   1843   1842   1841   1840   1839   1838   1837   1836   18

"I further reminded them of the two proverbs, which say: he who has a mind to eat a great deal, must eat but little; eating little makes life long, and, living long, he must eat much; and the other proverb was: that, what we leave after making a hearty meal, does us more good than what we have eaten.

But my arguments and proverbs were not able to prevent them teasing me upon the subject; therefore, not to appear obstinate, or affecting to know more than the physicians themselves, but above all, to please my family, I consented to the increase before mentioned; so that, whereas previous, what with bread, meat, the yolk of an egg, and soup, I ate as much as twelve ounces, neither more nor less, I now increased it to fourteen; and whereas before I drank but fourteen ounces of wine, I now increased it to sixteen."

Excerpt from: *Luigi Cornaro*

Graduate Student Parties, Wine and the Dean

When I was a student at the University of California at San Francisco, Harold Harper was the Graduate Dean . He took his class notes and turned them into to a best selling biochemistry book. He has passed on, but his book has lived in its 30th edition as *Harpers Illustrated Biochemistry*. Harold was Catholic, prominent in the Knights of Columbus, and would talk to the Pope about science. Harold often told me that I should try to bring science and religion together.

In 1972, the graduate tuition was $345 per year. Harold felt this should be used for the students and not frittered away on faculty nonsense. At the time, I was the Editor-in-Chief for the student newspaper, the *Synapse*. A good friend, Robert Solem, was President of the Graduate Student Union. We decided that to improve graduate student morale, we needed to have more student mixers, so we were off to see Harold about funding the purchase of food and wine. Harold was always generous and quickly wrote a check for the events, feeling it was a good use of tuition money.

If graduate students took a half bottle of wine home to help with writing their thesis, this was OK.

Sophia Ann Custer Pickart

My longest-lived family member that I can find over the past 319 years is Sophia Ann Custer Pickart who died near Winona, Minnesota, my home town, at age 103 in 1926.

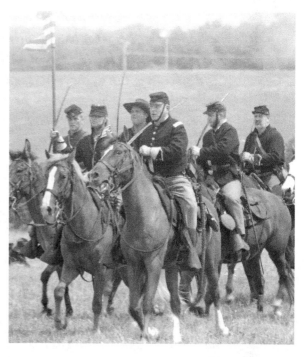

She ate mainly farm vegetables and took care of herself until the day she died. Family records say that on her 102nd birthday, she read the many cards and letters that she received without the benefit of glasses, her eyesight being nearly perfect.

Both she and her cousin George Armstrong Custer had ancestors from the Mohawk Valley in New York.

Custer, in the American Civil War, was a general at age 22 and a major general at age 24. Custer led cavalry charges *from the front* of the horse cavalry and was famous for "Custer's Luck" which lasted until Little Big Horn when his unit was wiped out by Sioux Tribes. I also have Mohawk Nation ancestors from New York.

Questions? Email: ghkcopperpeptides@gmail.com

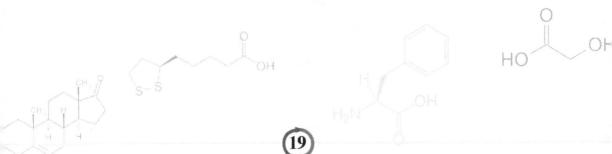

19

THE SCIENCE BEHIND SRCPs
GHK, Human Gene Expression & Health-Enhancing Actions

In 1962, I started my research on human aging by studying the production of the plasma proteins fibrinogen and albumin at the *University of Minnesota*. By 1964, I had evidence that there was an activity in human plasma that would make liver cells from older persons function like younger cells. This ultimately led me to discover the copper binding peptide GHK in 1973 during my PhD thesis work at the *University of California at San Francisco* (UCSF).

However, even though many university laboratories found and published important health positive actions of GHK on the regeneration of skin, wounds, boney tissue, the stomach and intestinal linings, nerves, and so on, GHK was basically rejected by the medical research establishment. At UCSF, I was told that GHK could no longer be researched at the school. My last grant application to NIH was disapproved as "of no possible medical value". GHK just did not fit into the one-dimensional theories regarding tissue regeneration.

In the year 2010, 46 years after I discovered the "GHK effect", what really saved the GHK ideas was the data from the Broad Gene Institute in Boston where the effect of GHK on human gene expression was measured. GHK was found to affect 31% of human genes by increasing or decreasing, by at least 50%, their production of messenger RNA (m-RNA) which is used to make our thousands of human proteins and peptides. When used by university researchers to treat diseases, the Broad computer system is set up to recommend possible therapeutic molecules as useful. GHK was chosen as the best therapeutic molecule from 1,309 bioactive molecules for the treatment of both aggressive metastatic colon cancer and COPD (chronic obstructive pulmonary disease). GHK activates many genes that promise to promote health in tissues of the body and various disease conditions.

Since 2010, research on GHK has increased and as of March 2017, at least 220 companies in the USA are selling copper peptides for skin care.

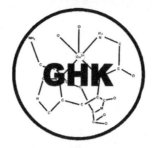

GHK

STRONGLY AFFECTS 32% OF HUMAN GENES
59% UP | 41% DOWN

Stem Cells
• Increases growth factor secretion

COPD Lungs
(Chronic Obstructive Pulmonary Disease
• Shuts down destructive genes
• Restores normal collagen development
• Activates TGF-beta repair pathway
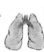

Skin Remodeling (Humans)
Six placebo controlled studies on 270+ subjects
• Increases keratinocyte proliferation
• Improves appearance, firmness,
  elasticity, and skin thickness
• Improves wrinkles, mottled
  hyperpigmentation & photodamage
• Increases skin collagen
• Tightens protective skin barrier proteins
• Improves skin clarity

Cancer Metastasis
• Turns on programmed cell death
• Inhibits cell replication
• Induces growth controlling gene expression
• GHK + ascorbic acid suppresses cancers

Stomach Lining
• Prevents ulcer
  development (Rats)
• Heals established gastric
  ulcers (Rats, Pigs)
 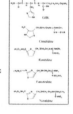

Wound Healing
— Heals:
• Rats, mice, pigs, rabbits, humans, dogs and
  Guinea pigs
— Heals:
• Surgical wounds
• Burn wounds
• Ischemic wounds
• Wound chambers
• Punch biopsy
• Dog paws
• Skin transplants
— Accelerates:
• Increased re-epithelialization, wound closure,
  wound strength, granulation tissue, collagen,
  elastin, proteoglycans, glycosaminoglycans,
  decorin, and subcutaneous fat cells

Intestinal Repair
• Blocks duodenal ulcer development (Rats)
• Heals intestinal ulcers (Rats)
• Heals ulcers of Crohn's disease (Humans)

Bone
• Repairs bone injuries (Pigs, Rats)
• Improves endoprosthesis attachment
  i.e. hip replacements, etc. (Pigs)
*"Produced vivid osteogenic activity at
the interface of trabecular bone and
metal stem."* — Milan Adam, Prague

Stem Cells?

Liver Protection
• Blocks lethal CCl4 (dichloromethane)-
  induced hepatic damage (Rats)

Hair Follicle Enlargement
• Increases hair growth (Humans)
• Improves hair transplant "take" (Humans)
• Reduces chemotherapeutic hair loss (Rats)
• Increases hair recovery after chemotherapy (Rats)
• Increases stem cells production? (Cell culture)

Injury Recovery
• Increases resistance to bacterial
  infection (Mice)
• Increases erythropoeitin levels of
  red blood cells (Rats)

Ultraviolet Radiation

Block UV Damage
• Blocks damage to skin cells

Anti-Pain and Anti-Anxiety Effects
• Analgesic and Anxiolytic actions (Rats)
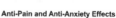

Self Confidence
• Seen in animals and humans
  (Rats, Human cage fighters)

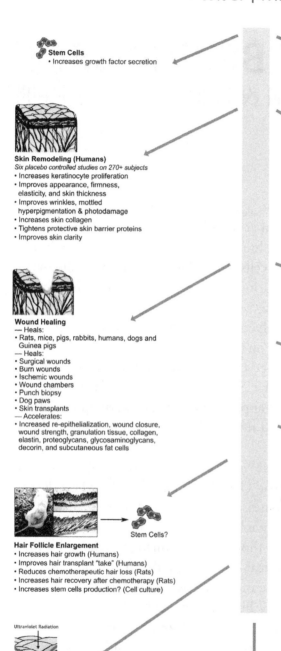

GHK & YOUR SKIN   My early observations in 1988, which showed that GHK reverses skin damage accumulated during aging and thickens skin, gathered dust for a decade. Finally, starting in 1998, more extensive human studies started to validate my observations. At present, GHK undoubtedly has more scientific support data than any peptide used in today's cosmetic practice. Its efficacy was confirmed in several placebo-controlled independent trials:

The best direct evidence supporting this remodeling role came from a series of placebo-controlled facial studies in women that gave evidence of skin remodeling.

◆ Abdulghani at the *Robert Wood Johnson Medical School* compared the effect on the skin's production of collagen after using creams containing copper-peptides, vitamin C, or retinoic acid. Volunteers applied the various creams to their thighs daily for one month. The study found that after one month, copper-peptides stimulated more new collagen production than retinoic acid or vitamin C (Abdulghani et al 1998).

◆ A GHK eye cream, tested on 41 women for twelve weeks with mild to advanced photodamage, was compared to a placebo control and an eye cream containing vitamin K. The GHK cream performed better than both controls in terms of reducing lines and wrinkles, improving overall appearance, and increasing skin density and thickness (Leyden et al C 2002, *University of Pennsylvania*).

◆ In another 12 week facial study of 67 women between 50-59 years with mild to advanced photodamage, a GHK cream was applied twice daily and improved skin laxity, clarity, firmness and appearance, reduced fine lines, coarse wrinkles and mottled hyperpigmentation, and increased skin density and thickness. The result was assessed visually by a trained technician (wrinkles, pigmentation, laxity, roughness, overall appearance) as well as using ballistometer (to determine firmness of the skin) and ultrasound (to measure skin density). The GHK cream also strongly stimulated dermal keratinocyte proliferation as determined by histological analysis of biopsies. At the same time, GHK-containing cream proved to be very safe. GHK complex at 20 times the use level was proven to be non-allergenic. It also did not produce eye irritation (Leyden et al A 2002; Leyden et al B 2002; Finkey et al 2005, *University of Pennsylvania, University of California at San Francisco*).

◆ GHK containing liquid foundation and cream concealer was tested in an 8 week study. It improved skin appearance and tightness, increased skin elasticity and epidermal thickness (Appa et al 2002, *Neutrogena Corporation*).

◆ GHK in a SPF 20 skin cream containing Octinoxate (7.5%), Octisalate (5%), and Zinc Oxide (1.9%) improved skin tone and texture in an 8 week study (Stephens et al 2003, *Dallas Research Center Texas*).

◆ After laser resurfacing, a 2% GHK cream improved cosmetic outcome as measured by greater patient satisfaction (Miller et al 2006, *Facial Aesthetic Concepts San Clemente California*).

◆ Krüger et al confirmed with their pilot study for topical application of copper tripeptide complexes in aged skin an increase in skin thickness in the range of the epidermis and dermis, improved skin humidity, a significant smoothing of the skin by stimulating collagen synthesis, increased skin elasticity, a significant improvement in skin contrast and an increased production of collagen I (N.Krüger et al 2003).

◆ Badenhorst et al reported that after 8 weeks, in a controlled double-blind study, GHK reduced wrinkle volume by 55.8% and wrinkle depth by 32.8%. It also increased elastin and collagen production (Badenhorst et al 2016).

Breakdown-Resistant Regenerative Copper Peptides for Infected Wounds

During early open clinical trials at the *University of Reims*, Bernard Kalis (dermatology) and Marc Leutenegger (diabetology) treated 60 patients and found that GHK creams accelerated healing of skin ulcers (Aupaix et al 1990).

Unfortunately these special creams that I developed, which showed great promise to cure skin ulcers, were never tested in larger FDA clinical trials since the pharmaceutical company funding the controlled study on venous stasis ulcers decided to develop their own formula which failed to reach clinical significance.

A later open study in one hospital used a GHK gel on 120 diabetic patients, after their skin ulcers were surgically excised of dead or infected tissue to reduce bacterial contamination. The percentage of closure of plantar ulcers was three times faster than with standard care. The incidence of ulcer infections significantly lessened (7% incidence compared with 34% for vehicle) (Mulder et al 1994). But a larger study of 530 patients with diabetic ulcers also failed. The high quality of skin ulcer care and infection control at Mulder's *Wound Healing Institute in Aurora, Colorado* apparently does not exist in most hospitals.

GHK-copper and powerful growth factors such as Transforming Growth Factor beta (TGF-B) and Platelet Derived Growth Factor (PDGF) are potent wound healing agents on fresh wounds. But they all failed to be effective at healing diabetic ulcers and bedsores. This was puzzling until some friends from the University of Texas at Galveston told me that their testing of liquids covering such wounds found that they were usually filled with powerful bacteria that destroy the healing molecules in minutes.

My idea was that small peptides produced by enzymatic breakdown would be resistant to further bacterial breakdown. Such small peptides might heal infected wounds if pre-loaded with copper 2+ ions. After testing a variety of commercially available mixture of peptides produced by enzymatic breakdown of proteins, I found several types that worked well on healing and called these Second-Generation Skin Remodeling Peptides.

Howard Maibach's group (*University of California, San Francisco*) tested the second-generation copper peptides in four small placebo-controlled human studies. They found that creams made from the new copper complexes produced significantly faster

SKIN REMODELING: MESSAGES FROM THE MOLECULE

Skin remodeling was once thought of as simply the removal of scar tissue associated with the early stages of healing and its replacement by normal skin. But experiments on GHK reveal remodeling as a far more complex and coordinated process. GHK possesses a diverse multiplicity of actions connected with skin remodeling.

skin healing and reduced redness and inflammation after mild skin injuries brought on by tape stripping, acetone burns (removal of skin lipids), 24-hour detergent irritation, and nickel allergy inflammation (Zhai et al 1998 A, B, C; Zhai et al 1999, Pickart 1995).

In the year 2000, I tested the breakdown resistant peptide copper complexes on infected wounds with a local veterinarian. The creams were designed to virtually "glue" the copper peptides to the skin. Mixtures of peptides have been used as glues for over 8,000 years. Long ago, skin and bones of animals were boiled to produce a glue of peptides. The word "collagen" itself is from Greek κόλλα or kolla, meaning glue.

We tested on dogs after spaying operations and on horses whose wounds (usually from running into barbed wire fences) on the area immediately above the hooves often developed sores in our wet western Washington State winters. The dogs healed about 2 days sooner than normal. But the most important result was that even the infected sores above the horses' hooves healed rapidly, despite the chronic heavy bacterial contamination of the area. No animal was ever hurt in any way, and their owners were not charged any extra fees. At this point, I was slowly modifying application creams for better results.

I was looking forward to setting up new studies on human bedsores and diabetic ulcers. However, the US FDA heard about the studies and strongly insisted that I stop these "unlawful studies" on the animals or face legal actions. I talked with lawyers about this and was told that getting a decision from a Federal Court would cost $2 million. So I had to stop these studies. Medical treatments for diabetic ulcers and bedsores are still expensive, based on primitive science and only marginally effective.

STIMULATION OF HAIR GROWTH
GHK-Cu does stimulate hair growth as was confirmed in animal and human experiments. But more lipid-like analogs of GHK, such as AGH and GHKVFV-Cu give even better results and produced effects comparable to that of minoxidil.

In humans, GHKVFV-Cu almost doubled follicle size after 3–4 months of treatment, and caused an 80% increase in the number of actively growing hair follicles. In addition, hair follicles became more robust and displayed increased DNA synthesis and cell proliferation. In cultured human hair follicles, AHK-Cu increased follicular cell growth while decreasing programmed cell death or apoptosis (Fors et al 1991, Pickart 1993, 2004, Patt et al 1996), Pyo et al 2007) *Seoul National University, Korea).*

Only the surface of what the GHK molecule can truly do for human tissues has been scratched...

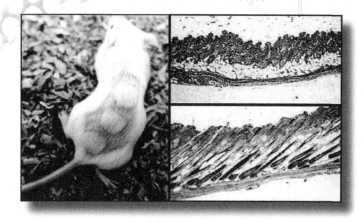

NORMAL HAIR FOLLICLES

ENLARGED HAIR FOLLICLES:
(After injection of GHK-Cu)

A 25 day-old mouse was shaved and injected intradermally in three spots with GHK-Cu. Twelve days later, hair growth was stimulated at the injection sites.

In 1997, Procyte Corporation released a study which compared the hair growth effects in men after using a GHK-Cu analog, "AHK-Cu", with minoxidil. AHK-Cu at 2.5% increased hair count by 97 non-vellus hairs while 2% minoxidil increased count by 73 non-vellus hair after 3 months.

Improved Hair Transplantation

In addition to stimulating hair growth, SRCPs have been shown to improve human hair transplantation. When used in the post-operative regimen, GraftCyte®, a SRCP product sold by ProCyte, results in faster healing of transplants and earlier regrowth of the hair shafts. Perez-Meza (*Mexico City, Mexico*) et al found the GraftCyte® system provided enhanced healing of the transplanted follicles and more immediate hair growth. In their study, patients saw new hair growth in six weeks, versus the normal 10 to 14 weeks. In most cases, skin crusting after transplantation is reduced from 10 to 14 days to five days (Perez-Meza et al 1998).

A second study of GraftCyte® by Gary Hitzig (*New York City, New York*), involving 30 hair transplant patients, found that GraftCyte® reduced the shedding of transplanted hair from 30 percent with saline to 10 percent with GraftCyte®. The healing time of the transplanted grafts was cut in half. Regrowth of new hair from the transplants occurred in six to eight weeks with saline and four to six weeks with GraftCyte®. Patient satisfaction after transplantation rose from 80 percent to 95 percent (Hitzig 2000).

Accelerated Hair Regrowth after Chemotherapy

Awa and Nogimori (*Kaken Pharmaceuticals, Japan*) found that mice pre-treated with AHK-Cu blocked the hair loss induced by the cancer chemotherapy drugs cytosine, arabinoside, and doxorubicin. If the mice were first treated with chemotherapeutic drugs to induce hair loss, subsequent treatment with AHK-Cu accelerated the recovery of lost hair (Awa et al 1995). At Skin Biology, the second-generation SRCPs also strongly stimulated hair growth in mice. To enhance the uptake of SRCPs into the hair follicles, natural penetrating agents, such as emu oil and squalane from olives, pushed more SRCPs into the follicle area.

Anti-Cancer Actions of GHK and 2nd Generation Copper Peptides

A major worry when using cosmetics for many years is their safety. Promoting skin repair and growth activates many systems and could cause cancer. This was found for both Transforming Growth Factor beta (TGF-B) and Platelet Derived Growth Factor (PDGF) which are potent wound healing proteins but also induce cancer in mice.

Happily, GHK, which repairs skin, possesses potent anti-cancer properties. In 2010, Hong et al used Broad Institute's Connectivity Map to find molecules that could inhibit metastatic colon cancer. The Broad computers selected GHK, from 1,309 bioactive molecules, as the best choice (Hong 2010).

Furthermore, there is a control system in cells called Programmed Cell Death which prevents cancers, but the cancer cells turn it off. But Matalka et al demonstrated that GHK at 1 to 10 nanomolar reactivates this system and inhibits the growth of cancerous human SH-SY5Y neuroblastoma cells and human U937 histiocytic lymphoma cells. In contrast, GHK promoted healthy fibroblast growth in their system (Matalka 2012).

Following this, in 1986 I tested GHK-copper 2+ on the growth of a muscle sarcoma in mice using a method developed by Linus Pauling's group in 1983. This involved using a small copper peptide, GHK-copper 2+ plus ascorbic acid (vitamin C), and had spectacular results in suppressing the cancer without even upsetting the mice. But this was unpublishable work because of the hostility to Pauling by "cancer experts". But in 2014, I was able to publish this work with an extensive analysis of GHK's actions on gene expression related to cancer growth.

GHK and Gene Expression in Apoptosis Proteins

GENES	Percent Change in Gene Expression	Comment
CASP 1	432	Caspase proteins activate programmed cell death.
CASP 3	65	
CASP 6	23	
CASP 7	48	
CASP 8	399	
CASP 10	195	
NLRP1	249	Apoptosis caspase recruitment domain
CARD10	173	Apoptosis signaling gene
BCL2L14	153	Apoptosis facilitator

GHK and Gene Expression in Cancer Suppressors

GENES	Percent Change in Gene Expression	Comment
USP29	1056	Ubiquitin specific peptidase 29, May stabilize P53 tumor suppressor
IFNA21	955	Combined treatment of IFN-alpha and IL-21 increases anti-cancer effects
TP73	938	Tumor suppressor
TP63	Uncertain	Tumor suppressor Gene probes are inconsistent; however, TP63 was induced by GHK in keratinocyte cells in skin equivalent organ culture
LEFTY2	935	Inhibition of pancreatic cancer cells
IL25	891	Inhibits breast cancer cell growth
IL15	875	Induces natural killer cells Anti-tumor and anti-viral
D4S234E	731	p53-responsive gene, induces apoptosis in response to DNA damage
MTUS2	474	Microtubule associated tumor suppressor
C13orf18	352	Inhibits cervical cancer cells
ING2	337	Functions in DNA repair and apoptosis
CTNNA1	336	Suppresses cancer invasion of tissues
CDKN1C	277	Breast cancer inhibitor
PAWR	199	Induces apoptosis in cancer cells
APC	195	Suppresses colon cancer
PTEN	165	Cancer suppressor
NRG1	164	Cancer suppressor
NF1	143	Neurofibromin 1
ATM	107	Senses DNA damage
ING4	107	Cancer suppressor
DCN	44	Suppresses cancer growth and metastasis In rat wound chamber experiments, GHK increased mRNA for decorin 302%.
BRCA1	44	Cancer suppressor

GHK and Gene Expression in Cancer Enhancers

GENES	Percent Change in Gene Expression	Comment
ABCB1	-1537	Increases drug resistance in cancer cells
STAT5	-982	Signals cancer cells to grow
FGFR2	-904	FGFR2 inhibitors reduce some cancers
FAIM2	-749	Prevents apoptosis
IGF1	-522	Risk factor for cancer
TNF	-115	May promote cell cancer invasion

Recently, I patented a non-toxic method that appears to remove melanomas in "Grey" horses and basal skin cancers in humans using the breakdown resistant copper peptides (Pickart Patent 2017).

GHK Increases the Ubiquitin/Proteasome Cell Cleansing System

The Ubiquitin Proteasome System (UPS) functions in the removal of damaged or mis-folded proteins. Aging is a natural process that is characterized by a progressive accumulation of unfolded, mis-folded, or aggregated proteins, and this is considered to impair cell functions. The UPS is responsible for the removal of damaged or mis-folded proteins. A well functioning UPS correlates with visible skin benefits. Recent work has demonstrated that proteasome activation by either genetic means or use of compounds retards aging (Pickart et al 2015).

Ubiquitin is also called *"The Kiss of Death Protein"*. It attaches itself to damaged proteins. Then the damaged proteins are taken to the proteasomes, that are like the little garbage disposal unit in your sink, and are broken down.

Ubiquitin
This small protein attaches to damaged proteins:

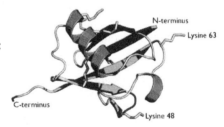

Proteasome
The proteasome is like an open-ended barrel. The damaged protein is pulled in one end, chopped up, and the pieces come out the other end. Graphic of a proteasome:

SIDE VIEW

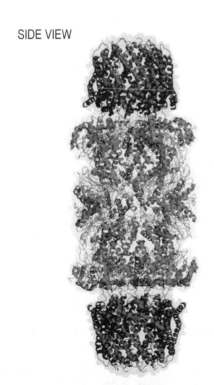

BOTTOM VIEW

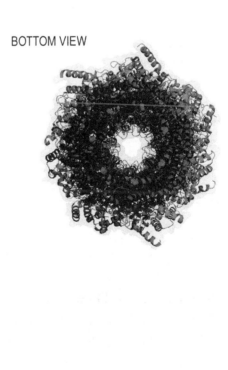

According to the Broad Institute's data, GHK increases gene expression in 41 UPS genes while suppressing 1 UPS gene (at 50% plus or minus). Thus, GHK should have a very positive effect on this system.

Ubiquitin/Proteasome System and GHK

UP	GENE TITLE	Percent Change in Gene Expression
1	ubiquitin specific peptidase 29, USP29	1056
2	ubiquitin protein ligase E3 component n-recognin 2, UBR2	455
3	gamma-aminobutyric acid (GABA) B receptor, 1 /// ubiquitin D, GABBR1 /// UBD	310
4	ubiquitin specific peptidase 34, USP34	195
5	parkinson protein 2, E3 ubiquitin protein ligase (parkin), PARK2	169
6	ubiquitin-conjugating enzyme E2I (UBC9 homolog, yeast), UBE2I	150
7	ubiquitin protein ligase E3 component n-recognin 4, UBR4	146
8	ubiquitin protein ligase E3B, UBE3B	116
9	ubiquitin specific peptidase 2, USP2	104
10	ubiquitin-like modifier activating enzyme 6, UBA6	104

Percent Change in Gene Expression	Genes UP	Genes DOWN
50 - 99%	31	1
100 - 199%	7	0
200 - 299%	0	0
300 - 399 %	1	0
400 - 499 %	1	0
500% +	1	0
Total	41	1

⚛ GHK Repairs DNA Damage ⚛

DNA damage is a major problem for cells. Normal cellular metabolism releases compounds that damage DNA such as reactive oxygen species, reactive nitrogen species, reactive carbonyl species, lipid peroxidation products and alkylating agents, among others, while hydrolysis cleaves chemical bonds in DNA. It is estimated that each normally functioning cell in humans suffers at least 10,000 DNA damaging incidents daily (De Bont & van Larebeke 2004).

Radiation therapy is considered to stop cell replication by damaging cellular DNA. A study of cultured primary human dermal fibroblast cell lines from patients who had undergone radiation therapy for head and neck cancer found that the procedure slowed the population doubling times for the cells. But treatment with one nanomolar GHK-Cu restored population doubling times to normal. The GHK-Cu treated irradiated cells also produced significantly more basic fibroblast growth factor and vascular endothelial growth factor than untreated irradiated cells (Pollard et al 2005, *Stanford University*).

GHK is primarily stimulatory for gene expression of DNA Repair genes (47 UP, 5 DOWN), suggesting an increased DNA repair activity).

GHK is Primarily Stimulatory on DNA Repair Genes

Percent Change in Gene Expression	Genes UP	Genes DOWN
50% - 100%	41	4
100% - 150%	2	1
150% - 200%	1	0
200% - 250%	2	0
250% - 300%	1	0

Most Affected DNA Repair Genes

UP	GENE TITLE	Percent Change in Gene Expression
1	poly (ADP-ribose) polymerase family, member 3, PARP3	253
2	polymerase (DNA directed), mu, POLM	225
3	MRE11 meiotic recombination 11 homolog A MRE11A	212
4	RAD50 homolog (S. cerevisiae), RAD50	175
5	eyes absent homolog 3 (Drosophila), EYA3	128
6	retinoic acid receptor, alpha, RARA	123
DOWN		
1	cholinergic receptor, nicotinic, alpha 4, CHRNA4	-105

GHK Has Powerful Anti-oxidation Properties Plus Anti-COPD Actions

Every time skin is exposed to UV-radiation, it has to deal with reactive oxygen species, and other types of highly damaging free radicals, which can impair the skin barrier, damage proteins and DNA, and cause premature skin aging or photodamage. Most antioxidant therapies focus on one damaging molecule, but an effective anti-oxidant must neutralize many diverse oxidants. GHK acts on many types of such molecules.

The use of GHK-Cu in mice protected their lung tissue from induced acute lung injury (ALI) and suppressed the infiltration of inflammatory cells into the lung.

The GHK-Cu also increased superoxide dismutase (SOD) activity while decreasing TNF-1 and IL-6 production through the blocking activation of NFkB's p65 and p38 MAPK. P38 protein kinases are responsive to stress stimuli, ultraviolet irradiation, heat shock, and are involved in cell differentiation, apoptosis, and autophagy while p65 activation has been found to be correlated with cancer development (Park et al 2016).

Like the lung cells above, GHK may also help as a treatment for the lung cells during COPD (Chronic Obstructive Pulmonary Disease). In 2012, Campbell et al identified 127 genes associated with COPD (Campbell et al 2012).

The Broad computers selected GHK, out of 1,309 compounds, as the best molecule to treat the disease. When COPD affected fibroblasts were grown in cell culture, the addition of 10 nanomolar GHK switched their gene expression patterns from tissue destruction to tissue repair. This led to a healthy organization of the actin cytoskeleton and restored collagen contraction.

GHK also blocks lethal ultraviolet radiation damage to cultured skin keratinocytes by inactivating reactive carbonyl species such as 4-hydroxynonenal, acrolein, malondialdehyde, and glyoxal. This protection was found at a relatively high level of GHK, 20 mg/ml or 0.2 %, but this concentration can be easily added to protective sunscreens. This would be a great improvement over the toxic chemicals used in most current sunscreens.

In chemical studies, GHK totally blocked copper 2+ oxidation of low-density lipoproteins. In comparison, superoxide dismutase (SOD1) was only 20% as active. Free iron atoms cause tissue oxidation, but GHK-Cu produced an 87% inhibition of iron release from ferritin by apparently blocking iron's exit channels from the protein.

Studies of gene expression found more evidence of GHK's anti-oxidant activities.

SEE FOLLOWING PAGE

Gene Expression that Suggests Antioxidant Activity

GENES	Percent Change in Gene Expression	Comment
TLE1	762	Inhibits the oxidative/inflammatory gene NF-κB.
SPRR2C	721	This proline-rich, antioxidant protein protects outer skin cells from oxidative damage from ROS. When the ROS level is low, the protein remains in the outer cell membrane, but when the ROS level is high, the protein clusters around the cell's DNA to protect it.
ITGB4	609	Upregulation of ITGB4 promotes wound repair ability and antioxidative ability.
APOM	403	Binds oxidized phospholipids and increases the antioxidant effect of HDL.
PON3	319	Absence of PON3 (paraoxonase 3) in mice resulted in increased rates of early fetal and neonatal death. Knockdown of PON3 in human cells reduced cell proliferation and total antioxidant capacity.
IL18BP	295	The protein encoded by this gene is an inhibitor of the pro-inflammatory cytokine IL18. IL18BP abolished IL18 induction of interferon-gamma (IFN-gamma), IL8, and activation of NF-κB in vitro. Blocks neutrophil oxidase activity.
HEPH	217	Inhibits the conversion of $Fe(2+)$ to $Fe(3+)$. HEPH increases iron efflux, lowers cellular iron levels, suppresses reactive oxygen species production, and restores mitochondrial transmembrane potential.
GPSM3	193	Acts as a direct negative regulator of NLRP3. NLRP3 triggers the maturation of the pro-inflammatory cytokines IL-1β and IL-18.
FABP1	186	Reduces intracellular ROS level. Plays a significant role in reduction of oxidative stress.
PON1	149	PON1 (paraoxonase 1) is a potent antioxidant and a major anti-atherosclerotic component of high-density lipoprotein.
MT3	142	Metallothioneins (MTs) display in vitro free radical scavenging capacity, suggesting that they may specifically neutralize hydroxyl radicals. Metallothioneins and metallothionein-like proteins isolated from mouse brain act as neuroprotective agents by scavenging superoxide radicals.
PTGS2	120	Produces cyclooxygenase-II (COX-II) which has antioxidant activities.
SLC2A9	117	The p53-SLC2A9 pathway is a novel antioxidant mechanism. During oxidative stress, SLC2A9 undergoes p53-dependent induction, and functions as an antioxidant by suppressing ROS, DNA damage and cell death.
NFE2L2	56	Nuclear respiratory factor 2 helps activate antioxidant responsive element regulated genes which contribute to the regulation of the cellular antioxidant defense systems.
PTGS1	50	Produces cyclooxygenase-I (COX-I) which has antioxidant activity.
TNF	-115	GHK suppresses this pro-oxidant TNF gene.
IL17A	-1018	This cytokine can stimulate the expression of IL6 and cyclooxygenase-2 (PTGS2/COX-2), as well as enhance the production of nitric oxide (NO). High levels of this cytokine are associated with several chronic inflammatory diseases including rheumatoid arthritis, psoriasis and multiple sclerosis (From NCBI GENE entry).

During World War II, physicians discovered that after burns to the skin, when hair follicles appeared at the edge of the healing wound, scar-free healing followed. If no follicles were observed, healing was incomplete and the scar remained. Likewise, when I studied the morphology of experimental wounds treated with GHK, the wound edge was always filled with enlarged hair follicles possessing greatly enlarged sebaceous glands. Yet there was no logical connection between hair follicles and skin repair. Then in 2000, a research group in Paris broadened our understanding of healing skin when they found that stem cells for skin are secreted from enlarged sebaceous glands protruding from the enlarged hair follicles.

Skin's stem cells are its "gold reserve"— a resource for renewal and rejuvenation. When skin is damaged (either by accident or by cosmetic procedures such as lasers or chemical peels), it recruits and activates these hidden reserves, prompting stem cells to multiply and differentiate into cells needed for repair. It was long believed that in aged skin, stem cells undergo senescence, losing their ability to repair damage.

However, today there is accumulating evidence that stem cells in aged skin resemble Sleeping Beauty—even though they appear dormant and inactive, they remain eternally young and can be activated with the right stimulus. Just as Sleeping Beauty needed a kiss from Prince Charming to rise from her slumber, GHK is that Prince Charming, awakening the skin's stem cells.

In 1995, Godet and Marie (*Lariboisiére Hospital, Paris France*) found GHK increases replication of human mesenchymal stem cells (A.K.A. Marrow Stromal Cells) (Godet & Marie 1995). Later, Tony Peled et al (*Gamida Cell in Jerusalem, Israel*) reported that GHK (without copper) stabilized undifferentiated hematopoietic stem cells from human donors or from neonatal umbilical cord blood. In contrast, GHK-Cu increased cell copper by 2,162 % above the control value and increased stem cell differentiation (Peled et al 2002, 2005, Patent 2005). This increased cell differentiation may be a factor in GHK's anti-cancer actions.

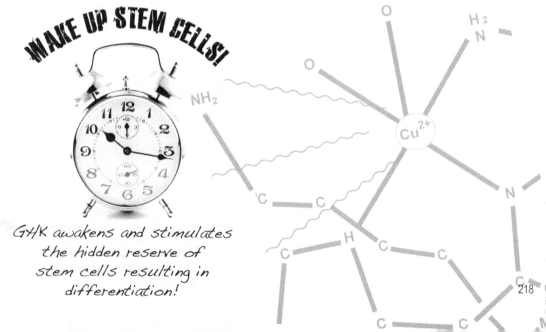

GHK awakens and stimulates the hidden reserve of stem cells resulting in differentiation!

In 2009, a group of researchers from the *Seoul National University (Republic of Korea)* demonstrated that GHK is able to "re-charge" skin stem cells. In particular, after GHK addition, skin stem cells produced more p63 protein, which is considered to be an "anti-senescence protein". They also acquired a shape that is typical for stem cells in younger skin and restored their ability to proliferate in response to skin damage (Kang et al 2009).

These recently discovered GHK effects on skin's stem cells may explain the dramatic, almost miraculous results that GHK based cosmetics produce in aged and photo-damaged skin.

Despite all the hype over stem cells, the reality is less attractive, and the failure rate remains very high. But some recent results suggests that GHK may improve stem cell successes. Mesenchymal stem cells are, in theory, a dream treatment. They are an intermediate type of cell, not too dangerous (e.g. causing cancer) and still able to rebuild organs such as the heart. They also are easy to isolate from excess body fat such as belly fat. But they also have a high failure rate in treatments.

Recently, Jose et al reported that GHK added to cultured mesenchymal cells induced an increased production of critical growth factors needed for effective regeneration, such as vascular endothelial growth factor, and the alpha-6 and beta-1 integrins (Jose et al 2014). This could improve the clinical performance of the stem cells.

HAIR FOLLICLES and STEM CELLS
Human Hair: 98% Vellus Hairs
2% Terminal Hairs

Vellus Hair Follicles

Produces nearly invisible, fine, short hairs on the skin
(4.8 - 4.9 million on body)

SRCPs increase follicle size ⟶

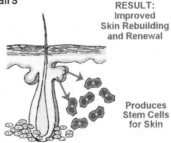

RESULT:
Improved
Skin Rebuilding
and Renewal

Produces
Stem Cells
for Skin

Terminal Hair Follicles

Produces long, thick, visible hairs on the skin
(100,000 - 150,000 on body)

SRCPs increase follicle size ⟶

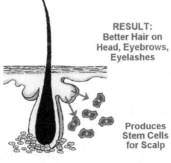

RESULT:
Better Hair on
Head, Eyebrows,
Eyelashes

Produces
Stem Cells
for Scalp

SRCPs increase follicle size, but vellus follicles are __not__ changed into terminal (long-hair) follicles. The use of SRCP facial products does __not__ result in increased facial hair.

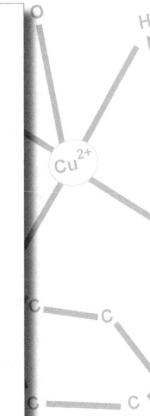

GHK has potent effects on the healing of stomach ulcers and intestinal inflammations. It reduces stomach acidity and increases the production of gastric mucous. GHK healed experimental stomach ulcers and intestinal damage in rats (Pickart Patent A 1988, Pickart Patent B 1991, Pickart Patent C 1992). GHK protected intestinal mucosal tissue from lipid peroxidation by oxygen-derived free radicals (Alberghina et al 1992, *University of Cantania, Italy*). GHK-Cu has potent effects on the healing of stomach ulcers and intestinal inflammations.

Reduction of Stomach Ulcers

Effects of GHK-Cu on gastric acidity, mucous production and the development of ulcers:

Shay gastric ulcer model (95% ethanol) in rats

Dosage of GHK	Stomach pH	Rats with visible gastric	Gastric mucous production
none	2.3	72%	Unobservable
1 milligram	3.8	33%	++
3 milligrams	4.7	none	++++
10 milligrams	6.7	none	++++

Inflammatory Bowel Disease and Crohn's Disease

Ten patients with refractory inflammatory bowel disease were successfully treated with rectally administered solutions of GHK. After the 12 week treatment, there was a 60% reduction in severity as measured by endoscopy, histopathology, and symptomatology scores (Levine et al 1995, *University of Washington*). Recently, GHK loaded Zn-pectinate microparticles in a form of coated tablets were proposed as a possible treatment for inflammatory bowel disease (Ugurlu 2011, *Marmara University*).

Bone Regeneration

Bone

Osteoporosis becomes an increasing problem as we age. We don't know if GHK would help, but it does strongly enhance bone regeneration in animal models (Pickart Patent A 1991). GHK accelerates the healing of bones by increasing the formation of healing granulation tissue in damaged bones. GHK has also been shown to increase collagen synthesis by bone chondrocytes from chickens and pigs, increase the growth of human marrow stromal cells, and promote the attachment of human osteoblastic cells (Godet et al 1995).

Milan Adam's group at the *Medical University in Prague* developed a GHK gel that was shown to promote the filling of bone defects in femurs and bone attachment to cementless endoprostheses. The GHK gel, when used with cementless endoprotheses, produced vivid osteogenic activity at the interface of bone and metal stem. Such gels may aid in the establishment and retention of artificial joints (Pickart Patent A 1991, Pesakova et al 1995, Adam et al A 1995, Adam et al B 1995, Pohunkova et al 1996, Adam et al 1997).

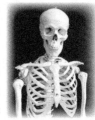

More recently, the combination of GHK, thymogen, and dalargin produced healing of tubular bone fractures in rats at very low concentrations (Cherdakov et al 2010).

Protection of Damaged Liver

Liver Protection

GHK improves liver organ cultures. It also increases repair of liver damage in rats (Pickart & Thaler 1973, *University of California, San Francisco*; Fouad et al 1981, *Max Planck Institute, Germany*; Globa et al 1996, *Russian Academy of Sciences, Moscow*; Kawase et al 1999 A, B) (*Kagama University, Japan*). Researchers at *Kursk Medical University in Russia* found that in rats, GHK increased the replication of hepatocytes (liver cells) while decreasing hepatic immune reactivity (delayed hypersensitivity reaction).

Pretreatment with GHK prevented acute lethal damage to the liver caused by tetrachloromethane (carbontetrachloride), and restored normal liver functions and immune responsiveness (Smakhtin et al 2002, Smakhtin et al 2003).

GHK's Reversal of Cortisone Repair Inhibition

Use of cortisone on skin often results in long-term thinning. It's called steroid atrophy, and the effects may become permanent. Steroid atrophy of the skin is seen as skin wrinkling, "broken capillaries," and skin weakness. Topical cortisone products to the face may also damage your eyes as it gravitates to the eye area. This can cause the cornea to become dangerously thin. Cortisone can also cause cortisone-specific cataracts.

Cortisone also slows or stops wound repair. In my studies, GHK-Cu would reverse this inhibition in mice, rats, and pigs (Pickart Patent 1992).

Suppression of Infections

A testing lab (*Panlabs*) found that GHK suppresses infections (Staphylococcus aureus, Streptococcus, and Pseudomonas aeruginosa) in mice during unpublished safety studies at Procyte in 1989. Later, a group at *Aristotle University* rediscovered these anti-bacterial actions (Liakopoulou-Kyriakides et al 1997).

When fibrinogen is increased, it decreases blood flow through microcirculation, preventing oxygen and nutrient flow to the tissues. Decreased circulation contributes to skin aging by impairing skin repair and renewal, since these processes are dependent on adequate nutrition and oxygenation.

In 1962, I started my research on the production of the plasma protein fibrinogen, which is converted into a semi-solid gel during blood clotting. Fibrinogen was a backwater of research at the time. Today, many studies have found the level of fibrinogen in your blood is the best predictor of mortality and also of cardiovascular disease (CVD). By 1964, I had evidence that a natural factor in blood plasma would suppress fibrinogen production in the body. By 1973, I identified this as GHK.

Studies in Germany and Scotland have found that fibrinogen levels are the top risk factor for CVD.

The Prospective Cardiovascular Münster (PROCAM) study followed 5,389 men for 10 years. It found that the incidence of coronary events in the top third of the plasma fibrinogen levels was 2.4-fold higher than in the bottom third. Individuals in the top third of levels of low-density lipoprotein (LDL) cholesterol who also had high plasma fibrinogen concentrations had a 6.1-fold increase in coronary risk. Unexpectedly, individuals with low plasma fibrinogen had a low incidence of coronary events even when serum LDL cholesterol was high.

The Scottish Heart Health Study followed 10,359 men and women for 2 years, and fibrinogen was the was the single most powerful risk factor for CVD risk or death and more predictive than lipoprotein cholesterol. The increase in (relative risk) between the highest and lowest fibrinogen levels was:

- *301% for men and 342% for women (CVD death)*
- *259% for men and 220% for women (Death from any cause)*

Why does GHK suppress fibrinogen? GHK suppresses the production of Interleukin-6, a main positive regulator of fibrinogen production, both in cell cultures and in mice.

But more importantly, GHK strongly suppresses (-475%) the gene for the beta chain of fibrinogen. A suppression of the fibrinogen beta chain will effectively inhibit fibrinogen synthesis since equal amounts of all three polypeptide chains are needed to produce fibrinogen.

The Brain and Nerves

When skin healing is inadequate, the healed area is often devoid of sensory abilities. In cell cultures, both Monique Sensenbrenner's lab (*University of Strasbourg, France*) and Gertrude Lindler's lab (*Karl Marx University, Berlin Germany*) found that GHK stimulates nerve outgrowth, an essential attribute of skin repair (Sensenbrenner et al 1975; Lindner et al 1979).

Ahmed and colleagues at the *Neurochemistry Lab in Chennai, India* wrote that when severed nerves within a rat are placed in a collagen tube impregnated with GHK, there is an increased nerve outgrowth (Ahmed et al 2005).

When we searched for GHK's gene activation effects on neurons, we came up with 408 genes that were more than 50% UP and 230 genes that were more than 50% down. So GHK has a huge effect on neurons, but we don't know exactly what this means. With time, we will be able to analyze the huge amount of data. Below are the top 10 increased and the top 10 decreased (Pickart et al 2017).

GHK and Genes Associated with Neurons (Increased)

UP	Gene Title	Percent Change in Gene Expression
1	opioid receptor, mu 1, OPRM1	1294
2	protein p73, TP73	938
3	potassium voltage-gated channel, Shal-related subfamily, member 1, KCND1	845
4	solute carrier family 8 (sodium/calcium exchanger), member 2, SLC8A2	737
5	contactin associated protein-like 2, CNTNAP2	581
6	stathmin-like 3, STMN3	500
7	latrophilin 3, LPHN3	494
8	angiopoietin 1, ANGPT1	487
9	synapsin III, SYN3	478
10	dipeptidyl-peptidase 6, DPP6	448

GHK and Genes Associated with Neurons (Decreased)

DOWN	Gene Title	Percent Change in Gene Expression
221	paired-like homeodomain 3, PITX3	-541
222	notch 3, NOTCH3	-547
223	discs, large (Drosophila) homolog-associated protein 1, DLGAP1	-547
224	slit homolog 1 (Drosophila), SLIT1	-553
225	bassoon (presynaptic cytomatrix protein), BSN	-563
226	cadherin, EGF LAG seven-pass G-type receptor 1 (flamingo homolog, Drosophila), CELSR1	-647
227	calcium channel, voltage-dependent, beta 4 subunit, CACNB4	-672
228	necdin homolog (mouse), NDN	-729
229	endothelin receptor type B, EDNRB	-768
230	cholinergic receptor, muscarinic 2, CHRM2	-1049

WHAT DOES ALL OF THIS NERVE DATA MEAN?

Mad Hatter: "Why is a raven
like a writing-desk?"
"Have you guessed the riddle yet?"
the Hatter said, turning to Alice again.
"No, I give it up," Alice replied: "What's the answer?"
"I haven't the slightest idea," said the Hatter.

—Lewis Carrol

It's not really that bad. Young medical
students have 2.5 times more GHK
than medical school faculty. So it may
be good for your brain.

Anti-Anxiety and Anti-Pain

Anxiety and pain are serious issues in patients with dementia and other disabling mental conditions. The clearest evidence that GHK positively affects the brain function is from studies on Anxiety (anxiolytic) and Pain (analgesic) which prove that GHK rapidly and strongly affects brain perception and function.

Several years ago, a trainer of cage fighters (Mixed Martial Arts) called to ask about the safety of GHK. He said that fighters were injecting themselves with 1 milligram GHK for more self confidence, which is the opposite of anxiety.

I thought this was a fad, but later Russian Universities were reporting that GHK had potent anti-anxiety (anxiolytic) and anti-pain actions in rats and mice.

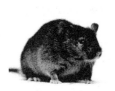

When rats are afraid, they try to hide. But within 12 minutes after intraperitoneal injection of GHK into rats in a testing cage built as a maze, the amount of time the rats spent exploring more open and lighted areas of the maze increased, and the time spent immobile (the freeze reaction) decreased, which indicated a reduction of fear and anxiety (Bobyntsev et al 2015).

The same occurred in a grassy field, where the rats spent less time hiding under the grass and had the confidence to explore the area. These actions were induced 12 minutes after the injection of 0.5 micrograms/kilogram body weight. If scaled up for human weight, this suggests that a similar effect could be induced in humans with 35 micrograms GHK (Chernysheva et al 2014).

Anti-pain effects measured how long it took for mice to lick their paws after being placed on a mildly hot heated plate. Here, GHK reduced pain at a dose of 0.5 milligrams/kilogram.

Studies of GHK passage through the skin by Howard Maibach's laboratory suggest that it may be possible to easily pass an adequate amount of GHK-Cu through the skin to reduce anxiety and possibly pain (Hostynek et al 2010). People do tell us that GHK-Cu does reduce certain types of pain.

A manual search of genes affected by GHK found that seven anti-pain genes increased and two genes decreased.

Adequate copper is also needed in the body for effective anti-pain actions. Opiate peptides often possess both anti-pain and wound healing properties (Stein et al 2013). When healthy human males were fed a low copper diet (1 mg/day of copper) for 11 weeks, their opiate levels dropped by 80%. As soon as copper was restored (with a diet containing 3 mg/day of copper), the levels returned to normal (Bhathena et al 1986).

GHK and Genes Associated with Pain

UP	Gene	Percent Change in Gene Expression	Comments
1	OPRMI	1294	Opioid mu 1-High Affinity for enkephalins and beta-endorphins
2	OPRL1	246	Receptor for neuropeptide nociceptin
3	CCKAR	190	Cholecystokinin A receptor, cholecystokinin affects satiety, release of beta-endorphin and dopamine
4	CNR1	172	Cannabinoid receptor, pain-reducing
5	SIGMAR1	155	Non-opioid receptor
6	PNOC	150	Prepronociceptin, complex interactions with pain and anxiety induction
7	OXT	136	Oxytocin, bonding protein—gene also increases human chorionic gonadotropin

DOWN	Gene	Percent Change in Gene Expression	Comments
1	AMPA 3/ GRIA3	-122%	Glutamate receptor, retrograde endocannabinoid signaling, nervous system
2	OPRK1	-199%	Reduced cocaine effects

Ghk Suppresses Insulin and Insulin-Like Systems

Suppression of insulin and insulin-like genes extended the lifespan of roundworms from 3 to 10 fold. Experiments show that mutations that reduce insulin/IGF-1 signaling decelerate aging and extend lifespan in many organisms, including fruit flies, mice, and possibly humans. GHK increases two, and suppresses six, insulin system genes including the important insulin and IGF-1 genes.

GHK and Insulin/Insulin-like Genes

UP	Gene Title	Percent Change in Gene Expression
1	insulin-like 6, INSL6	188
2	insulin-like growth factor binding protein 3, IGFBP3	62

DOWN		
1	insulin receptor-related receptor, INSRR	-437
2	insulin, INS	-289
3	insulin-like INSL3	-188
4	insulin-like growth factor IGF1	-147
5	insulin-like binding protein 7, IGFBP7	-110
6	insulin-like 5, INSL5	-101

NFkB is believed to be a major factor of the diseases of human aging, with either a causative or intensifying action. Many synthetic inhibitors of NFkB have been tested and appear to block NFkB action but have serious negative side effects.

GHK-Cu blocks the activation of NFkB as mentioned above. It could be administered to humans with a transdermal skin patch and encapsulated in liposomes or taken as a drink with a fruit juice as is done with fragile peptides such as Glutathione (Park et al 2016).

Diseases in Which Activation of NFkB Has Been Implicated:

Ageing
Allergies
Headaches
Pain
Complex Regional Pain Syndrome
Cardiac Hypertrophy
Muscular Dystrophy (type 2A)
Muscle wasting
Catabolic disorders
Diabetes mellitus, Type 1
Diabetes mellitus, Type 2
Obesity
Fetal Growth Retardation
Hypercholesterolemia
Atherosclerosis
Heart Disease
Chronic Heart Failure
Ischemia/reperfusion
Stroke
Cerebral aneurysm
Angina Pectoris
Pulmonary Disease
Cystic Fibrosis
Acid-induced Lung Injury
Pulmonary hypertension
Chronic Obstructive Pulmonary Disease (COPD)
Hyaline Membrane

Kidney Disease
Glomerular Disease
Alcoholic Liver Disease
Leptospirosis renal disease
Gut Diseases
Peritoneal endometriosis
Skin Diseases
Nasal sinusitis
Anhidrotic Ecodermal Dysplasia-ID
Behcet's Disease
Incontinentia pigmenti
Tuberculosis
Asthma
Arthritis
Crohn's Disease
Colitis (rat)
Ocular Allergy
Glaucoma
Appendicitis
Paget's Disease
Pancreatitis
Periodonitis
Endometriosis
Inflammatory Bowel Disease
Inflammatory Lung Disease
Sepsis
Silica-induced

Sleep Apnea
AIDS (HIV-1)
Autoimmunity
Antiphospholipid Syndrome
Lupus
Lupus nephritis
Chronic Disease Syndrome
Familial Mediterranean Fever
Hereditary Periodic Fever Syndrome
Psychosocial Stress Diseases
Neuropathological Diseases
Familial amyloidotic polyneuropathy, inflammatory neuropathy
Traumatic brain injury
Spinal cord injury
Parkinson Disease
Multiple Sclerosis
Rheumatic Disease
Alzheimers Disease
Amyotropic lateral sclerosis
Huntington's Disease
Retinal Disease
Cataracts
Hearing loss
Many Cancers

From Dr. Thomas Gilmore, Boston University
For references, go to: https://www.bu.edu/nf-kb/physiological-mediators/diseases

Questions? Email: ghkcopperpeptides@gmail.com

(20)

THE ESSENTIALS OF NUTRITIONAL COPPER
YOUR BODY'S PROTECTIVE AND ANTI-AGING METAL

In the 1930's, farmers in Western Australia were puzzled, observing a strange affliction in newborn lambs—they would lose their coordination, had difficulty standing, and subsequently died. Later, it was determined that the condition (swayback) was caused by copper deficiency. Australian soil is low on copper. Native wildlife adapted to this condition, but sheep, while grazing on copper-deficient grass did not receive sufficient copper for the lambs to develop normal nervous systems and brains.

Sheep are different from humans, however, copper is just as essential for our bodies. If you look at the list of ingredients of some of the high potency multivitamins, especially those designed for elderly people, pregnant women or for sport nutrition, you will find that they contain copper along with zinc and magnesium.

Many people ask, is there any difference in the effects of nutritional copper and GHK-Cu? GHK and other copper peptides need copper 2+ to be most active. In some studies, GHK alone is active, but GHK can gain copper from easily available copper 2+ (not tightly bound in proteins) in the human body. This is about 10% of the total copper in the blood serum and mainly bound to the protein albumin. There is a chemical called bathocuproine that strongly binds copper 2+, and it totally abolishes GHK's effects. Also, studies of skin keratinocytes found that using copper 2+ (greater than 1.3 micromolar) in the growth medium will not promote the changes needed (more beta 1 integrin, protein p63, and proliferating nuclear cell antigen) for stem cell production, but the addition of 1 micromolar GHK activates the entire process (Choi et al 2012).

UPTAKE OF COPPER FROM COPPER PEPTIDES
Copper is an essential micronutrient, which means that even though we need very little of it, our body cannot function properly without it.

Numerous safety studies in animals have failed to find a rise in blood copper levels after six months of application of copper peptides to the skin of rats and rabbits. There were no negative effects observed in the animals. Use GHK-Cu and other skin regenerating copper peptides to stimulate skin renewal and to obtain other beneficial effects. But you still should provide your body with additional copper from foods or supplements.

How Much Copper Do You Need?

The US Food and Nutrition Board gives the estimated amount of a nutrient per day considered necessary for the maintenance of good health. This is commonly called the RDA (Recommended Daily Allowance) and has been set at 0.9 mg per day of copper for adults. But keep in mind that these are the same people who recommended the now discredited high carbohydrate, low-fat diet that only seems to increase the death rate. They also recommended low levels of salt intake that increase both the death rate and incidence of CVD (cardiovascular heart disease).

Low Copper / Low GHK → **NO** REGENERATION

Low Copper / Adequate GHK → **LOW** REGENERATION

Adequate Copper / Low GHK → **LOW** REGENERATION

Adequate Copper / Adequate GHK → **STRONG** REGENERATION

It is difficult to understand the currently recommended RDA of copper. For example, in 1985 a human study by the US Department of Agriculture found that men "consuming a typical American diet containing either fructose or starch", but low in copper, could not maintain health on a diet with 1.03 mgs of copper daily. Twenty-four men started on the study, but within 6 weeks, four men experienced serious heart issues ranging from heart arrhythmias to myocardial infarction, and the study was stopped (Reiser et al 1985).

In experimental settings, researchers gave healthy volunteers 4-8 mg of copper a day for 1 to 3 months without any adverse effects. Even this high dosage didn't change the plasma concentration (Harvey et al 2003, Turnlund et al 2005). In a multicenter European study performed in 2000, researchers investigated the effect of extra copper on oxidative processes in the blood cells of middle aged people. Again, even 7 mg per day of copper taken during the 6-week period did not produce any side-effects. Moreover, it improved anti-oxidant defense (Rock et al 2000). Chambers et al studied the effects of copper deficiency and excess. This study came to the conclusion that to prevent copper deficiency, 2.6 mg of copper is needed per day. But keep in mind, this 2.6 is the minimal amount of copper, not the optimal amount (Chambers et al 2010).

What is most obvious is that the US Government advisers do not read the scientific literature.

Actual human studies find that 4 to 6 mg of copper appears to the healthiest. Many scientists who study copper and its health benefits take 4 mg daily. Studies in humans have found that daily supplemental copper, ranging from 4 to 7 mg, promotes positive actions, such as reducing damaging cellular oxidation, lowering LDL levels, and increasing HDL levels. Such high intakes may reduce the risk of some degenerative diseases, but do not exceed 10 mgs per day (but even this number has no science behind it).

My best guess is that we need a copper-to-zinc ratio of about 4 to 1, perhaps 16 mgs zinc and 4 mgs copper. Too much zinc drives copper out of the body (Reiser et al 1985). The richest sources of copper are red wine, chocolate, cocoa, legumes, nuts (especially Brazilian nuts), seaweed, oysters and other shellfish, fish, liver and organ meats, well water in certain regions (depending on copper content in soil) or soft, acidic water that has passed through copper pipes. Or you can take 2 to 4 mgs of copper daily with a supplement such as copper glycinate.

Copper Deficient Skin

Impaired collagen synthesis:
Lax skin / wrinkles

Disruption of anti-oxidant defense:
Accelerated aging

Increased glycation of proteins:
Brittle collagen / wrinkles

Delayed
wound healing

Impaired pigment synthesis:
Graying of hairs

Increased
inflammation

 Youth
STEM CELLS

Adequate GHK and Copper 2+
Stem cells are converted to
differentiated cells for tissue repair

 HEALTHY TISSUES

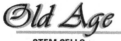 *Old Age*
STEM CELLS

Inadequate GHK and Copper 2+
Stem cells fail to differentiate
adequate cells for tissue maintenance

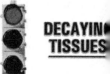 DECAYING TISSUES

COPPER & ZINC   First of all, copper levels may be lower in people who routinely consume too much zinc—this is due to zinc interfering with copper absorption (Klevay 2001). Most people are aware of the importance of zinc.

Of course, commercial food manufacturers use this knowledge to increase sales—almost all processed food products in the United States are generously fortified with zinc and iron. In addition, all vitamin/mineral complexes contain zinc and iron. As a result, people who consume large amounts of processed foods and regularly take vitamin/mineral supplements may actually get too much iron and zinc, thereby putting themselves at risk of copper deficiency.

COPPER DEFICIENCY AND DISEASES   Copper deficiency can contribute to a host of major health problems, including cancer, cardiovascular disease, atherosclerosis, aortic aneurysms, osteoarthritis, rheumatoid arthritis, osteoporosis, chronic conditions involving bone and connective tissue, brain defects in newborns, obesity, graying of hair, sensitivity to pain, Alzheimer's disease, reproductive problems, depression, and fatigue; reduction in the pleasure-producing brain enkephalins, and impaired brain function (Pickart et al 2017).

The first evidence for the essential role copper plays in the human body was obtained in 1928. When rats were kept on an iron-free milk diet, they developed severe anemia. Surprisingly, iron supplementation alone couldn't reverse this condition. It turned out that not only iron, but also copper deficiency, contributed to the observed symptoms of anemia. Since then, copper/iron supplements have been used to correct anemia in malnourished infants (Hart et al 2002). When pregnant rats were kept on a marginally copper-deficient diet, their offspring had behavioral problems, due to copper deficiency in the brain (Prohaska & Hoffman 1996).

The majority of the data on the symptoms of severe copper deficiency came from animal studies, studies in malnourished children, or studies on the rare genetic abnormalities such as Wilson's disease or Menkes syndrome. The main sign of severe copper deficiency in animals and humans is anemia that is unresponsive to iron therapy and is accompanied by severe abnormalities in bone marrow. Other symptoms include low white cell count in blood, increased incidence of infections, impaired growth and low weight in infants, bone abnormalities (fractures of long bones and ribs, osteoporosis, spur formation, formation of bone tissue outside of bones), impaired collagen synthesis, impaired melanin synthesis, hypotonia, and heart problems (including heart failure) (Elsherif et al 2003, Cartwright & Wintrobe 1964). These symptoms coincide with low levels of copper in plasma and are reversed by copper supplementation (Uauy et al 1998).

Another factor that can lower copper is the high consumption of fructose, sucrose, and other refined sugars (Klevay 2010). If you regularly consume foods high in sugar, you may need more copper in your diet.

The popularity of bariatric surgery as a fast means to eliminate obesity also puts many people at risk of copper deficiency, since it lowers copper absorption in the intestine (Ernst et al 2009). But even more marginal copper deficiency often has health damaging effects.

A New *Ethereal* Understanding of GHK and Copper

Controls or influences about 32% of human genes

Increases anti-inflammatory proteins
Increases anti-oxidant proteins

Suppresses inflammatory proteins

Protects tissues from oxygen radicals and reactive carbonyl species

Blocks the release of oxidizing iron

Suppresses bacterial infections

Shifts many genes in aggressive, metastatic colon cancer and chronic obstructive pulmonary disease to more healthy function

Produces biologically younger skin

Accelerates healing of wounds, bones, stomach, intestine healing, and hair growth

Improves hair transplants

Breaks the "Hayflick Limit" on maximum cell generations

Increases anti-senescence protein p63

Blocks proteins that shut down DNA during aging

Repairs cellular DNA damage

Understanding of Copper Before GHK

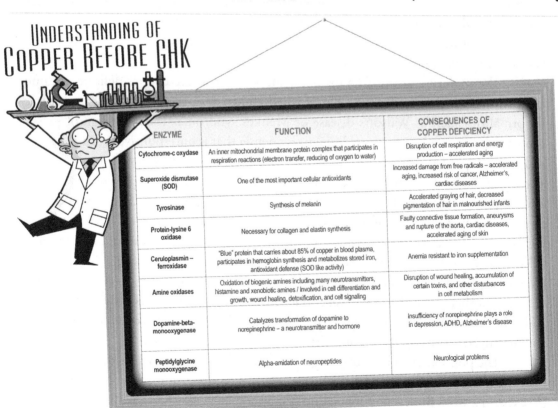

ENZYME	FUNCTION	CONSEQUENCES OF COPPER DEFICIENCY
Cytochrome-c oxydase	An inner mitochondrial membrane protein complex that participates in respiration reactions (electron transfer, reducing of oxygen to water)	Disruption of cell respiration and energy production – accelerated aging
Superoxide dismutase (SOD)	One of the most important cellular antioxidants	Increased damage from free radicals – accelerated aging, increased risk of cancer, Alzheimer's, cardiac diseases
Tyrosinase	Synthesis of melanin	Accelerated graying of hair, decreased pigmentation of hair in malnourished infants
Protein-lysine 6 oxidase	Necessary for collagen and elastin synthesis	Faulty connective tissue formation, aneurysms and rupture of the aorta, cardiac diseases, accelerated aging of skin
Ceruloplasmin – ferroxidase	"Blue" protein that carries about 85% of copper in blood plasma, participates in hemoglobin synthesis and metabolizes stored iron, antioxidant defense (SOD like activity)	Anemia resistant to iron supplementation
Amine oxidases	Oxidation of biogenic amines including many neurotransmitters, histamine and xenobiotic amines / Involved in cell differentiation and growth, wound healing, detoxification, and cell signaling	Disruption of wound healing, accumulation of certain toxins, and other disturbances in cell metabolism
Dopamine-beta-monooxygenase	Catalyzes transformation of dopamine to norepinephrine – a neurotransmitter and hormone	Insufficiency of norepinephrine plays a role in depression, ADHD, Alzheimer's disease
Peptidylglycine monooxygenase	Alpha-amidation of neuropeptides	Neurological problems

Is There Such Thing As "Too Much Copper"?

One of the fascinating things about copper is the precision with which this essential mineral is regulated in the body.

In one study of copper transport in the blood, scientists tried to create an elevated level of copper in plasma, injecting dogs and healthy human volunteers with high doses of copper. To their amazement, all excess copper magically disappeared from the blood shortly after injection!

For example, 50 mg of copper injected in healthy human volunteers (which amounts to 55 times the recommended 0.9 mg of copper a day) completely cleared from the blood in just 4 hours (Gubler et al 1953).

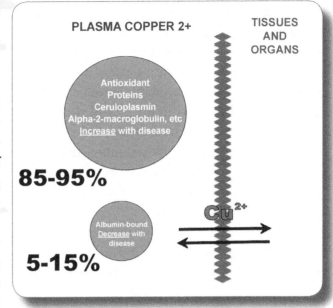

The only dietary source of copper that a person should worry about is in contaminated water, since it supplies inorganic copper, not bio-complexes of copper.

However, nowadays such problems do not exist, unless we are talking about extremely poor quality of drinking water (Araya et al 2001).

As you can see, our bodies are well equipped with a system of copper balancing proteins and peptides that regulate copper absorption and elimination, swiftly correcting copper excess. For the majority of us, the issue of copper deficiency is much more worrisome than that of copper excess.

More Support for a Copper-Rich Diet

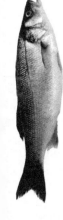

While CuZnSOD requires two metals, copper and zinc, only copper seems to regulate the antioxidant activity. Restricting dietary copper quickly impairs the catalytic function of CuZnSOD in numerous tissues. However, when we supplement our diets with copper, our CuZnSOD activity is quickly restored (Harris 1992).

Animal studies have found that a reduced copper intake increases cellular oxidation which promotes a wide variety of the types of degenerative diseases associated with aging. On the other hand, higher dietary copper reduces cellular oxidation.

CONFUSION OVER COPPER AND DISEASE Many studies of diseases have erroneously claimed that high copper was the disease cause, e.g. arthritis, cancer, heart disease. Deeper biochemical studies in humans and animals have repeatedly demonstrated that this conclusion was wrong.

Nearly 90% of copper in blood serum is bound to ceruloplasmin and other protective proteins. During stress or illness, the body increases the copper-rich anti-oxidant proteins as a protective mechanism. Because metabolically active copper, mainly bound to albumin, is technically difficult to measure, most copper and disease studies report only the total level of copper in the blood serum, which is mostly copper bound to protective proteins. When more advanced methods allowed researchers to measure copper with more precision, it became clear that many major illnesses are associated with copper deficiency, not excess (Sorenson 1985, Sorenson 1987, Sorenson 1989, Frieden 1986, Sorenson et al 1989).

When copper supplements are given to animals and humans, the additional dietary copper has been found to lower carcinogenesis and tumor growth, inhibit the development of cardiovascular problems, and reverse many arthritic effects.

LOW TISSUE COPPER CAUSES:

INCREASED:	DECREASED:
Cardiovascular Disease	Immune System Function
Sensitivity to Pain	Anti-oxidant Activity
Aortic Aneurysms	Energy Production
Diabetes	DHEA
Anemia	HDL
Arthritis	
Blood Pressure	
Cholesterol	
LDL	
Obesity	
Damaging Oxidations	
Tissue Inflammation	
Atherogenic Blood Lipids	
Protein Glycation	
Cancers	
Osteoporosis	
Fatigue	
Psychosis	
Alzheimer's Brain Plaques	
Emphysema, COPD	

DO YOU REALIZE? "AGEs" stands for Advanced Glycosylation End-products. These are substances that form a harmful waste that can prematurely age skin. Copper has been linked to reducing protein glycation. Low tissue copper has been linked to degenerative diseases.

Did You Know? GHK and other copper peptides need copper 2+ to be active. This copper is most effective if combined with the copper peptide. GHK can gain copper from easily available copper 2+ (not tightly bound in proteins) in the human body. This is about 10% of the total copper in the blood serum and mainly bound to the protein albumin. There is a chemical called bathocuproine that strongly binds copper 2+, and it totally abolishes GHK's effects. Also, studies of skin keratinocytes find that using copper 2+ (greater than 1.3 micromolar) will not promote the formation reactions for the production of proteins that are critical for skin regeneration (beta 1 integrin, protein P63, proliferating cell nuclear antigen and stem cell formation). But the addition of 1 micromolar GHK activates the entire process.

So, GHK needs either pre-loaded copper or a good source on easily available copper.

COPPER & CANCER The Centers for Disease Control states that copper has not been shown to cause cancer in people or animals. In fact, evidence mounts daily revealing copper's ability to help fight cancer.

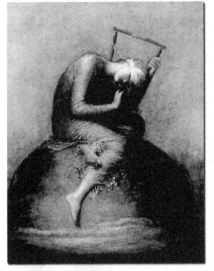

As an example, let us consider colon cancer, the second most deadly form of cancer in the U.S. APC, a gene known to suppress the formation of tumors, mutates during the development of colon cancer. Individuals possessing these mutations develop numerous intestinal polyps (precancerous lesions).

A species of mice that has a mutation similar to APC was studied. As with APC, the mutation causes intestinal polyps and colon cancer. Nutritionist Cindy D. Davis of the Human Nutrition Research Center in North Dakota found that when these mice were fed a copper-deficient diet (20% lower than normal), they developed a significantly higher incidence of small intestine tumors and mass than mice fed adequate dietary copper. Davis says these results have important implications because 80% of the population in the United States does not ingest adequate amounts of copper (Davis & Johnson 2002).

Copper complexes cause some types of cancer cells to revert to non-cancerous growth patterns. John R. J. Sorenson of University of Arkansas for Medical Sciences and his colleagues treated rats which had solid tumors with various copper complexes (such as copper salicylate) and found that this treatment decreased tumor growth and increased survival rates. While these copper complexes did not kill cancer cells, they often caused them to revert to the growth patterns of normal (differentiated) cells.

In another study, Sorenson found that numerous copper complexes with superoxide dismutase activity retarded the spontaneous development of cancers in mice (Oberley et al 1984). Copper stimulates the production of the tumor-suppressor protein p53, which inhibits the growth of tumors in the body (Greene et al 1987, Narayanan et al 2001).

We found the combination of GHK-copper 2+ and vitamin C to possess potent anti-cancer activities in mice. See more in Chapter 19: The Science Behind SRCPs.

COPPER AND CARDIOVASCULAR DISEASE
If we want a healthy heart, we need to control our good and bad cholesterol. That's where copper comes to the rescue.

Human and animal studies demonstrate that copper deficiency increases plasma cholesterol, "bad" LDL cholesterol, and blood pressure while decreasing "good" HDL cholesterol, thus increasing the risk of cardiovascular disease (Klevay 1987; Klevay & Halas 1991; Klevay 1996, 2000A, 2000B, 2002, 2004).

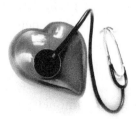

Investigators have found that copper complexes can minimize damage to the aorta and heart muscle following myocardial infarction. Severe copper deficiency results in heart abnormalities and damage (cardiomyopathy) in some animals (Trumbo et al 2001).

A multi-center study found that copper supplementation of 3 to 6 mg daily increased the resistance of red blood cells to damaging oxidation, indicating that relatively high intakes of copper do not increase the susceptibility of LDL or red blood cells to oxidation (Rock et al 2000). Rats on a copper-deficient diet had a decrease in aortic integrity that produced eventual aneurysm (Greene et al 1987).

COPPER & LUNG FUNCTION Copper deficiency causes emphysema and COPD (chronic obstructive pulmonary disease) (Nut. Review 1983, review with no author). In healthy, non-smoking humans, higher levels of copper were associated with better lung function (Sparrow et al 1982).

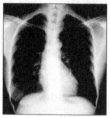

Copper deficiency in rats produced emphysematous lung destruction (O'Dell et al 1978, Mizuno et al 2012). In hamsters and pigs, a copper-deficient, zinc-supplemented diet produced emphysema (Soskel et al 1982, 1984). Copper-deficient hamsters developed lung injury (Soskel et al 1984). In fibroblasts from the affected lungs of patients, GHK at 10 nanomolar shifted the cellular gene expression patterns from tissue destruction to tissue repair (Campbell 2012). For the possible usage of GHK for COPD, see more in Chapter 19: The Science Behind SRCPs.

COPPER & IMMUNE SYSTEM FUNCTION In order to prevent disease, we need to boost our immune system to fight off those pesky germs such as viruses, bacteria and parasites. Copper can help.

A medical publication in 1867 reported that, during the Paris cholera epidemics of 1832, 1849, and 1852, workers exposed to copper salts did not develop cholera. Immune impairment can be detected as early as one week after the start of a diet low in copper; conversely, the addition of adequate copper rapidly reverses the immune suppression within one week (Bala & Failla 1992).

The immune system turned out to be so sensitive to copper deficiency that decreased function of immune cells is now considered an accurate indicator of marginal copper deficiency (Bonham et al 2002).

Human and animal studies show that copper deficiency leads to low interleukin 2, decreased proliferation of T-cells and a reduced number of neutrophils. In addition, even marginal copper deficiency affects a neutrophil's ability to ingest and kill microorganisms such as Candida albicans (yeast infection of the skin). Similar changes can be detected in macrophages (Percival 1998).

Animals deficient in copper have an increased susceptibility to bacterial pathogens such as salmonella and listeria (Bala & Failla 1992). A study of 11 infants with copper deficiencies found that the ability of their white blood cells to engulf pathogens increased after one month of copper supplementation (Heresi et al 1985). Adult men on a low-copper diet (0.66 mg of copper a day for 24 days, and then 0.38 mg a day for another 40 days) showed a decreased ability of their mononuclear cells to respond to antigens (Kelley et al 1995).

Abnormally low numbers of white blood cells are a clinical indicator of copper deficiency in humans, and the functionality of macrophages decreases in even marginally copper-deficient rats (Babu & Failla 1990, Bala & Failla 1992).

COPPER & ARTHRITIS No one likes those achy joints that wake us up from blissful slumber. Copper can help minimize the painful inflammation.

John R. J. Sorenson led the scientific groundwork for the use of copper complexes to treat arthritic and other chronic degenerative diseases. He found that copper complexes combined with more than 140 anti-inflammatory agents, such as aspirin and ibuprofen, to be far more active than these compounds without copper.

Studies show copper aspirinate to be more effective in the treatment of rheumatoid arthritis than aspirin alone. Studies also reveal that copper prevents or even cures the ulceration of the stomach often associated with aspirin therapy (Sorenson 1982).

In 1885, the French physician, Luton, effectively treated arthritic patients with a salve of hogs lard and 30% neutral copper acetate that he applied to the skin over affected

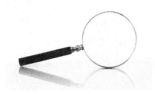

joints. He also had his patients take pills containing 10 mg of copper acetate.

Studies of rheumatoid arthritis exemplify the paradox that has so confounded researchers regarding copper and its effects on various diseases. For example, between 1940 and 1970, patients with rheumatoid arthritis were found to have higher than normal serum copper levels. Similar results were discovered for various inflammatory diseases in both humans and animals. Yet, in seeming contradiction, copper complexes were successfully used to treat numerous conditions characterized by arthritic changes and inflammation.

Subsequent research concluded that an increase in serum copper is a physiological response to inflammation, rather than a cause of inflammation. The rise in copper is due to an elevation of the ceruloplasmin in serum, a protein with strong anti-inflammatory activity.

Copper deficiency increases the severity of experimentally induced inflammation (Sorenson & Hangarter 1977, Sorenson 1977, Giampaolo et al 1982, Dollwet & Sorenson 1985, Sorenson 1988).

Recent studies found that patients with severe rheumatoid arthritis are often copper deficient. According to dietary studies, they typically ingest too much fat and not enough fiber, zinc, magnesium and copper. Their consumption of copper was significantly lower than in a typical American diet (Kremer & Bigaouette 1996).

COPPER & MENTAL HEALTH Brain tissue is exceptionally rich in copper and for a good reason. First, brain health and safety depends on the antioxidant enzyme Cu,Zn-SOD. This enzyme protects it against aggressive free radicals of oxygen, which brain cells—highly metabolically active cells—produce in abundance. Faulty SOD due to insufficient copper can have dire consequences, instantly increasing oxidative brain damage. Besides this, copper is essential for a number of other brain enzymes that are involved in the making of important nerve mediators and hormones (Lutsenko et al 2010).

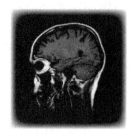

Several neurological conditions have been associated with copper deficiency. Among them is Alzheimer's disease that plagues not only America's seniors, but recently has begun to manifest itself at earlier and earlier ages: 40s-50s.

Copper's role in Alzheimer's has long puzzled researchers. In this condition, there is focal accumulation of an amyloid beta protein, which traps copper and other metal ions. Only recently has it been discovered that copper deficient brains are prone to beta-amyloid accumulation (Hung et al 2009). Another study demonstrated that copper deficiency increased cell secretion of amyloid-beta. The exact mechanism of this paradox is not yet fully understood, but it is clear that copper deficiency may increase the brain's susceptibility to Alzheimer's (Cater et al 2008). Today, there is more and more evidence that copper deficiency in the diet (as well as an excess of zinc) may be the leading cause of Alzheimer's disease (Klevay 2008).

Another neurological symptom of copper deficiency is myelopathy or "human swayback"—a disease similar to that which occurs in sheep grazing on Australian soil lacking copper. Its symptoms include spastic gait or foot dragging and loss of coordination (Kumar 2006).

It is also interesting to note that neurological symptoms often follow bariatric surgery for obesity, which reduces absorption of copper in the intestine. These symptoms may range from neuropathy to encephalopathy and sometimes are irreversible (Kazemi et al 2010).

Human studies have concluded that higher tissue copper protects the brain tissue. In one interesting, placebo-controlled study, 68 Alzheimer's disease (AD) patients (34 control, 34 high copper) were put on 8 mgs daily copper (a high amount) for 1 year. There was no negative finding. Additional copper caused the AD predictive protein marker of CSF Abeta42 to be lower in persons developing a possible anti-AD effect (Kessler et al 2008).

A study of 60 human brains with age-associated brain dysfunction found the healthiest brain areas had the most copper (Exley et al 2012). In brain plaques from persons with Alzheimer's disease, iron and aluminum appear to cause plaque formation while copper and zinc do not (Exley

> **Did You Know?** Most of the body's copper binds into proteins where it plays an important role in biological activities such as antioxidant effects, energy generation, and tissue regeneration. In fact, over a dozen important enzymes in the human body require **copper**. Our brain contains more copper than any other organ except the liver, where copper stores are tapped on as needed. This fact suggests that copper plays a role in brain functions.

2006). Low serum copper in Alzheimer's patients correlates with low cognitive ability (Pajont et al 2005).

Animal studies are in conflict. Laboratory animals are highly inbred, and different animal strains may give different results and may not reflect human results. Two mouse studies found more copper reduced brain plaque formation (Bayer et al 2003, Phinney et al 2003), and one study said that copper salts, when added to water, increased plaque formation in a strain of mice (Singh 2013). But copper is never taken in as pure copper ion; rather, it is chelated to other molecules such as proteins.

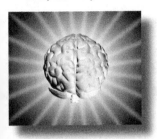

On the other hand, some researchers are rejecting the theory that sticky plaques in the brain are responsible. "The plaque is not the main culprit in terms of toxicity," said Alzheimer's doctor and researcher Scott McGinnis of Harvard Medical School. "If you say Alzheimer's, everyone immediately thinks that it's the plaques that actually cause the disease. That couldn't be further from the truth," Andrew Dillin, of the Salk Institute in California and the Howard Hughes Medical Institute, recently told reporters in London at a conference on aging. "The data actually suggests these plaques are a form of protection that the body tries to put on. So this is a sign that your brain was trying to do something very useful and helpful to you, and the remnant was the formation of amyloid plaques."

COPPER & OSTEOPOROSIS Osteoporosis is a common consequence of low copper (Klevay & Wildman 2002). Two hundred years ago, German physician Rademacher established that copper supplements accelerated the healing of broken bones in his patients.

Inadequate dietary copper causes osteoporosis in humans and numerous animal species. Copper deficiency is also associated with scoliosis, skeletal abnormalities, and increased susceptibility to fractures. Too little dietary copper lowers bone calcium levels.

A study of elderly subjects found a decreased loss of bone-mineral density from the lumbar spine after copper supplementation of 3 mg daily for two years. Healthy adult males on a low-copper intake (0.7 mgs daily) for six weeks exhibited an increased rate of bone breakdown (Dollwet & Sorenson 1988, Conlan et al 1990, Janas et al 1993, Baker et al 1999).

ULCER HEALING ACTIVITIES OF COPPER COMPLEXES Gastric ulcers are no fun—especially when they give you a stomach ache and kill the pleasure of a hot spicy meal. So next time, add some copper rich oysters, and perhaps you'll ward off ulcers.

Studies demonstrate that copper complexes, such as copper aspirinate and copper tryptophanate, markedly increase the healing rate of gastric ulcers while non-steroidal anti-inflammatory drugs, such as ibuprofen and enefenamic acid, suppress ulcer healing.

As a result, these copper complexes promote normal wound healing while at the same time retaining anti-inflammatory activity (Sorenson & Hangartes 1977, Sorenson 1977, Dollwet & Sorenson 1985, Sorenson 1988, Sorenson et al 1982, Alzuet et al 1994, Morgant et al 2000, Lemoine et al 2002, Viossat et al 2005).

ANTI-CONVULSANT ACTIVITIES OF COPPER COMPLEXES It is important to remember that the brain contains more copper than any other organ with the exception of the liver. This is where copper reserves are tapped into as it is needed by the body. This fact suggests that copper plays a role in brain function.

Since humans and animals are prone to brain seizures when deficient in copper, studies have shown anti-convulsant drugs to more effectively prevent seizures when complexed with copper.

COPPER & PREGNANCY Research at the US Department of Agriculture's Grand Forks Human Nutrition Research Center found that even marginal copper deficiency in pregnant rats produces brain damage and neurological defects in their offspring.

The copper-deficient newborn rats have structural abnormalities in the areas of the brain involved in learning and memory and those responsible for coordination and movement. These abnormalities resulted in behavioral changes; for example, the young rats lacked the normal startle reflex as a response to unexpected noises. The copper deficit permanently affected the young rats and could not be corrected by a high-copper diet.

Another study reported that copper deficiency during pregnancy can result in numerous gross structural and biochemical abnormalities, which seem to arise because the copper deficiency reduces free radical defense mechanisms, connective tissue metabolism, and energy production (Ebbs et al 1941, Morten et al 1976, Keen et al 1998, Lonnerdal 1998, Hawk et al 2003, Penland & Prohaska 2004).

DOES THE COPPER IN WINE HELP THE FRENCH LIVE LONGER?
The French enjoy fine wine, fine dining and live long, happy lives. It is indeed a 'French Paradox' that they have healthy hearts while enjoying buttery croissants, Bernaise sauce, and mouth watering Duck A L'Orange—all dripping with fats. Red wine contains an abundance of copper. The copper in wine comes from the skin of the grapes which retain copper from the sulfates used by French vintners. Red wine from France contains about 0.2 mg of copper per liter. So go pour yourself a glass from the wine fountain of youth. Isn't it nice to know you may be sipping your way to a longer life?

COPPER & LOVE This magic molecule not only provides a door to the future but also offers a window to the past. Ancients believed in copper's power to heal. They wrote that copper was the metal of healing and of love. Throughout this chapter, we have assessed the healing properties of copper—the power of this metal elixir. However, according to the ancients, copper not only heals, it is also the metal of love. Is this mythology? Maybe not.

Today's research has confirmed that copper attracts the molecules that make us feel euphoric pleasure by releasing endorphins. Chemically speaking, love translates into endorphins, serotonin, dopamine, oxytocin, and other brain chemicals. Increased tissue copper has been found to increase brain enkephalins (Bhathena et al 1986). Sorenson determined that copper complexes reduce pain and may activate opioid receptors (Okuyama et al 1987).

Not surprisingly, copper deficiency (even if marginal) can alter the balance of brain chemicals. When healthy males were fed a low copper diet (1 mg per day) for 11 weeks, their plasma opiates level dropped by 80%. As soon as copper was restored (with a diet containing 3 mg per day), it returned to normal (Bhathena et al 1986).

Copper not only contributes to euphoric attraction, it can also play a part in sustaining relationships. During early stages of romantic love, the blood level of NGF (Nerve Growth Factor) nearly doubles. It was also apparent that those who reported the most intense feelings also had the highest NGF levels. But NGF then declines over a year's time as passion cools. In wound models, GHK-Cu increases production of NGF.

In addition to feel-good endorphins and NGF levels enhanced by copper, sexual hormones can also boost our sex drives. The hormone DHEA works well with copper to both increase our interest in sex and to lower stress. DHEA converts into the sexual hormones, testosterone and estrogen, which not only promote sex drive but protect against the damaging actions of cortisol.

DHEA levels sharply decrease with age while cortisol remains relatively constant. Too much cortisol can result in physical problems and stress-related illnesses. The combination of too much stress and decreased sexual hormones can dampen our mood for romance. DHEA is widely used as a dietary supplement to help prevent deleterious changes that occur with age. Klevay and Christopherson found that copper deficiency in rats decreased DHEA in serum by approximately 50 percent. The researchers suggest that eating a higher-copper diet increases the DHEA level in the body (Klevay & Christopherson 2000).

So what about the Metal of Love? While an endorphin-induced sense of euphoric pleasure, coupled with feeling less stress and high personal sexual hormones, may not be love, it is still a good approximation.

THE MORAL NEED FOR BEAUTY
"My Skin Is My Hobby" — Why We Obsess Over Skincare

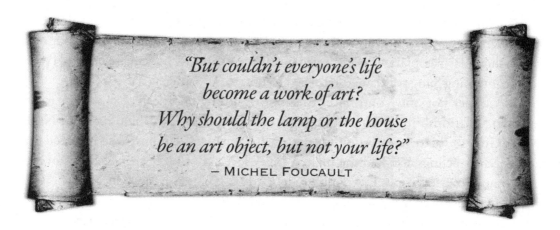

*"But couldn't everyone's life
become a work of art?
Why should the lamp or the house
be an art object, but not your life?"*
— MICHEL FOUCAULT

Do you delight in your quest for beauty, or do you feel vain? I once knew a woman who lamented with me in jest. As she applied shiny lacquer to plump her lips, she laughed: "I'm vain. I sit here at my vanity table full of vanity items and primp myself in vain." And indeed her vanity table was adorned with exotic bottles of colorful lotions and cosmetic potions (many of which were useless concoctions as we've discussed earlier).

However, I assured her that her quest for beautiful skin and hair was not only natural, it was a moral need that she inherited from women throughout the ages. It was in her genes. And like many people, she was a bit embarrassed about the price tag of her costly cosmetics. Maybe this was what Shakespeare meant by "unthrifty loveliness" in Sonnet 4. "I feel shallow," she added. However that didn't stop her from applying a lavish coat of mascara. I reassured her that there was nothing shallow about the quest for beauty.

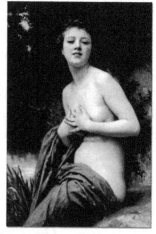

Women decorate their homes and receive praise, yet they feel uncomfortable, even a bit embarrassed, about the many hours they spend primping and pruning to look their best. The pursuit of beauty is nothing to be ashamed of.

After all, glowing skin and shiny hair have always been linked with good health. So in a sense, the quest for beauty is really the quest for health in all its wonderful aspects. Good health aside, who can deny the pleasure we receive as we gaze upon men and women who put themselves together well? It's not about looking like a supermodel but rather about taking the time to enhance your own unique assets, to look and feel your very best. It may take a little time, but aren't you worth it?

COSMETICS, JEWELRY, TECHNOLOGY, ART, AND SYMBOLISM

So OK, maybe your vanity table brims over with a plethora of lipsticks, mascara, blushers, foundation, nail polish, dream creams, perfume, and oh so many other products. Dare I say more? It can be a challenge just to sort through this colorful stockpile, let alone actually make yourself up. But don't let that turn into unease about your personal vanity.

There are those in our society who equate the obsession with self-beauty as some type of moral defect or evil. On the contrary, to deeply care about the beauty of the human body is an essential part of a tight matrix of behaviors that bring out the best in human nature. The most valued possessions of early humans were cosmetic body paints such as red ochre (a form of iron ore), jewelry such as necklaces made from small seashells or fox teeth, a technology that created finely crafted tools such as arrowheads, spear points, implements for food preparation and sewing, symbolic figurative art objects, and geometric forms. The behaviors that created these objects rose from the deepest recesses of the human psyche. We cannot function properly without them. Red lipstick and computer microprocessors arise from the same deep human drives and needs.

The human body itself has been a vessel for artistic expression for hundreds of thousands of years. In all civilizations where art, science, and culture have flourished, women and men found ways to embellish their beauty. And like poetry, which reveals inner truth through metaphor, outer beauty can reflect the beauty within. It's our moral right and need to look and feel our best.

It's In Your Genes

Mutual grooming, rubbing, and caressing of skin thrive amongst all social beings. Some birds and primates spend up to 90 percent of their time grooming themselves or others. We humans also love the rub—that special sprucing touch. We share an innate drive for beauty buried deep in our genes. When a masseuse melts your stress away, when you receive an amazing manicure, spend a day adding waves to your hair, or pamper yourself with beauty and pleasure, your body increases its level of "happiness hormones." These endorphins

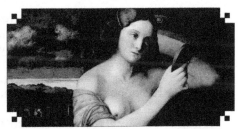

All early human cultures were obsessed with personal beauty.

enhance your sense of well being. To skyrocket this happiness several notches higher, have someone else groom you. Being pampered by another heightens the pleasure by increasing endorphins even further.

All early human cultures were obsessed with personal beauty. Many presented their bodies as a colorful palette. They painted their skin and pierced various body parts, some inserting bones, feathers, and shells in the punctured skin. Young and old alike decorated their bodies.

Ninety-nine percent of our ancestors lived in small, nomadic bands of hunters and gatherers, and our psychological drives still reflect this. In ancient times, physical attributes and body decor attracted partners, contributing to the reproduction of our species.

Our ancestors were drawn to smooth skin, lush and shiny hair, and bodies often adorned with body art. These qualities continue to appeal today and guarantee the future of our species.

BODY PAINTING: THE FIRST MAKE-UP
The first make-up, body painting, depicts a fundamental behavior driven by the deep desire for luxury and beauty. Body art is not just the latest fashion. In fact, if the impulse to create art is one of the defining signs of humanity, the body may well have been the first canvas.

• Archaeological findings suggest Japanese inhabitants were already decorating their bodies in the Neolithic Jomon period (c.10,000-300 B.C.E.).

• In Egypt, during the time of the pharaohs, upper-class women used face powders and other make-up, perfume, paintbrushes, and polished silver or copper mirrors.

• For thousands of years, Maasai warriors applied body decoration and art to express their cultural characteristics.

• In Papua, New Guinea, traditional ceremonial face paint consists of black powdered charcoal. The Huli Wigmen, who live in vibrant valleys, accentuate the nose and mouth with bright colors and apply white clay to emphasize the eye and beard.

• In ancient Athens, noblewomen and courtesans applied white lead carbonate hydroxide foundation with brushes. The Roman poet Ovid wrote that the naked breasts of the Greek women were "rosy buds enhanced with a tincture of gold."

• The ancient Celts wore blue body paint from "woad," a type of mustard plant.

• Native Americans used pigments of brown, red, yellow, black, blue, green and white.

• In India, extracts of henna plant have been used for centuries as a reddish-yellow hair dye and to decorate the hands and feet.

• In China, during the Chou dynasty of 600 B.C.E., members of the emperor's family wore gold and silver nail polish. Later, these colors changed to red and black. Well-manicured nails represented the difference between the aristocrats and the working classes.

• In an ancient Peruvian grave, a mummified woman was found perfectly preserved with her light brown hair carefully combed and braided. Her legs, from knee to ankle, were painted red, as was the fashion for beauties of Peru in her time. Buried along with her was her toilet powder (a fine powder, perhaps scented, for spreading on the body after bathing) for use in the afterlife.

Cultures dating back at least 285,000 years collected red ochre. In Africa, people have worn necklaces and painted their bodies for more than 75,000 years. Skeletons sprinkled with red ochre and found in graves date as far back as the Paleolithic Period, when ice sheets covered Northern Europe and hunters and gatherers roamed the landscape. This ancient burial ritual suggests that body painting already had a long-established practice among the living. Minerals from the earth, chiefly ochre in shades ranging from red to yellow and pyrolusite (manganese) in shades of black and white, were used as pigments. The examples on the previous page illustrate the practice of body painting recorded throughout the world.

THE ANCIENT ART OF TATTOO The legacy of the tattoo originated over thousands of years ago. The word tattoo stems from the Tahitian word "tatau," meaning to inflict wounds.

In the centuries before modern-day tattoo needles, the tattooing process required enduring considerable pain and sometimes took several years to complete. The risk of death by infection loomed as a great concern. Yet, devotees paid this painfully high price for beauty and acceptance. Tribal tattoos marked rites of passage such as puberty, marriage, or a first successful hunt. In Polynesia, tattoo patterns symbolized prosperity and conferred prestige. The following illustrates additional examples of the art of tattoo throughout history:

• In 1000 B.C.E., Egyptian and Nubian dancers were tattooed on the thigh and pubic areas.

• Japanese aristocrats distinguished themselves with tiny tattoos near the eye. Japanese tattooists followed the lines of the muscle movements so that when the person moved, the pictures would "come alive."

• Roman soldiers gave the name "Picts" to Gallic warriors who went to battle naked in order to display their fearsome tattoos.

• The Maoris of New Zealand reserved tattoos for both nobles and free people.

QUOTABLE QUOTES: *Not one great country can be named, from the polar regions in the north to New Zealand in the south, in which the aboriginals do not tattoo themselves.* —Charles Darwin, *Voyage of the Beagle*

The First Beauty Parlors

Paleolithic statues show elaborate hair styling and braiding dating back more than 30,000 years. Early cultures worldwide used elaborate top-knots, braids, and other forms of hair styling to attract others. Roman women washed their hair with bleach made from dried nuts and acid, hoping to turn it yellow. In the 1700's, French hairstyles often topped four feet, and the women used wool, paste, glue, and wires to hold their hair in place.

THE POWER OF HUMAN BEAUTY

Of all the forms of beauty, it is the allure of the human form that most excites us. The human figure has always been a common object of visual art and chemical attraction. The earliest known depictions of the human body originate from Europe and date between 25,000 and 12,000 years ago. Carved from stone and ivory, these Venus figurines represent the female form and may have been associated with fertility.

Attraction and fertility are interrelated and fill us with pleasure. When our eyes gaze upon an exceptionally beautiful person, our thought process alters, our breathing changes, our hormones surge, and our brain releases endorphins that fill our body with a sense of bliss. Beauty may even have a positive impact on our health; one Danish/German study found that men who had survived one heart attack had a 50 percent reduction in new heart attacks after daily viewing of pictures with nude women.

Studies show that more attractive people are judged by others to have good personalities, to be kinder and warmer, to have happier marriages, to have a more positive outlook on life, to be more likely to live longer than average, and to be more satisfied with their lives.

QUOTABLE QUOTES: *For the women of my court, hairstyle remains the most important thing, the subject is inexhaustible.*
—Louis XIV

Beyond the way others perceive you, can sprucing up your appearance really make a difference in your life? The answer is yes. The more attractive you look, the more attention you will attract from others and this, in turn, builds your sense of self-confidence. The attention you receive in the form of admiring glances and prolonged conversations might even have a positive impact on your health. Researchers have found that when babies are massaged, they gain weight as much as 50 percent faster than un-massaged infants, leading one to conclude that adults also physically thrive from positive attention.

Beauty and Progressive Cultures

Creative ideas and a love of physical beauty are two sides of the same coin. Historically, the areas of the world where the public has been the most attracted to the concept of physical beauty are the areas where culture, art, science, and basic human freedoms have thrived. Conversely, the areas where physical beauty has been frowned upon or suppressed are the areas where freedom of thought, belief, and other personal liberties have been stifled.

In a sense, an obsession with personal beauty helps ignite the events that raise a society's standard of living, cure disease, and promote freedom. The statues of Athens helped create the logic of Socrates, Plato, and Aristotle. Renaissance Florence found the blend of beauty, art, science, religion, and economic activity that is still our best social model for building a successful and uplifting society. There even appears to be a connection between the number of nude statues and paintings in an area and its economic progress. For example, the most economically vibrant region of the United States is the very tolerant and self-absorbed San Francisco Bay Area.

In 2002, the per-capita income of the Bay Area was $67,000. In comparison, the second-most prosperous area was Boston at $51,000. The free-living and life-loving culture of the Bay Area attracts and energizes the creative types of people who build a prosperous culture.

Many who love to primp and preen, dress to impress, and beguile us with their glowing skin are highly intelligent, cultured, creative, and prosperous. They epitomize the synergy, the special dance that unites their quest for beauty and art, that swirls us around the dance floor of life, unfolding nuances of our human nature.

So the next time you reach into that jam-packed drawer of cosmetics, creams, and other concoctions, remember that you are carrying on a tradition that has been passed down through at least 75,000 years and probably much longer: The Universal Quest for Beauty in all its wonderful forms.

At the same time, you are also maintaining innate human drives that produce art, science, prosperity, happiness, freedom, and civilized behavior. In revealing how the science of SRCPs is helping men and women turn back the clock, it is my hope that this book will help you reach your personal beauty goals as well.

QUOTABLE QUOTES: *Fair tresses man's imperial race insnare,*
and Beauty draws us with a single hair.
—Alexander Pope

Many people have contacted me reflecting on the extraordinary blend of personal beauty and cultural progress. As one woman so aptly stated: "My skin is my hobby". Here are a few other comments from individuals thinking about how beauty has affected their lives:

"My skin is my hobby. My high point of the month is when Vogue Magazine comes out. I love looking at cosmetics in Bloomingdales. I enjoy going to art shows. I study quantum mechanics for entertainment. Every week I meet with my financial adviser." – RG, New York

"I am definitely what you would call a beauty 'addict'. I could open a drugstore with all the products I have purchased in the past few years. I also spend a good amount of time in front of a mirror, attempting to fit in all of my exfoliation, moisturizing, buffing, rebuilding, repairing, enhancing etc, etc... The irony of the situation is that my purpose for doing all these things is to eventually <u>decrease</u> the amount of time I have to do them...However, I do seem to find comfort in my beauty rituals, particularly if I see improvement over time. It makes the investment seem worth all the time, money, and energy spent." – WN, Wisconsin

"I feel totally consumed and obsessed with achieving the most beautiful and flawless skin I know that I have underneath the blemishes and scars. And as long as those imperfections persist, I will never stop the journey – no matter how rocky and tiresome it may become – to skin perfection....I enjoy skin care products, because these products make me feel that I am 'not letting my beauty fade without a fight.'...Having clear, beautiful, and flawless skin will allow me to reach my highest potential." – RO, Florida

"I love to get a group of us girlfriends together and dedicate the whole day to getting our nails done, or hair done, or a pedicure. Some type of bonding occurs between us and it is unforgettable... There's even something relaxing and enjoyable about doing my own nails. I find myself making designs and playing around with colors all the time." – CM, Washington

Beauty is related to life.

"Its opposite, is related to death.
Beauty is like a reflection of light, of sun,
of spring, of happiness, of strength and health.
The Beauty I'm thinking about, is not connected with
an idea of perfection. It's an idea of harmony, of peace.
And, for instance, beautiful and good
skin reflects light." – AM, Italy

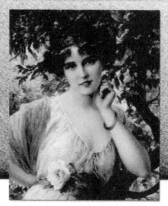

KEEP LEARNING!

GLOSSARY
ADDITIONAL INFORMATION · DEFINITIONS

Acne	Acne results due to a disruption in dead skin cell exfoliation in the opening of the oil gland.
Alpha Lipoic Acid	The most important single antioxidant. The best method to raise cellular glutathione which is considered to be the master antioxidant in the body.
Camphor	Produces a cooling effect similar to menthol leaves. Camphor is used in conjunction with menthol as an anti-inflammatory.
Citric Acid	Citric acid is used to adjust the acidity of products. Derived from citrus fruits.
Collagen	Collagen forms the structural network of our skin and is the most abundant protein in the body. As we age, collagen begins to deteriorate and causes the skin to become thinner and eventually sag.
Dermis	The dermis is a thick, supple and sturdy layer of connective tissue (a dense meshwork of collagen and elastin fibers) that makes up about 90 percent of the skin's thickness.
DHT	DHT (dihydrotestosterone) is considered a key contributing factor to the onset and progression of androgenic alopecia and benign prostatic hyperplasia.
DMAE	Dimethylaminoethanol is an organic compound with strong anti-inflammatory and aging reversal properties. It is a precursor to the chemical that stimulates nerve function and stimulates the muscles to contract and tighten under the skin.
Eczema	Eczema is often associated with dry skin which is also called xerosis, or xerotic eczema (xeros is Greek for "dry").
Elastin	Elastin is a stretchable protein that maintains the skin's elasticity and provides the matrix that holds individual skin cells in place.
Emu Oil	Traditionally used to help alleviate discomfort of arthritis, shingles, eczema, psoriasis and other inflammatory conditions. The fatty acid composition of human skin oil and emu oil are very similar.
Extracellular Matrix	A collection of extracellular molecules that are secreted by cells and provide structural and biochemical support to the surrounding cells.
Epidermis	The epidermis ("overskin") or top layer of the skin. The epidermis is the thinnest skin layer at a maximum 1 millimeter or as thin as a pencil line.
Free Radicals	Free radicals cause much of the tissue damage responsible for degenerative diseases. The absorption or detoxifying of free radicals would protect our bodies from many of those diseases.

GHK-Cu	GHK-Cu (glycyl-l-histidyl-l-lysine:copper(II)) is a Skin Remodeling Copper Peptide. The tripeptide, GHK, discovered by Dr. Pickart, is generated by proteolysis after tissue injury. Its high affinity for copper(II) allows it to obtain copper from carrier molecules such as albumin and form GHK-Cu.
Hydrolyzed Soy Protein	Hydrolyzed soy protein (glycine soja) derived from soybeans and broken down by water to form a complex with copper to produce copper peptides.
Lactic Acid	Lactic acid is an alpha hydroxy acid extracted from milk.
Leucine	An essential amino acid. Leucine is used by the body to repair bone, skin and muscle tissue.
Lipids	Lipids and fats in the skin provide the epidermal barrier to transcutaneous (through the skin) water loss.
Lutein	Lutein (from Latin lutea meaning "yellow") is one of over 600 known naturally occurring carotenoids. It is employed by organisms as an antioxidant and for blue light absorption.
Lycopene	Lycopene (solanum lycopersicum) is a tomato extract high in beta carotene, a natural source of vitamin A, which protects and strengthens the skin.
Olive Oil	Olive oil works as an emollient in our skin creams. It is an antioxidant and improves skin moisture. May also protect against UVB damage.
Psoriasis	A chronic skin disease, characterized by itching, scaling and inflammation. Psoriasis develops red patches of thick lesions covered with silvery scales.
Retinoic Acid	The acidic version of vitamin A or retinol. It reduces skin oil by shrinking sebaceous glands and unclogging hair follicles.
Retinyl Palmitate	A combination of retinol (pure vitamin A) and palmitic acid.
Rosacea	Classic rosacea manifests many tiny, visible red blood vessels in the central part of the face. Starts as a tendency to blush easily.
Salicylic Acid	First obtained from the bark of the willow tree, Salix. It is a beta hydroxy acid exfoliator and one of the best known skin renewal methods. Unlike alpha hydroxy acids, it can penetrate into the skin's pores to remove blemishes and reduce acne.
Saw Palmetto	A popular herbal remedy for a type of hair loss and baldness called androgenic alopecia, or male- and female-pattern baldness.
Sebaceous Glands	Clusters of cells that produce an oil called sebum. Two or more sebaceous glands secrete sebum via minuscule tubes in the hair follicle. Sebum helps waterproof the skin and hair.
Squalane	A natural biological oil obtained from olive oil.
SRCPs	Skin Remodeling Copper Peptides that repair and remodel skin. Its actions focus on being able to generate skin remodeling, the skin's renewal process that return it to a younger, healthier state.
Titanium Dioxide	Mineral used as a sunscreen ingredient in cosmetics. Protects skin from UVA and UVB radiation and is considered to have no risk of skin irritation.
Tocopherols	Tocopherols, tocotrienols and tocophersolan are different members of the vitamin E family. Both tocopherols and tocotrienols are fat-soluble antioxidants and have been exhaustively studied.
Ubiquinone (CoQ-10)	Coenzyme Q-10 (Ubiquinone, CoQ10) is a natural part of the body's cell protection function and energy synthesis. Studies have confirmed CoQ10 to be a powerful antioxidant for the skin and effective in reducing wrinkles.

REFERENCES
Scientific Sources for Chapter Information

[No Author] "Copper deficiency and developmental emphysema." Nutr Rev 41, no. 10 (1983): 318-20.

Abdulghani, AA, A Sherr, S Shirin, G Solodkina, EM Tapia, B Wolf, and AB Gottlieb. "Effects of topical creams containing vitamin C, a copper-binding peptide cream and melatonin compared with tretinoin on the ultrastructure of normal skin - a pilot clinical, histologic, and ultrastructural study " Dis Manag Clin Outcome 1, no. 4 (1998): 136-41.

Adam, M, H Pohunkova, O Cech, and J Vachal. A. "[the effect of collagenous gel on endoprosthesis anchoring]." Acta Chir Orthop Traumatol Cech 62, no. 6 (1995): 336-42.

Adam, M, O Cech, H Pohunkova, J Stehlik, and Z Klezl. B. "[the role of collagen implants containing the tripeptide gly-his-lys in bone healing process]." Acta Chir Orthop Traumatol Cech 62, no. 2 (1995): 76-85.

Adam, M, H Pohunkova, Z Klezl, V Pesakova, and O Cech. "[use of bioimplants to replace cartilage part II: Application of implants in animal experiments.]." Acta Chir Orthop Traumatol Cech 64, no. 4 (1997): 207-11.

Ahmed, MR, SH Basha, D Gopinath, R Muthusamy, and R Jayakumar. "Initial upregulation of growth factors and inflammatory mediators during nerve regeneration in the presence of cell adhesive peptide-incorporated collagen tubes." J Peripher Nerv Syst 10, no. 1 (2005): 17-30.

Ainsleigh, HG. "Beneficial effects of sun exposure on cancer mortality." Prev Med 22, no. 1 (1993): 132-40.

Alberghina, M, G Lupo, G La Spina, A Mangiameli, M Gulisano, D Sciotto, and E Rizzarelli. "Cytoprotective effect of copper(II) complexes against ethanol-induced damage to rat gastric mucosa." J Inorg Biochem 45, no. 4 (1992): 245-59.

Alzuet, G, S Ferrer, J Borras, and JR Sorenson. "Anticonvulsant properties of copper acetazolamide complexes." J Inorg Biochem 55, no. 2 (1994): 147-51.

Ambesi-Impiombato, FS, LA Parks, and HG Coon. "Culture of hormone-dependent functional epithelial cells from rat thyroids." Proc Natl Acad Sci U S A 77, no. 6 (1980): 3455-59.

Appa, Y, T Stephens, S Barkovic, and MB Finkey. "A clinical evaluation of a copper-peptide containing liquid foundation and cream concealer designed for improving skin condition." Paper presented at the American Academy of Dermatology: 60th Annual Meeting, New Orleans, LA, 2002: Abstract P66.

Araya, M, MC McGoldrick, LM Klevay, JJ Strain, P Robson, F Nielsen, M Olivares, F Pizarro, LA Johnson, and KA Poirier. "Determination of an acute no-observed-adverse-effect level (noael) for copper in water." Regul Toxicol Pharmacol 34, no. 2 (2001): 137-45.

Arul, V., D. Gopinath, K. Gomathi, and R. Jayakumar. "Biotinylated GHK peptide incorporated collagenous matrix: A novel biomaterial for dermal wound healing in rats." J Biomed Mater Res B Appl Biomater 73, no. 2 (2005): 383-91.

Arul, V, R Kartha, and R Jayakumar. "A therapeutic approach for diabetic wound healing using biotinylated GHK incorporated collagen matrices." Life Sci 80, no. 4 (2007): 275-84.

Aupaix, F, FX Maquart, L Salagnac, L Pickart, P Gillery, JP Borel, and B Kalis. "Effects of the tripeptide glycyl-histidyl-lysine on healing. Clinical and biochemical correlations." J Invest Dermatol 94 (1990): 390 (abst).

Autier, P, JF Doré, AM Eggermont, and JW Coebergh. "Epidemiological evidence that UVA radiation is involved in the genesis of cutaneous melanoma." Curr Opin Oncol 23, no. 2 (2011): 189-96.

Awa, T, K Nogimori, and RE Trachy. "Hairloss protection by peptide-copper complex in animal models of chemotherapy-induced alopecia." Journal of Dermatological Science 10, no. 1 (1995): 99.

Babu, U, and ML Failla. "Copper status and function of neutrophils are reversibly depressed in marginally and severely copper-deficient rats." J Nutr 120, no. 12 (1990): 1700-9.

Badenhorst T, Svirskis D, Merrilees M, Bolke L, Wu Z (2016) Effects of GHK-Cu on MMP and TIMP Expression, Collagen and Elastin Production, and Facial Wrinkle Parameters. J Aging Sci 4:166. doi: 10.4172/2329-8847.1000166.

Baker, A, L Harvey, G Majask-Newman, S Fairweather-Tait, A Flynn, and K Cashman. "Effect of dietary copper intakes on biochemical markers of bone metabolism in healthy adult males." Eur J Clin Nutr 53, no. 5 (1999): 408-12.

Bala, S, and ML Failla. "Copper deficiency reversibly impairs DNA synthesis in activated T lymphocytes by limiting interleukin 2 activity." Proc Natl Acad Sci U S A 89, no. 15 (1992): 6794-7.

Beaudry, VG, and LD Attardi. "SKP-ing TAp63: Stem cell depletion, senescence, and premature aging." Cell Stem Cell 5, no. 1 (2009): 1-2.

Beresford, SA, KC Johnson, C Ritenbaugh, NL Lasser, LG Snetselaar, HR Black, GL Anderson, AR Assaf, T Bassford, D Bowen, RL Brunner, RG Brzyski, B Caan, RT Chlebowski, M Gass, RC Harrigan, J Hays, D Heber, G Heiss, SL Hendrix, BV Howard, J Hsia, FA Hubbell, RD Jackson, JM Kotchen, AZ LaCroix, DS Lane, RD Langer, CE Lewis, JE Manson, KL Margolis, Y Mossavar-Rahmani, JK Ockene, LM Parker, MG Perri, L Phillips, RL Prentice, J Robbins, JE Rossouw, GE Sarto, ML Stefanick, L Van Horn, MZ Vitolins, J Wactawski-Wende, RB Wallace, and E Whitlock. "Low-fat dietary pattern and risk of colorectal cancer: The women's health initiative randomized controlled dietary modification trial." JAMA 295, no. 6 (2006): 643-54.

Beretta, G, E Arlandini, R Artali, JM Anton, and R Maffei Facino. "Acrolein sequestering ability of the endogenous tripeptide glycyl-histidyl-lysine (GHK): Characterization of conjugation products by ESI-MSn and theoretical calculations." J Pharm Biomed Anal 47, no. 3 (2008): 596-602.

Beretta, G, R Artali, L Regazzoni, M Panigati, and RM Facino. "Glycyl-histidyl-lysine (GHK) is a quencher of alpha,beta-4-hydroxy-trans-2-nonenal: A comparison with carnosine. Insights into the mechanism of reaction by electrospray ionization mass spectrometry, 1h nmr, and computational techniques." Chem Res Toxicol 20, no. 9 (2007): 1309-14.

Berwick, M. "The good, the bad, and the ugly of sunscreens." Clin Pharmacol Ther 89, no. 1 (2011): 31-3.

———. "Counterpoint: Sunscreen use is a safe and effective approach to skin cancer prevention." Cancer Epidemiol Biomarkers Prev 16, no. 10 (2007): 1923-4.

Bhathena, SJ, L Recant, NR Voyles, KI Timmers, S Reiser, JC Jr Smith, and AS Powell. "Decreased plasma enkephalins in copper deficiency in man." Am J Clin Nutr 43, no. 1 (1986): 42-6.

Boal, AK, and AC Rosenzweig. "Structural biology of copper trafficking." Chem Rev 109, no. 10 (2009): 4760-79.

Bobyntsev, I. I., et al. "Anxiolytic Effects of Gly-His-Lys Peptide and Its Analogs."Bulletin of experimental biology and medicine 158.6 (2015): 726.

———. "Effect of Gly-His-Lys peptide and its analogs on pain sensitivity in mice."Eksperimental'naia i klinicheskaia farmakologiia 78.1 (2014): 13-15.

———. "The tripeptide Gly-His-Lys influence on behavior of rats in the open field". Adv. Cur. Nat. Sci. 2014(12): 357-360).

Bonham, M, JM O'Connor, BM Hannigan, and JJ Strain. "The immune system as a physiological indicator of marginal copper status?" Br J Nutr 87, no. 5 (2002): 393-403.

Britton, A, A Singh-Manoux, and M Marmot. "Alcohol consumption and cognitive function in the Whitehall II study." Am J Epidemiol 160, no. 3 (2004): 240-7.

Bruce, B, GA Spiller, LM Klevay, and SK Gallagher. "A diet high in whole and unrefined foods favorably alters lipids, antioxidant defenses, and colon function." J Am Coll Nutr 19, no. 1 (2000): 61-7.

Cabrera, A, E Alonzo, E Sauble, YL Chu, D Nguyen, MC Linder, DS Sato, and AZ Mason. "Copper binding components of blood plasma and organs, and their responses to influx of large doses of (65)Cu, in the mouse." Biometals 21, no. 5 (2008): 525-43.

Camakaris, J, I Voskoboinik, and JF Mercer. "Molecular mechanisms of copper homeostasis." Biochem Biophys Res Commun 261, no. 2 (1999): 225-32.

Campbell, J. D., J. E. McDonough, J. E. Zeskind, T. L. Hackett, D. V. Pechkovsky, C. A. Brandsma, M. Suzuki, J. V. Gosselink, G. Liu, Y. O. Alekseyev, J. Xiao, X. Zhang, S. Hayashi, J. D. Cooper, W. Timens, D. S. Postma, D. A. Knight, L. E. Marc, H. C. James, and S. Avrum. "A gene expression signature of emphysema-related lung destruction and its reversal by the tripeptide GHK." Genome Med 4, no. 8 (2012): 67.

Canapp, SO Jr, JP Farese, GS Schultz, S Gowda, AM Ishak, SF Swaim, J Vangilder, L Lee-Ambrose, and FG Martin. "The effect of topical tripeptide-copper complex on healing of ischemic open wounds." Vet Surg 32, no. 6 (2003): 515-23.

Cangul, IT, NY Gul, A Topal, and R Yilmaz. "Evaluation of the effects of topical tripeptide-copper complex and zinc oxide on open-wound healing in rabbits." Vet Dermatol 17, no. 6 (2006): 417-23.

Cartwright, GE, and MM Wintrobe. "The question of copper deficiency in man." Am J Clin Nutr 15 (1964): 94-110.

Cater, MA, KT McInnes, QX Li, I Volitakis, S La Fontaine, JF Mercer, and AI Bush. "Intracellular copper deficiency increases amyloid-beta secretion by diverse mechanisms." Biochem J 412, no. 1 (2008): 141-52.

Cebrian, J, A Messeguer, RM Facino, and JM Garcia Anton. "New anti-RNS and -RCS products for cosmetic treatment." Int J Cosmet Sci 27, no. 5 (2005): 271-8.

Chambers, A, D Krewski, N Birkett, L Plunkett, R Hertzberg, R Danzeisen, PJ Aggett, TB Starr, S Baker, M Dourson, P Jones, CL Keen, B Meek, R Schoeny, and W Slob. "An exposure-response curve for copper excess and deficiency." J Toxicol Environ Health B Crit Rev 13, no. 7-8 (2010): 546-78.

Chang-Claude, J, S Hermann, U Eilber, and K Steindorf. "Lifestyle determinants and mortality in german vegetarians and health-conscious persons: Results of a 21-year follow-up." Cancer Epidemiolology, Biomarkers, & Prevention 14, no. 4 (2005): 963-68.

Cherdakov, V.Y., M.Y. Smakhtin, G.M. Dubrovin, V.T. Dudka, and I.I. Bobyntsev. "Synergetic antioxidant and reparative action of thymogen, dalargin and peptide gly-his-lys in tubular bone fractures." Exp Biol Med 4 (2010): 15-20.

Chernysheva O.I., Bobyntsev I.I., Dolgintsev M.E. The tripeptide Gly-His-Lys influence on behavior of rats in the test "open field. Adv. Cur. Nat. Sci. 2014 (12): 357-360.

Choi, EH, BE Brown, D Crumrine, S Chang, MQ Man, PM Elias, and KR Feingold. "Mechanisms by which psychologic stress alters cutaneous permeability barrier homeostasis and stratum corneum integrity." J Invest Dermatol 124, no. 3 (2005): 587-95.

Choi et al. "Stem cell recovering effect of copper-free GHK in skin." Journal of Peptide Science 18.11 (2012): 685-690.

Chowdhury, R., S. Warnakula, S. Kunutsor, F. Crowe, H. A. Ward, L. Johnson, O. H. Franco, A. S. Butterworth, N. G. Forouhi, S. G. Thompson, K. T. Khaw, D. Mozaffarian, J. Danesh, and E. Di Angelantonio. "Association of dietary, circulating, and supplement fatty acids with coronary risk: A systematic review and meta-analysis." Ann Intern Med 160, no. 6 (2014): 398-406.

Coastal, D. "The runner." (1984): 41.

Conlan, D, R Korula, and D Tallentire. "Serum copper levels in elderly patients with femoral-neck fractures." Age Ageing 19, no. 3 (1990): 212-4.

Cornaro, L. Discorsi della vita sobria [discourses on the sober life]1677.

Counts, D, E Hill, M Turner-Beatty, M Grotewiel, S Fosha-Thomas, and L Pickart. "Effect of lamin on full thickness wound healing." Fed Am Soc Exp Biol (1992): A1636.

Cutler, WB. Love cycles : The science of intimacy. 2 ed. New York: Athena Institute Press, 1996.

Davis, CD, and WT Johnson. "Dietary copper affects azoxymethane-induced intestinal tumor formation and protein kinase C isozyme protein and mRNA expression in colon of rats." J Nutr 132, no. 5 (2002): 1018-25.

De Spirt, S, W Stahl, H Tronnier, H Sies, M Bejot, JM Maurette, and U Heinrich. "Intervention with flaxseed and borage oil supplements modulates skin condition in women." Br J Nutr 101, no. 3 (2009): 440-5.

Dollwet, HH, and JR Sorenson. "Roles of copper in bone maintenance and healing." Biol Trace Elem Res 18 (1988): 39-48.

———. "Historic uses of copper compounds in medicine." Trace Elements in Medicine 2, no. 2 (1985): 80-87.

Downey, D, WF Larrabee, V Voci, and L Pickart. "Acceleration of wound healing using glycyl-histidyl-lysine copper (II)." Surg Forum 25 (1985): 573-75. Drug&CosmeticIndustry. (1997).

Dwivedi, C, X Guan, WL Harmsen, AL Voss, DE Goetz-Parten, EM Koopman, KM Johnson, HB Valluri, and DP Matthees. "Chemopreventive effects of alpha-santalol on skin tumor development in CD-1 and sencar mice." Cancer Epidemiol Biomarkers Prev 12, no. 2 (2003): 151-6.

Dwivedi, C, and Y Zhang. "Sandalwood oil prevent skin tumour development in CD1 mice." Eur J Cancer Prev 8, no. 5 (1999): 449-55.

Ebbs, JH, FF Tisdall, and WA Scott. "The influence of prenatal diet on the mother and child." J Nutr 22, no. 5 (1941): 515-26.

Ehrlich, HP. "Stimulation of skin healing in immunosuppressed rats." Paper presented at the Symposium on collagen and skin repair Reims, France, Sept 12-13 1991.

Elias, PK, MF Elias, RB D'Agostino, H Silbershatz, and PA Wolf. "Alcohol consumption and cognitive performance in the Framingham heart study." Am J Epidemiol 150, no. 6 (1999): 580-9.

Ellis, JA, M Stebbing, and SB Harrap. "Genetic analysis of male pattern baldness and the 5alpha-reductase genes." J Invest Dermatol 110, no. 6 (1998): 849-53.

Elserif, L, RV Ortines, JT Saari, and YJ Kang. "Congestive heart failure in copper-deficient mice." Exp Biol Med (Maywood) 228, no. 7 (2003): 811-7.

Ernst, B, M Thurnheer, and B Schultes. "Copper deficiency after gastric bypass surgery." Obesity (Silver Spring) 17, no. 11 (2009): 1980-1.

Fackelmann, K. "Melanoma madness: The scientific flap over sunscreens and skin cancer " Science News 153, no. 23 (1998): 360.

Farmer, KC, and MF Naylor. "Sun exposure, sunscreens, and skin cancer prevention: A year-round concern." Ann Pharmacother 30, no. 6 (1996): 662-73.

Finkley, MB, Y Appa, and S Bhandarkar. "Copper peptide and skin." In Cosmeceuticals and active cosmetics: Drugs vs. Cosmetics, edited by P Elsner and HI Maibach, 549-63. New York: Marcel Dekker, 2005.

Fouad, FM, M Abd-El-Fattah, R Scherer, and G Ruthenstroth-Bauer. "Effect of glucocorticoids, insulin and a growth promoting tripeptide on the biosynthesis of plasma proteins in serum-free hepatocyte cultures." Z Naturforsch C 36, no. 3-4 (1981): 350-52.

Frieden, E. "Perspectives on copper biochemistry." Clin Physiol Biochem 4, no. 1 (1986): 11-9.

Friedman, HS, and LR Martin. The longevity project: Surprising discoveries for health and long life from the landmark eight-decade study: Hudson Street Press, 2011.

Frost, PA, GB Hubbard, MJ Dammann, CL Snider, CM Moore, VL Hodara, LD Giavedoni, R Rohwer, MC Mahaney, TM Butler, LB Cummins, TJ McDonald, PW Nathanielsz, and NE Schlabritz-Loutsevitch. "White monkey syndrome in infant baboons (papio species)." J Med Primatol 33, no. 4 (2004): 197-213.

Gacheru, SN, PC Trackman, MA Shah, CY O'Gara, P Spacciapoli, FT Greenaway, and HM Kagan. "Structural and catalytic properties of copper in lysyl oxidase " J Biol Chem 265, no. 31 (1990): 19022-7.

Garcia-Sainz, JA, and JA Olivares-Reyes. "Glycyl-histidyl-lysine interacts with the angiotensin II AT1 receptor." Peptides 16, no. 7 (1995): 1203-7.

Garg, A, MM Chren, LP Sands, MS Matsui, KD Marenus, KR Feingold, and PM Elias. "Psychological stress perturbs epidermal permeability barrier homeostasis: Implications for the pathogenesis of stress-associated skin disorders." Arch Dermatol 137, no. 1 (2001): 53-9.

Garland, CF, FC Garland, and ED Gorham. "Re: Effect of sunscreens on UV radiation-induced enhancement of melanoma growth in mice." J Natl Cancer Inst 86, no. 10 (1994): 798-800.

———. "Rising trends in melanoma. An hypothesis concerning sunscreen effectiveness." Ann Epidemiol 3, no. 1 (1993): 103-10.

———. "Could sunscreens increase melanoma risk?" Am J Public Health 82, no. 4 (1992): 614-5.

Gehring, W. "The influence of biotin on nails of reduced quality." Aktuelle Dermatologie (Germany) 22, no. 1-2 (1996): 20-24.

Giampaolo, V, F Luigina, A Conforti, and R Milanino. "Copper and inflammation." In Inflammatory diseases and copper: The metabolic and therapeutic roles of copper and other essential metalloelements in humans, edited by JR Sorenson. Clifton, New Jersey: Humana Press, 1982.

Gilbert, R, G Salanti, M Harden, and S See. "Infant sleeping position and the sudden infant death syndrome: Systematic review of observational studies and historical review of recommendations from 1940 to 2002." Int J Epidemiol 34, no. 4 (2005): 874-87.

Gill, SE, and WC Parks. "Metalloproteinases and their inhibitors: Regulators of wound healing." Int J Biochem Cell Biol 40, no. 6-7 (2008): 1334-47.

Globa, AG, VA Vishnevskiĭ, VS Demidova, Olu Abakumova, and AA Karelin. "[accumulation of ATP in rat and human hepatocyte cell membranes exposed to certain growth factors and phosphatidylcholine]." Biull Eksp Biol Med 121, no. 3 (1996): 271-4.

Godet, D, and PJ Marie. "Effects of the tripeptide glycyl-l-histidyl-l-lysine copper complex on osteoblastic cell spreading, attachment and phenotype." Cell Mol Biol (Noisy-le-grand) 41, no. 8 (1995): 1081-91.

Gonzalez, S, A Wu, MA Pathak, M Sifakis, and DA Goukassian. "Oral administration of lutein modulates cell proliferation induced by acute UV-B radiation in the SHK-1 hairless mouse animal model." The Society for Investigative Dermatology, 63rd Annual Meeting (2002): Abstract 769.

Granstein, R, D Faulhaber, and W Ding. "Lutein inhibits UVB radiation-induced tissue swelling and suppression of the induction of contact hypersensitivity (CHS) in the mouse." 62nd Annual Meeting of the Society for Investigative Dermatology (2001): 497.

Greene, FL, LS Lamb, M Barwick, and NJ Pappas. "Effect of dietary copper on colonic tumor production and aortic integrity in the rat." J Surg Res 42, no. 5 (1987): 503-12.

Gubler, CJ, ME Lahey, GE Cartwright, and MM Wintrobe. "Studies on copper metabolism. IX. The transportation of copper in blood." J Clin Invest 32, no. 5 (1953): 405-14.

Gul, NY, A Topal, IT Cangul, and K Yanik. "The effects of topical tripeptide copper complex and helium-neon laser on wound healing in rabbits." Vet Dermatol 19, no. 1 (2008): 7-14.

Hanson, KM, E Gratton, and CJ Bardeen. "Sunscreen enhancement of UV-induced reactive oxygen species in the skin." Free Radic Biol Med 41, no. 8 (2006): 1205-12.

Harris, ED. "Basic and clinical aspects of copper." Crit Rev Clin Lab Sci 40, no. 5 (2003): 547-86.

———. "Copper as a cofactor and regulator of copper,zinc superoxide dismutase." J Nutr 122, no. 3 Suppl (1992): 636-40.

Hart, EB, H Steenbock, J Waddell, and CA Elvehjem. "Iron in nutrition. VII. Copper as a supplement to iron for hemoglobin building in the rat. 1928." J Biol Chem 277, no. 34 (2002): e22.

Harvey, LJ, G Majsak-Newman, JR Dainty, DJ Lewis, NJ Langford, HM Crews, and SJ Fairweather-Tait. "Adaptive responses in men fed low- and high-copper diets." Br J Nutr 90, no. 1 (2003): 161-8.

Hawk, SN, L Lanoue, CL Keen, CL Kwik-Uribe, RB Rucker, and JY Uriu-Adams. "Copper-deficient rat embryos are characterized by low superoxide dismutase activity and elevated superoxide anions." Biol Reprod 68, no. 3 (2003): 896-903.

Heinrich, U, C Gartner, M Wiebusch, O Eichler, H Sies, H Tronnier, and W Stahl. "Supplementation with beta-carotene or a similar amount of mixed carotenoids protects humans from UV-induced erythema." J Nutr 133, no. 1 (2003): 98-101.

Heinrich, Jurgen, et al. "Fibrinogen and factor VII in the prediction of coronary risk. Results from the PROCAM study in healthy men." Arteriosclerosis, Thrombosis, and Vascular Biology 14.1 (1994): 54-59.

Heresi, G, C Castillo-Durán, C Muñoz, M Arévalo, and L Schlesinger. "Phagocytosis and immunoglobulin levels in hypocupremic infants." Nutrition Research 5, no. 12 (1985): 1327-34.

Hill, PL, NA Turiano, MD Hurd, DK Mroczek, and BW Roberts. "Conscientiousness and longevity: An examination of possible mediators." Health Psychol 30, no. 5 (2011): 536-41.

Hirsch, A. Scentsational sex: The secret to using aroma for arousal: Element Books, 1998.

Hitzig, G. "Enhanced healing and growth in hair transplantation using copper peptides." Cosmetic Dermatol 13 (2000): 18-21.

Hobday, R. The healing sun: Sunlight and health in the 21st century: Findhorn Press, 2000.

Holick, M. "The UV advantage." (2003): 190.

Holstege, G. Paper presented at the European Society for Human Reproduction and Development, 2005.

Hong, Y, T Downey, KW Eu, PK Koh, and PY Cheah. "A 'metastasis-prone' signature for early-stage mismatch-repair proficient sporadic colorectal cancer patients and its implications for possible therapeutics." Clin Exp Metastasis 27, no. 2 (2010): 83-90.

Hostynek, JJ, F Dreher, and HI Maibach. "Human skin penetration of a copper tripeptide in vitro as a function of skin layer." Inflamm Res 60, no. 1 (2011): 79-86.

———. "Human skin retention and penetration of a copper tripeptide in vitro as function of skin layer towards anti-inflammatory therapy." Inflamm Res 59, no. 11 (2010): 983-8.

Howard, BV, L Van Horn, J Hsia, JE Manson, ML Stefanick, S Wassertheil-Smoller, LH Kuller, AZ LaCroix, RD Langer, NL Lasser, CE Lewis, MC Limacher, KL Margolis, WJ Mysiw, JK Ockene, LM Parker, MG Perri, L Phillips, RL Prentice, J Robbins, JE Rossouw, GE Sarto, IJ Schatz, LG Snetselaar, VJ Stevens, LF Tinker, M Trevisan, MZ Vitolins, GL Anderson, AR Assaf, T Bassford, SA Beresford, HR Black, RL Brunner, RG Brzyski, B Caan, RT Chlebowski, M Gass, I Granek, P Greenland, J Hays, D Heber, G Heiss, SL Hendrix, FA Hubbell, KC Johnson, and JM Kotchen. "Low-fat dietary pattern and risk of cardiovascular disease: The women's health initiative randomized controlled dietary modification trial." JAMA 295, no. 6 (2006): 655-66.

Huang, PJ, YC Huang, MF Su, TY Yang, JR Huang, and CP Jiang. "In vitro observations on the influence of copper peptide aids for the led photoirradiation of fibroblast collagen synthesis." Photomed Laser Surg 25, no. 3 (2007): 183-90.

Hung, YH, EL Robb, I Volitakis, M Ho, G Evin, QX Li, JG Culvenor, CL Masters, RA Cherny, and AI Bush. "Paradoxical condensation of copper with elevated beta-amyloid in lipid rafts under cellular copper deficiency conditions: Implications for Alzheimer disease." J Biol Chem 284, no. 33 (2009): 21899-907.

Hunt, JR, and RA Vanderpool. "Apparent copper absorption from a vegetarian diet." Am J Clin Nutr 74, no. 6 (2001): 803-7.

Ibrahim Z.A., El-Ashmawy A.A., Shora O.A. Therapeutic effect of microneedling and autologous platelet-rich plasma in the treatment of atrophic scars: A randomized study. J Cosmet Dermatol. 2017 May 14. doi: 10.1111/jocd.12356. [Epub ahead of print].

Itoh, S, K Ozumi, HW Kim, O Nakagawa, RD McKinney, RJ Folz, IN Zelko, M Ushio-Fukai, and T Fukai. "Novel mechanism for regulation of extracellular SOD transcription and activity by copper: Role of antioxidant-1." Free Radic Biol Med 46, no. 1 (2009): 95-104.

Jacob, RA, HH Sandstead, JM Munoz, LM Klevay, and DB Milne. "Whole body surface loss of trace metals in normal males." Am J Clin Nutr 34, no. 7 (1981): 1379-83.

Jonas, J, J Burns, EW Abel, MJ Cresswell, JJ Strain, and CR Paterson. "Impaired mechanical strength of bone in experimental copper deficiency." Ann Nutr Metab 37, no. 5 (1993): 245-52.

Jose, S., M. L. Hughbanks, B. Y. Binder, G. C. Ingavle, and J. K. Leach. "Enhanced trophic factor secretion by mesenchymal stem/stromal cells with glycine-histidine-lysine (GHK)-modified alginate hydrogels." Acta Biomater 10, no. 5 (2014): 1955-64.

Kang, YA, HR Choi, JI Na, CH Huh, MJ Kim, SW Youn, KH Kim, and KC Park. "Copper-GHK increases integrin expression and p63 positivity by keratinocytes." Arch Dermatol Res 301, no. 4 (2009): 301-6.

Kaur, M, C Agarwal, RP Singh, X Guan, C Dwivedi, and R Agarwal. "Skin cancer chemopreventive agent, {alpha}-santalol, induces apoptotic death of human epidermoid carcinoma A431 cells via caspase activation together with dissipation of mitochondrial membrane potential and cytochrome c release." Carcinogenesis 26, no. 2 (2005): 369-80.

Kawase, M, N Kurikawa, S Higashiyama, N Miura, T Shiomi, C Ozawa, T Mizoguchi, and K Yagi. A. "Effectiveness of polyamidoamine dendrimers modified with tripeptide growth factor, glycyl-l-histidyl-l-lysine, for enhancement of function of hepatoma cells." J Biosci Bioeng 88, no. 4 (1999): 433-7.

Kawase, M, N Miura, N Kurikawa, K Masuda, S Higashiyama, K Yagi, and T Mizoguchi. B. "Immobilization of tripeptide growth factor glycyl-l-histidyl-l-lysine on poly(vinylalcohol)-quarternized stilbazole (PVA-SbQ) and its use as a ligand for hepatocyte attachment." Biol Pharm Bull 22, no. 9 (1999): 999-1001.

Kazemi, A, T Frazier, and M Cave. "Micronutrient-related neurologic complications following bariatric surgery." Curr Gastroenterol Rep 12, no. 4 (2010): 288-95.

Keen, CL, JY Uriu-Hare, SN Hawk, MA Jankowski, GP Daston, CL Kwik-Uribe, and RB Rucker. "Effect of copper deficiency on prenatal development and pregnancy outcome." Am J Clin Nutr 67, no. 5 Suppl (1998): 1003S-11S.

Kelley, DS, PA Daudu, PC Taylor, BE Mackey, and JR Turnlund. "Effects of low-copper diets on human immune response." Am J Clin Nutr 62, no. 2 (1995): 412-6.

Keyes, WM, and AA Mills. "p63: A new link between senescence and aging." Cell Cycle 5, no. 3 (2006): 260-5.

Kimoto, E, H Tanaka, J Gyotoku, F Morishige, and L Pauling. "Enhancement of antitumor activity of ascorbate against ehrlich ascites tumor cells by the copper:Glycylglycylhistidine complex." Cancer Res 43, no. 2 (1983): 824-28.

Klevay, LM. "Metabolic interactions among dietary choletstrol, copper, and fructose." Am J Physiol Endocrinol Metab 298, no. 1 (2010): E138-9.

———. "Alzheimer's disease as copper deficiency." Med Hypotheses 70, no. 4 (2008): 802-7.

———. "Ischemic heart disease as deficiency disease." Cell Mol Biol (Noisy-le-grand) 50, no. 8 (2004): 877-84.

———. "Extra dietary copper inhibits LDL oxidation." Am J Clin Nutr 76, no. 3 (2002): 687-8; author reply 88.

———. "Iron overload can induce mild copper deficiency." J Trace Elem Med Biol 14, no. 4 (2001): 237-40.

———. A. "Cardiovascular disease from copper deficiency--a history." J Nutr 130, no. 2S Suppl (2000): 489S-92S.

———. B. "Dietary copper and risk of coronary heart disease." Am J Clin Nutr 71, no. 5 (2000): 1213-4.

———. "Trace elements, atherosclerosis, and abdominal aneurysms." Ann N Y Acad Sci 800 (1996): 239-42.

———. "Hypertension in rats due to copper deficiency." Nutr Rep Int 35 (1987): 999-1005.

Klevay, LM, and DM Christopherson. "Copper deficiency halves serum dehydroepiandrosterone in rats." J Trace Elem Med Biol 14, no. 3 (2000): 143-5.

Klevay, LM, and ES Halas. "The effects of dietary copper deficiency and psychological stress on blood pressure in rats." Physiol Behav 49, no. 2 (1991): 309-14.

Klevay, LM, and DM Medeiros. "Deliberations and evaluations of the approaches, endpoints and paradigms for dietary recommendations about copper." J Nutr 126, no. 9 Suppl (1996): 2419S-26S.

Klevay, LM, and RE Wildman. "Meat diets and fragile bones: Inferences about osteoporosis." J Trace Elem Med Biol 16, no. 3 (2002): 149-54.

Kohl, JV, and RT Francoeur. The scent of eros : Mysteries of odor in human sexuality. New York: Continuum Publishing Company, 1995.

Kremer, JM, and J Bigaouette. "Nutrient intake of patients with rheumatoid arthritis is deficient in pyridoxine, zinc, copper, and magnesium." J Rheumatol 23, no. 6 (1996): 990-4.

Krüger et al., Topische Applikation eines Kupfertripeptidkomplexes: Pilotstudie bei gealterter Haut., J Dtsch Dermatol Ges; 1(S1)., 2003; N.Krüger, et al., Zur Behandlung der Hautalterung: Spurenelemente in Form eines Kupfertripeptidkomplexes., Kosmetische Medizin; 1., 2003.

Kubecova, M, K Kolostova, D Pinterova, G Kacprzak, and V Bobek. "Cimetidine: An anticancer drug?" Eur J Pharm Sci 42, no. 5 (2011): 439-44.

Kumar, N. "Copper deficiency myelopathy (human swayback)." Mayo Clin Proc 81, no. 10 (2006): 1371-84.

Lane, TF, ML Iruela-Arispe, RS Johnson, and EH Sage. "SPARC is a source of copper-binding peptides that stimulate angiogenesis." J Cell Biol 125, no. 4 (1994): 929-43.

Larsen, HR. "Sunscreens: Do they cause skin cancer." Internat J of Alternative & Complementary Med 12 (1994): 17-19.

Lau, SJ, and B Sarkar. "The interaction of copper(II) and glycyl-l-histidyl-l-lysine, a growth-modulating tripeptide from plasma." Biochem J 199, no. 3 (1981): 649-56.

Laussac, JP, R Haran, and B Sarkar. "N.M.R. And e.P.R. Investigation of the interaction of copper(II) and glycyl-l-histidyl-l-lysine, a growth-modulating tripeptide from plasma." Biochem J 209, no. 2 (1983): 533-9.

Lee, A. J., et al. Plasma fibrinogen and coronary risk factors: the Scottish Heart Health Study. Journal of clinical epidemiology 43.9 (1990): 913-919.

Lee, A, and R Langer. "Shark cartilage contains inhibitors of tumor angiogenesis." Science 221, no. 4616 (1983): 1185-7.

Lee, J, S Jiang, N Levine, and RR Watson. "Carotenoid supplementation reduces erythema in human skin after simulated solar radiation exposure." Proc Soc Exp Biol Med 223, no. 2 (2000): 170-4.

Lemoine, P, B Viossat, G Morgant, FT Greenaway, A Tomas, NH Dung, and JR Sorenson. "Synthesis, crystal structure, EPR properties, and anti-convulsant activities of binuclear and mononuclear 1,10-phenanthroline and salicylate ternary copper(II) complexes." J Inorg Biochem 89, no. 1-2 (2002): 18-28.

Levine, DS, LM Patt, MA Koren, J Joslin, An open-labeL, pilot-study of prezatide copper-acetate (PCA) rectal solution in the treatment of distal inflammatory bowel-disease · Gastroenterology 108(4):A861-861, April 1995.

Leyden, J, G Grove, S Barkovic, and Y Appa. A. "The effect of tripeptide to copper ratio in two copper peptide creams on photoaged facial skin." Paper presented at the American Academy of Dermatology: 60th Annual Meeting, New Orleans, LA, 2002: Abstract P67.

Leyden, J, T Stephens, MB Finkey, Y Appa, and S Barkovic. B. "Skin care benefits of copper peptide containing facial cream." Paper presented at the American Academy of Dermatology: 60th Annual Meeting, New Orleans, LA, 2002: Abstract P68.

Leyden, J, T Stephens, MB Finkey, and S Barkovic. C. "Skin care benefits of copper peptide containing eye creams." Paper presented at the American Academy of Dermatology: 60th Annual Meeting, 2002: Abstract P69.

Li H., Low Y.S., Chong H.P., Zin M.T., Lee C.Y., Li B., Leolukman M., Kang L. Microneedle-Mediated Delivery of Copper Peptide Through Skin. Pharm Res. 2015 Aug;32(8):2678-89. doi: 10.1007/s11095-015-1652-z. Epub 2015 Feb 19.

Liakopoulou-Kyriakides, M, C Pachatouridis, L Ekateriuiadou, and VP Papageorgiou. "A new synthesis of the tripeptide gly-his-lys with antimicrobial activity." Amino Acids 13, no. 2 (1997): 155-61.

Lindner, G, G Grosse, W Halle, and P Henklein. "Uber die wirkung eines synthetischen tripeptids auf in vitro kultiviertes nervengewebe [the effect of a synthetic tripeptide nervous tissue cultured in vitro]." Z Mikrosk Anat Forsch 93, no. 5 (1979): 820-8.

Linnane, AW, C Zhang, N Yarovaya, G Kopsidas, S Kovalenko, P Papakostopoulos, H Eastwood, S Graves, and M Richardson. "Human aging and global function of coenzyme q10." Ann N Y Acad Sci 959 (2002): 396-411; discussion 63-5.

Lipotec, S.A. "ALDENINE® PBC CODE: P10-PD050." www.reverseskinaging.com/lipotec-aldenine.html.

Lonnerdal, B. "Copper nutrition during infancy and childhood." Am J Clin Nutr 67, no. 5 Suppl (1998): 1046S-53S.

Lopez, A, DE Sims, RF Ablett, RE Skinner, LW Leger, CM Lariviere, LA Jamieson, J Martinez-Burnes, and GG Zawadzka. "Effect of emu oil on auricular inflammation induced with croton oil in mice." Am J Vet Res 60, no. 12 (1999): 1558-61.

Lutsenko, S, A Bhattacharjee, and AL Hubbard. "Copper handling machinery of the brain." Metallomics 2, no. 9 (2010): 596-608.

Manot, L. "Effects du tripeptide GHK-Cu sur le coeur isole de rat." Universite de Reims Champagne-Ardenne, 1997.

Maquart, FX, G Bellon, B Chaqour, J Wegrowski, L. M Patt, RE Trachy, JC Monboisse, F Chastang, P Birembaut, P Gillery, and et al. "In vivo stimulation of connective tissue accumulation by the tripeptide-copper complex glycyl-l-histidyl-l-lysine-Cu2+ in rat experimental wounds." J Clin Invest 92, no. 5 (1993): 2368-76.

Maquart, FX, G Bellon, S Pasco, and JC Monboisse. "Matrikines in the regulation of extracellular matrix degradation." Biochimie 87, no. 3-4 (2005): 353-60.

Maquart, FX, P Gillery, JC Monboisse, L Pickart, M Laurent, and JP Borel. "Glycyl-l-histidyl-l-lysine, a triplet from the a2 (I) chain of human type I collagen, stimulates collagen synthesis by fibroblast cultures." Ann N Y Acad Sci 580 (1990): 573-75.

Maquart, FX, L Pickart, M Laurent, P Gillery, JC Monboisse, and JP Borel. "Stimulation of collagen synthesis in fibroblast cultures by the tripeptide-copper complex glycyl-l-histidyl-l-lysine-Cu2+." FEBS Lett 238, no. 2 (1988): 343-6.

Maquart, FX, A Simeon, S Pasco, and JC Monboisse. "Regulation de l'activite cellulaire par la matrice extracelulaire: Le concept de matrikines [regulation of cell activity by the extracellular matrix: The concept of matrikines]." French J Soc Biol 193, no. 4-5 (1999): 423-8.

Masuda, A, S Akiyama, M Kuwano, and N Ikekawa. "Potentiation of antifungal effect of amphotericin B by squalene, an intermediate for sterol biosynthesis." J Antibiot (Tokyo) 35, no. 2 (1982): 230-4.

Matalka, L.E., A. Ford, and M.T. Unlap. "The tripeptide, GHK, induces programmed cell death in sh-sy5y neuroblastoma cells." J Biotechnol Biomater 2, no. 5 (2012): 1-4.

Mazurowska, L, and M Mojski. "Biological activities of selected peptides: Skin penetration ability of copper complexes with peptides." J Cosmet Sci 59, no. 1 (2008): 59-69.

———. "ESI-MS study of the mechanism of glycyl-l-histidyl-l-lysine-Cu(II) complex transport through model membrane of stratum corneum." Talanta 72, no. 2 (2007): 650-4.

McCormack, MC, KC Nowak, and RJ Koch. "The effect of copper tripeptide and tretinoin on growth factor production in a serum-free fibroblast model." Arch Facial Plast Surg 3, no. 1 (2001): 28-32.

Miller, DM, D DeSilva, L Pickart, and SD Aust. "Effects of glycyl-histidyl-lysyl chelated Cu(II) on ferritin dependent lipid peroxidation." Adv Exp Med Biol 264 (1990): 79-84.

Miller, TR, JD Wagner, BR Baack, and KJ Eisbach. "Effects of topical copper tripeptide complex on CO2 laser-resurfaced skin." Arch Facial Plast Surg 8, no. 4 (2006): 252-9.

Mizuno, S., M. Yasuo, H. J. Bogaard, D. Kraskauskas, A. Alhussaini, J. Gomez-Arroyo, D. Farkas, L. Farkas, and N. F. Voelkel. "Copper deficiency induced emphysema is associated with focal adhesion kinase inactivation." PLoS One 7, no. 1 (2012): e30678.

Moan, J, and A Dahlback. "The relationship between skin cancers, solar radiation and ozone depletion." Br J Cancer 65, no. 6 (1992): 916-21.

Morgant, G, NH Dung, JC Daran, B Viossat, X Labouze, M Roch-Arveiller, FT Greenaway, W Cordes, and JR Sorenson. "Low-temperature crystal structures of tetrakis-mu-3,5-diisopropylsalicylatobis-dimethylformamidodico pper(II) and tetrakis-mu-3,5-diisopropylsalicylatobis-diethyletheratodicopp er(II) and their role in modulating polymorphonuclear leukocyte activity in overcoming seizures." J Inorg Biochem 81, no. 1-2 (2000): 11-22.

Morganti, P, C Bruno, and G Colelli. "[gelatin-cystine, keratogenesis and structure of the hair]." Boll Soc Ital Biol Sper 59, no. 1 (1983): 20-5.

Morganti, P, C Bruno, F Guarneri, A Cardillo, P Del Ciotto, and F Valenzano. "Role of topical and nutritional supplement to modify the oxidative stress." Int J Cosmet Sci 24, no. 6 (2002): 331-9.

Morton, MS, PC Elwood, and M Abernethy. "Trace elements in water and congenital malformations of the central nervous system in south wales." Br J Prev Soc Med 30, no. 1 (1976): 36-9.

Mulder, GD, L. M Patt, L Sanders, J Rosenstock, MI Altman, ME Hanley, and GW Duncan. "Enhanced healing of ulcers in patients with diabetes by topical treatment with glycyl-l-histidyl-l-lysine copper." Wound Repair Regen 2, no. 4 (1994): 259-69.

Narayanan, VS, CA Fitch, and CW Levenson. "Tumor suppressor protein p53 mRNA and subcellular localization are altered by changes in cellular copper in human Hep G2 cells." J Nutr 131, no. 5 (2001): 1427-32.

Nassar A., Ghomey S., El Gohary Y., El-Desoky F. Treatment of striae distensae with needling therapy versus microdermabrasion with sonophoresis. J. Cosmet. Laser Ther. 2016 Oct;18(6):330-4. doi: 10.1080/14764172.2016.1175633. Epub 2016 Jun 2.

Naughton, BA, GK Naughton, P Liu, GB Zuckerman, and AS Gordon. "The influence of pancreatic hormones and diabetogenic procedures on erythropoietin production." J Surg Research 21, no. 2 (1982): 97-103.

O'Dell, B. L., K. H. Kilburn, W. N. McKenzie, and R. J. Thurston. "The lung of the copper-deficient rat. A model for developmental pulmonary emphysema." Am J Pathol 91, no. 3 (1978): 413-32.

Oberley, LW, SW Leuthauser, RF Pasternack, TD Oberley, L Schutt, and JR Sorenson. "Anticancer activity of metal compounds with superoxide dismutase activity." Agents Actions 15, no. 5-6 (1984): 535-8.

Okuyama, S, S Hashimoto, H Aihara, WM Willingham, and JR Sorenson. "Copper complexes of non-steroidal antiinflammatory agents: Analgesic activity and possible opioid receptor activation." Agents Actions 21, no. 1-2 (1987): 130-44.

Paffenbarger, RS Jr, AL Wing, and RT Hyde. "Physical activity as an index of heart attack risk in college alumni." Am J Epidemiol 108, no. 3 (1978): 161-75.

Park, JH, and MS Tallman. "Managing acute promyelocytic leukemia without conventional chemotherapy: Is it possible?" Expert Rev Hematol 4, no. 4 (2011): 427-36.

Park Jeong-Ran, et al. "The tri-peptide GHK-Cu complex ameliorates lipopolysaccharide-induced acute lung injury in mice."Oncotarget 7.36 (2016): 58405.

Pauling, L. "Orthomolecular psychiatry. Varying the concentrations of substances normally present in the human body may control mental disease." Science 160, no. 825 (1968): 265-71.

Peled, T, E Fibach, and A Treves. "Methods of controlling proliferation and differentiation of stem and progenitor cells ". U.S. Patent 6,962,698: Gamida Cell Ltd. (Jerusalem, IL), Hadasit Medical Research Services and Development, Ltd. (Jerusalem, IL), filed Aug 17, 1999, and issued Nov 08, 2005.

Peled, T, E Glukhman, N Hasson, S Adi, H Assor, D Yudin, C Landor, J Mandel, E Landau, E Prus, A Nagler, and E Fibach. "Chelatable cellular copper modulates differentiation and self-renewal of cord blood-derived hematopoietic progenitor cells." Exp Hematol 33, no. 10 (2005): 1092-100.

Peled, T, E Landau, E Prus, AJ Treves, A Nagler, and E Fibach. "Cellular copper content modulates differentiation and self-renewal in cultures of cord blood-derived CD34+ cells." Br J Haematol 116, no. 3 (2002): 655-61.

Penland, JG, and JR Prohaska. "Abnormal motor function persists following recovery from perinatal copper deficiency in rats." J Nutr 134, no. 8 (2004): 1984-8.

Percival, SS. "Copper and immunity." Am J Clin Nutr 67, no. (5 Suppl) (1998): 1064S-68S.

Perez-Meza, D, M Leavitt, and R Trachy. "Clinical evaluation of graftcyte moist dressings on hair graft viability and quality of healing." Int J Cos Surg 6, no. 1 (1998): 80-84.

Pesakova, V, J Novotna, and M Adam. "Effect of the tripeptide glycyl-l-histidyl-l-lysine on the proliferation and synthetic activity of chick embryo chondrocytes." Biomaterials 16, no. 12 (1995): 911-5.

Pickart, L. "The human tri-peptide GHK and tissue remodeling." J Biomater Sci Polym Ed 19, no. 8 (2008): 969-88.

———. "Formula of love." Cosmetics & Medicine (Russia) 2 (2005): 24-33.

———. "Compositions and methods for skin tanning and protection." U.S. Patent 5,698,184: Skin Biology, Inc., filed Aug 23, 1996, and issued Dec 16, 1997.

———. "Non-toxic skin cancer therapy with copper peptide." U.S. Patent 9,586,989: Skin Biology, Inc., issued Mar 7, 2017.

———. A. "Metal-peptide compositions and methods for stimulating hair growth." U.S. Patent 5,550,183: ProCyte Corporation, Inc., filed Mar 07, 1995, and issued Aug 27, 1996.

———. B. "Tissue protective and regenerative compositions." U.S. Patent 5,554,375: Skin Biology, Inc., filed Jan 06, 1995, and issued Sept 10, 1996.

———. "Tissue protective and regenerative compositions." U.S. Patent 5,382,431: Skin Biology, Inc, filed Sept 29, 1992, and issued Jan 17, 1995.

———. "Cosmetic and skin treatment compositions." U.S. Patent 5,348,943: ProCyte Corporation, Inc., filed Aug 03, 1992, and issued Sept 20, 1994.

———. "GHK-copper 2+ strongly lowers blood pressure in goats." Unpublished Safety Study, 1993.

———. "Method for stimulating hair growth using GHL-Cu complexes." U.S. Patent 5,177,061: ProCyte Corporation, filed Sept 22, 1989, and issued Jan 05, 1993.

———. A. "Cosmetic and skin treatment compositions." U.S. Patent 5,135,913: ProCyte Corporation, Inc., filed Jun 16, 1988, and issued Aug 04, 1992.

———. B. "Method of using copper(II) containing compounds to accelerate wound healing." U.S. Patent 5,164,367: ProCyte Corporation, Inc., filed Mar 26, 1990, and issued Nov 17, 1992.

———. C. "Methods and compositions for healing ulcers ". U.S. Patent 5,145,838: Skin Biology, Inc., filed Jun 10, 1991, and issued Sept 08, 1992.

———. A. "Methods and compositions for healing bone using gly his lys: Copper." U.S. Patent 5,059,588: ProCyte Corporation, Inc., filed Oct 13, 1989, and issued Oct 22, 1991.

———. B. "Methods and compositions for healing ulcers." U.S. Patent 5,023,237: ProCyte Corporation, Inc., filed Aug 30, 1989, and issued Jun 11, 1991.

———. "Method of healing wounds in horses." U.S. Patent 4,937,230: ProCyte Corporation, inc., filed Dec 04, 1987, and issued Jun 26, 1990.

———. A. "Methods and compositions for preventing ulcers ". U.S. Patent 4,767,753: Skin Biology, Inc., filed May 11, 1987, and issued Aug 30, 1988.

———. B. "Use of GHL-Cu as a wound-healing and anti-inflammatory agent." U.S. Patent 4,760,051: filed Jan 24,1985, and issued Jul 26, 1988.

———. "Chemical derivatives of GHL-Cu." U.S. Patent 4,665,054: Bioheal, Inc., filed Feb 08, 1985, and issued May 12, 1987.

———. "Iamin: A human growth factor with multiple wound-healing properties." In Biology of copper complexes, edited by JR Sorenson, 273-85. Clifton, NJ: Humana Press, 1987.

———. "Suppression of growth of a fibrosarcoma in mice with gly-his-lys: Cu 2+ and ascorbic acid." Unpublished, 1985.

———. "A tripeptide in human plasma that increases the survival of hepatocytes and the growth of hepatoma cells." University of California, San Francisco, 1973.

Pickart, L, D Downey, S Lovejoy, and B Weinstein. "Gly-l-his-l-lys:Copper(II) - a human plasma factor with superoxide dismutase-like and wound-healing properties." In Superoxide and superoxide dismutase in chemistry, biology and medicine, edited by G Rotilio, 555-58: Elsevier Science, 1986.

Pickart, Loren, Jessica Michelle Vasquez-Soltero, and Anna Margolina. "The Effect of the Human Peptide GHK on Gene Expression Relevant to Nervous System Function and Cognitive Decline." Brain Sciences 7.2 (2017): 20.

———. A. "GHK peptide as a natural modulator of multiple cellular pathways in skin regeneration." Biomed Res Int 2015 (2015).

———. B. "Resetting Skin Genome Back to Health Naturally with GHK." Textbook of Aging Skin; Farage, M.A., Miller, K.W., Maibach, H.I., Eds.; Springer: Berlin/Heidelberg, Germany, 2015; pp. 1–19. (2015).

———. C. "GHK peptide as a natural modulator of multiple cellular pathways in skin regeneration." Biomed Res Int 2015 (2015).

———. D. "GHK and DNA: Resetting the human genome to health." Biomed Res Int 2014 (2014): 151479.

———. E. "GHK-Cu may prevent oxidative stress in skin by regulating copper and modifying expression of numerous antioxidant genes." Cosmetics 2.3 (2015): 236-247.

———. F. "The human tripeptide GHK-Cu in prevention of oxidative stress and degenerative conditions of aging: Implications for cognitive health." Oxid Med Cell Longev 2012 (2012): 324832.

Pickart, L., J. M. Vasquez-Soltero, F. D. Pickart, and J. Majnarich. B. "GHK, the human skin remodeling peptide, induces anti-cancer expression of numerous caspase, growth regulatory, and DNA repair genes." Journal of Analytical Oncology 3, no. 2 (2014): 79-87.

Pickart, L, JH Freedman, WJ Loker, J Peisach, CM Perkins, RE Stenkamp, and B Weinstein. "Growth-modulating plasma tripeptide may function by facilitating copper uptake into cells." Nature 288, no. 5792 (1980): 715-7.

Pickart, L, WH Goodwin, W Burgua, TB Murphy, and DK Johnson. "Inhibition of the growth of cultured cells and an implanted fibrosarcoma by aroylhydrazone analogs of the gly-his-lys-Cu(II) complex." Biochem Pharmacol 32, no. 24 (1983): 3868-71.

Pickart, L, and S Lovejoy. "Biological activity of human plasma copper-binding growth factor glycyl-l-histidyl-l-lysine." Methods Enzymol 147 (1987): 314-28.

Pickart, L, and A Margolina. "GHK-copper peptide in skin remodeling and anti-aging." SOFW Journal 136 (2010): 10-20.

Pickart, L, and F Pickart. "A possible mechanism whereby skin remodeling may suppress cancer metastasis genes." In Society for the Advancement of Wound Care and the Wound Healing Society, A8-A62. Dallas, Texas: Wound Repair and Regeneration 2011. Pickart, L, and MM Thaler. "Tripeptide in human serum which prolongs survival of normal liver cells and stimulates growth in neoplastic liver." Nat New Biol 243, no. 124 (1973): 85-7.

Pickart, L, and M Millard. "Effect of transition metals on recovery from plasma of the growth-modulating tripeptide glycylhistidyllysine." J Chromatogr 175, no. 1 (1979): 65-73.

Podda, M, MG Traber, C Weber, LJ Yan, and L Packer. "UV-irradiation depletes antioxidants and causes oxidative damage in a model of human skin." Free Radic Biol Med 24, no. 1 (1998): 55-65.

Pohunkova, H, J Stehlik, J Vachal, O Cech, and M Adam. "Morphological features of bone healing under the effect of collagen-graft-glycosaminoglycan copolymer supplemented with the tripeptide gly-his-lys." Biomaterials 17, no. 16 (1996): 1567-74.

Politis, MJ, and A Dmytrowich. "Promotion of second intention wound healing by emu oil lotion: Comparative results with furasin, polysporin, and cortisone." Plast Reconstr Surg 102, no. 7 (1998): 2404-7.

Pollard, JD, S Quan, T Kang, and RJ Koch. "Effects of copper tripeptide on the growth and expression of growth factors by normal and irradiated fibroblasts." Arch Facial Plast Surg 7, no. 1 (2005): 27-31.

Poole, TJ, and BR Zetter. "Stimulation of rat peritoneal mast cell migration by tumor-derived peptides." Cancer Res 43, no. 12 Pt 1 (1983): 5857-61.

Porter, RH, and J Winberg. "Unique salience of maternal breast odors for newborn infants." Neurosci Biobehav Rev 23, no. 3 (1999): 439-49.

Procyte Corp., Press Release. Procyte, Redmond, WA. (1997).

Prohaska, JR, and RG Hoffman. "Auditory startle response is diminished in rats after recovery from perinatal copper deficiency." J Nutr 126, no. 3 (1996): 618-27.

Purba, MB, A Kouris-Blazos, N Wattanapenpaiboon, W Lukito, E Rothenberg, B Steen, and ML Wahlqvist. A. "Can skin wrinkling in a site that has received limited sun exposure be used as a marker of health status and biological age?" Age Aging 30, no. 3 (2001): 227-34.

Purba, MB, A Kouris-Blazos, N Wattanapenpaiboon, W Lukito, EM Rothenberg, BC Steen, and ML Wahlqvist. B. "Skin wrinkling: Can food make a difference?" J Am Coll Nutr 20, no. 1 (2001): 71-80.

Pyo, HK, HG Yoo, CH Won, SH Lee, YJ Kang, HC Eun, KH Cho, and KH Kim. "The effect of tripeptide-copper complex on human hair growth in vitro." Arch Pharm Res 30, no. 7 (2007): 834-9.

Rabenstein, DL, JM Robert, and S Hari. "Binding of the growth factor glycyl-l-histidyl-l-lysine by heparin." FEBS Lett 376, no. 3 (1995): 216-20.

Raju, KS, G Alessandri, and PM Gullino. "Characterization of a chemoattractant for endothelium induced by angiogenesis effectors." Cancer Res 44, no. 4 (1984): 1579-84.

Raju, KS, G Alessandri, M Ziche, and PM Gullino. "Ceruloplasmin, copper ions, and angiogenesis." J Natl Cancer Inst 69, no. 5 (1982): 1183-8.

Rao, MS, B Hattiangady, and AK Shetty. "The window and mechanisms of major age-related decline in the production of new neurons within the dentate gyrus of the hippocampus." Aging Cell 5, no. 6 (2006): 545-58.

Reiser, S., J. C. Smith, Jr., W. Mertz, J. T. Holbrook, D. J. Scholfield, A. S. Powell, W. K. Canfield, and J. J. Canary. "Indices of copper status in humans consuming a typical american diet containing either fructose or starch." Am J Clin Nutr 42, no. 2 (1985): 242-51.

Rittschof, D, and JH Cohen. "Crustacean peptide and peptide-like pheromones and kairomones." Peptides 25, no. 9 (2004): 1503-16.

Rock, E, A Mazur, JM O'Connor, MP Bonham, Y Rayssiguier, and JJ Strain. "The effect of copper supplementation on red blood cell oxidizability and plasma antioxidants in middle-aged healthy volunteers." Free Radic Biol Med 28, no. 3 (2000): 324-9.

Rong, Y., L. Chen, T. Zhu, Y. Song, M. Yu, Z. Shan, A. Sands, F. B. Hu, and L. Liu. "Egg consumption and risk of coronary heart disease and stroke: Dose-response meta-analysis of prospective cohort studies." BMJ 346 (2013): e8539.

Saari, JT, AM Bode, and GM Dahlen. "Defects of copper deficiency in rats are modified by dietary treatments that affect glycation." J Nutr 125, no. 12 (1995): 2925-34.

Sage, EH, and RB Vernon. "Regulation of angiogenesis by extracellular matrix: The growth and the glue." J Hypertens Suppl 12, no. 10 (1994): S145-52.

Sang S, Chu YF. "Whole grain oats, more than just a fiber: Role of unique phytochemicals." Mol. Nutr. Food. Res. 2017 9. [Epub ahead of print]

Saxen, L, PC Holmberg, M Nurminen, and E Kuosma. "Sauna and congenital defects." Teratology 25, no. 3 (1982): 309-13.

Schaal, B, G Coureaud, D Langlois, C Ginies, E Semon, and G Perrier. "Chemical and behavioural characterization of the rabbit mammary pheromone." Nature 424, no. 6944 (2003): 68-72.

Schagen, S, R Voegeli, D Imfeld, T Schreier, and CC Zouboulis. "Lipid regulation in SZ95 sebocytes by glycyl-histidyl-lysine." Paper presented at the 16th European Academy of Dermatology and Venereology Congress, Vienna, May 16-20 2007.

Scher, RK. "Foods which contain biotin." Prevention 46 (1994): 122.

Schlesinger, DH, L Pickart, and MM Thaler. "Growth-modulating serum tripeptide is glycyl-histidyl-lysine." Experientia 33, no. 3 (1977): 324-5.

Schlumpf, M, B Cotton, M Conscience, V Haller, B Steinmann, and W Lichtensteiger. "In vitro and in vivo estrogenicity of UV screens." Environ Health Perspect 109, no. 3 (2001): 239-44.

Schlumpf, M, K Kypke, M Wittassek, J Angerer, H Mascher, D Hascher, C Vokt, M Birchler, and W Lichtensteiger. "Exposure patterns of UV filters, fragrances, parabens, phthalates, organochlor peticides, PBDEs, and PCBs in human milk: Correlation of UV filters with use of cosmetics." Chemosphere 81, no. 10 (2010): 1171-83.

Schmidt, SP, JR Resser, RL Sims, DL Mullins, and DJ Smith. "The combined effects of glycyl-l-histidyl-l-lysine copper (II) and cell-tak on the healing of linear incision wounds." Wounds 6 (1994): 62-67.

Senoo, M, F Pinto, CP Crum, and F McKeon. "p63 is essential for the proliferative potential of stem cells in stratified epithelia." Cell 129, no. 3 (2007): 523-36.

Sensenbrenner, M, GG Jaros, G Moonen, and P Mandel. "Effects of synthetic tripeptide on the differentiation of dissociated cerebral hemisphere nerve cells in culture." Neurobiology 5, no. 4 (1975): 207-13.

Simeon, A, H Emonard, W Hornebeck, and FX Maquart. B. "The tripeptide-copper complex glycyl-l-histidyl-l-lysine-Cu2+ stimulates matrix metalloproteinase-2 expression by fibroblast cultures." Life Sci 67, no. 18 (2000): 2257-65.

Simeon, A, F Monier, H Emonard, P Gillery, P Birembaut, W Hornebeck, and FX Maquart. "Expression and activation of matrix metalloproteinases in wounds: Modulation by the tripeptide-copper complex glycyl-l-histidyl-l-lysine-Cu2+." J Invest Dermatol 112, no. 6 (1999): 957-64.

Simeon, A, Y Wegrowski, Y Bontemps, and FX Maquart. A. "Expression of glycosaminoglycans and small proteoglycans in wounds: Modulation by the tripeptide-copper complex glycyl-l-histidyl-l-lysine-Cu(2+)." J Invest Dermatol 115, no. 6 (2000): 962-8.

Singh, I., A. P. Sagare, M. Coma, D. Perlmutter, R. Gelein, R. D. Bell, R. J. Deane, E. Zhong, M. Parisi, J. Ciszewski, R. T. Kasper, and R. Deane. "Low levels of copper disrupt brain amyloid-beta homeostasis by altering its production and clearance." Proc Natl Acad Sci U S A 110, no. 36 (2013): 14771-6.

Smakhtin, MIu, AI Konoplia, LA Sever'ianova, and IA Shveinov. "[pharmacological correction of immuno-metabolic disorders with the peptide gly-his-lys in hepatic damage induced by tetrachloromethane]." Patol Fiziol Eksp Ter (Russia), no. 2 (2003): 19-21.

Smakhtin, MY, LA Sever'yanova, AI Konoplya, and IA Shveinov. "Tripeptide gly-his-lys is a hepatotropic immunosuppressor." Bull Exp Biol Med 133, no. 6 (2002): 586-7.

Sobel, N, V Prabhakaran, CA Hartley, JE Desmond, GH Glover, EV Sullivan, and JD Gabrieli. "Blind smell: Brain activation induced by an undetected air-borne chemical." Brain 122 (Pt 2) (1999): 209-17.

Sorenson, JR. "Copper complexes offer a physiological approach to treatment of chronic diseases." Prog Med Chem 26 (1989): 437-568.

———. "Antiinflammatory, analgesic, and antiulcer activities of copper complexes suggest their use in a physiologic approach to treatment of arthritic diseases." Basic Life Sci 49 (1988): 591-4.

———. "Biology of copper complexes." Experimental Biology and Medicine 16 (1987).

———. "A role for copper in mediating oxidative damage associated with degenerative disease processes seems to be more imaginary than real." Med Biol 63, no. 1 (1985): 40-1.

———. Inflammatory diseases and copper: The metabolic and therapeutic roles of copper and other essential metalloelements in humans, Experimental biology and medicine. Clifton, New Jersey: Humana Press, 1982.

———. "Evaluation of copper complexes as potential anti-arthritic drugs." J Pharm Pharmacol 29, no. 7 (1977): 450-2.

Sorenson, JR, and W Hangarter. "Treatment of rheumatoid and degenerative diseases with copper complexes: A review with emphasis on copper-salicylate." Inflammation 2, no. 3 (1977): 217-38.

Sorenson, JR, K Ramakrishna, and TM Rolniak. "Antiulcer activities of D-penicillamine copper complexes." Agents Actions 12, no. 3 (1982): 408-11.

Sorenson, JR, LS Soderberg, MV Chidambaram, DT de la Rosa, H Salari, K Bond, G.L Kearns, RA Gray, CE Epperson, and ML Baker. "Bioavailable copper complexes offer a physiologic approach to treatment of chronic diseases." Adv Exp Med Biol 258 (1989): 229-34.

Soskel, N. T., S. Watanabe, E. Hammond, L. B. Sandberg, A. D. Renzetti, Jr., and J. D. Crapo. "A copper-deficient, zinc-supplemented diet produces emphysema in pigs." Am Rev Respir Dis 126, no. 2 (1982): 316-25.

Soskel, N. T., S. Watanabe, and L. B. Sandberg. "Mechanisms of lung injury in the copper-deficient hamster model of emphysema." Chest 85, no. 6 Suppl (1984): 70S-73S.

Sparrow, D., J. E. Silbert, and S. T. Weiss. "The relationship of pulmonary function to copper concentrations in drinking water." Am Rev Respir Dis 126, no. 2 (1982): 312-5.

Steenvoorden, DP, and G Beijersbergen van Henegouwen. "Protection against UV-induced systemic immunosuppression in mice by a single topical application of the antioxidant vitamins C and E." Int J Radiat Biol 75, no. 6 (1999): 747-55.

Stein, Christoph, and Sarah Küchler. "Targeting inflammation and wound healing by opioids."Trends in pharmacological sciences 34.6 (2013): 303-312.

Stenn, KS, AG Messenger, and HP Baden, eds. the molecular and structural biology of hair, Annals of the new york academy of sciences. New York, NY: New York Academy of Sciences, 1991.

Stephens, TJ, ML Sigler, MB Finkley, and Y Appa. "Skin benefits of an SPF 20 copper peptide containing face cream." Paper presented at the 61st Annual American Academy of Dermatology Meeting, San Francisco, CA, 2003.

Stern, RS, and N Laird. "The carcinogenic risk of treatments for severe psoriasis. Photochemotherapy follow-up study." Cancer 73, no. 11 (1994): 2759-64.

Stolarz-Skrzypek, K, T Kuznetsova, L Thijs, V Tikhonoff, J Seidlerová, T Richart, Y Jin, A Olszanecka, S Malyutina, E Casiglia, J Filipovský, K Kawecka-Jaszcz, Y Nikitin, and Staessen JA; European Project on Genes in Hypertension (EPOGH) Investigators. "Fatal and nonfatal outcomes, incidence of hypertension, and blood pressure changes in relation to urinary sodium excretion." JAMA 305, no. 17 (2011): 1777-85.

Storm, HM, SY Oh, BF Kimler, and S Norton. "Radioprotection of mice by dietary squalene." Lipids (United States) 28, no. 6 (1993): 555-9.

Stromberg, BE, PB Khoury, and EJ Soulsby. "Development of larvae of ascaris suum from the third to the fourth stage in a chemically defined medium." Int J Parasitol 7, no. 2 (1977): 149-51.

Su, X, M Paris, YJ Gi, KY Tsai, MS Cho, YL Lin, JA Biernaskie, S Sinha, C Prives, LH Pevny, FD Miller, and ER Flores. "TAp63 prevents premature aging by promoting adult stem cell maintenance." Cell Stem Cell 5, no. 1 (2009): 64-75.

Sugimoto, Y, I Lopez-Solache, F Labrie, and V Luu-The. "Cations inhibit specifically type I 5 alpha-reductase found in human skin." J Invest Dermatol 104, no. 5 (1995): 775-8.

Swaim, SF, DM Bradley, JS Spano, and et al. "Evaluation of multipeptide copper complex medications on open wound healing in dogs." J Am Anim Hosp Assoc 29 (1993): 519-25.

Swaim, SF, DM Vaughn, SA Kincaid, NE Morrison, SS Murray, MA Woodhead, CE Hoffman, JC Wright, and JR Kammerman. "Effect of locally injected medications on healing of pad wounds in dogs." Am J Vet Res 57, no. 3 (1996): 394-9.

Tavera-Mendoza, LE, and JH White. "Cell defenses and the sunshine vitamin." Sci Am 297, no. 5 (2007): 62-5, 68-70, 72.

Taylor, RS, KE Ashton, T Moxham, L Hooper, and S Ebrahim. "Reduced dietary salt for the prevention of cardiovascular disease: A meta-analysis of randomized controlled trials (Cochrane review)." Am J Hypertens 24, no. 8 (2011): 843-53.

Thornfeldt, CR. "Chronic inflammation is etiology of extrinsic aging." J Cosmet Dermatol 7, no. 1 (2008): 78-82.

Timpe, ED, RE Trachy, and I Dumwiddle. "Evaluation of telogen hair follicle stimulation using an in vivo model: Results with peptide copper complexes." In Dermatologic research techniques, edited by HI Maibach, 241-54. Boca Raton: CRC Press, 1996.

Traber, MG, M Podda, C Weber, J Thiele, M Rallis, and L Packer. "Diet-derived and topically applied tocotrienols accumulate in skin and protect the tissue against ultraviolet light-induced oxidative stress." Asia Pacific J Clin Nutr 6, no. 1 (1997): 63-67.

Trachy, RE, TD Fors, L Pickart, and H Uno. "The hair follicle-stimulating properties of peptide copper complexes. Results in C3H mice." Ann N Y Acad Sci 642 (1991): 468-9.

Trachy, RE, L Patt, G Duncan, and B Kalis. A. "Phototrichogram analysis of hair follicle stimulation: A pilot clinical study with a peptide-copper complex." In Dermatologic research techniques, edited by H. I. Maibach, 217-26: CRC Press, 1996.

Trachy, RE, U Uno, S Packard, and L Patt. B. "Quantitative assessment of peptide-copper complex-induced hair follicle stimulation using the fuzzy rat." In Dermatologic research techniques, edited by HI Maibach, 227-39. Boca Raton: CRC Press, 1996.

Trumbo, P, AA Yates, S Schlicker, and M Poos. "Dietary reference intakes for vitamin A, vitamin K, boron, chromium, copper, iodine, iron, manganese, molybdenum, nickel, silicon, vanadium, and zinc." J Am Diet Assoc 101, no. 3 (2001): 294-301.

Turnlund, JR, WR Keyes, SK Kim, and JM Domek. "Long-term high copper intake: Effects on copper absorption, retention, and homeostasis in men." Am J Clin Nutr 81, no. 4 (2005): 822-8.

Uauy, R, M Olivares, and M Gonzalez. "Essentiality of copper in humans." Am J Clin Nutr 67, no. 5 Suppl (1998): 952S-59S.

Uğurlu, T, M Türkoğlu, and T Ozaydın. "In vitro evaluation of compression-coated glycyl-l-histidyl-l-lysine-Cu(II) (GHK-Cu(2+))-loaded microparticles for colonic drug delivery." Drug Dev Ind Pharm 37, no. 11 (2011): 1282-9.

Uno, H. The histopathology of hair loss. Kalamazoo, MI: The Upjohn Company, 1988.

Uno, H, and S Kurata. "Chemical agents and peptides affect hair growth." J Invest Dermatol 101, no. 1 Suppl (1993): 143S-47S.

Vinci, C, V Caltabiano, AM Santoro, AM Rabuazzo, M Buscema, R Purrello, E Rizzarelli, R Vigneri, and F Purrello. "Copper addition prevents the inhibitory effects of interleukin 1-beta on rat pancreatic islets." Diabetologia 38, no. 1 (1995): 39-45.

Viossat, B, FT Greenaway, G Morgant, JC Daran, NH Dung, and JR Sorenson. "Low-temperature (180 K) crystal structures of tetrakis-mu-(niflumato) di(aqua)dicopper(II) N,N-dimethylformamide and N,N-dimethylacetamide solvates, their EPR properties, and anticonvulsant activities of these and other ternary binuclear copper(II)niflumate complexes." J Inorg Biochem 99, no. 2 (2005): 355-67.

Wegrowski, Y, FX Maquart, and JP Borel. "Stimulation of sulfated glycosaminoglycan synthesis by the tripeptide-copper complex glycyl-l-histidyl-l-lysine-Cu2+." Life Sci 51, no. 13 (1992): 1049-56.

Williams, DM. "Copper deficiency in humans." Semin Hematol 20, no. 2 (1983): 118-28.

Williams, RJ. Biochemical individuality: The basis for the genetotrophic concept New York: Wiley, 1956.

Winberg, J, and RH Porter. "Olfaction and human neonatal behaviour: Clinical implications." Acta Paediatr 87, no. 1 (1998): 6-10.

Wise, JA, RJ Morin, R Sanderson, and K Blum. "Changes in plasma carotenoid, alpha-tocopherol, and lipid peroxide levels in response to supplementation with concentrated fruit and vegetable extracts: A pilot study." Current Therapeutic Research 57, no. 6 (1996): 445-61.

Zemtsov, A, M Gaddis, and VM Montalvo-Lugo. "Moisturizing and cosmetic properties of emu oil: A pilot double blind study." Australas J Dermatol 37, no. 3 (1996): 159-61.

Zeitter S, Sikora Z2, Jahn S2, Stahl F3, Strauß S2, Lazaridis A2, Reimers K, Vogt PM, Aust MC. Microneedling: matching the results of medical needling and repetitive treatments to maximize potential for skin regeneration. Burns. 2014 Aug;40(5):966-73. doi: 10.1016/j.burns.2013.12.008. Epub 2014 Feb 7.

Zetter, BR, N Rasmussen, and L Brown. "Methods of laboratory investigation: An in vivo assay for chemoattractant activity." Lab Invest 53, no. 3 (1985): 362-8.

Zhai, H, YC Chang, M Singh, and HI Maibach. "In vivo nickel allergic contact dermatitis: Human model for topical therapeutics." Contact Dermatitis 40, no. 4 (1999): 205-8.

Zhai, H, YH Leow, and HI Maibach. A. "Human barrier recovery after acute acetone perturbation: An irritant dermatitis model." Clin Exp Dermatol 23, no. 1 (1998): 11-3.

Zhai, H, N Poblete, and HI Maibach. B. "Sodium lauryl sulfate damaged skin in vivo in man: A water barrier repair model." Skin Res Tech 4, no. 1 (1998): 24-27.

———. C. "Stripped skin model to predict irritation potential of topical agents in vivo in humans." Int J Dermatol 37, no. 5 (1998): 386-9.

Ziegler, TA, and RB Forward, Jr. "Larval release behaviors in the caribbean spiny lobster, panulirus argus: Role of peptide pheromones." J Chem Ecol 33, no. 9 (2007): 1795-805.

INDEX
ALPHABETICAL GUIDE TO WORDS FREQUENTLY USED

Made in the USA
Columbia, SC
05 January 2024

29932793R00143